No Longer Property of
EWU Libraries

No Longer Property of
EWU Libraries

The Patella

A Team Approach

Ronald P. Grelsamer, MD

Chief
Hip and Knee Reconstruction
Maimonides Medical Center
Brooklyn, New York

Staff Orthopaedic Surgeon
The Hospital for Joint Diseases
Beth Israel Medical Center
New York, New York

Member of the International Patellofemoral Study Group

Jenny McConnell, PT, GDMT, MBiomedE

Director
McConnell & Clements Physiotherapy
Sydney, Australia

Director
McConnell Institute
Marina del Rey, California

AN ASPEN PUBLICATION®
Aspen Publishers, Inc.
Gaithersburg, Maryland
1998

CALS
RD561
,G74
1998

The authors have made every effort to ensure the accuracy of the information herein. However, appropriate information sources should be consulted, especially for new or unfamiliar procedures. It is the responsibility of every practitioner to evaluate the appropriateness of a particular opinion in the context of actual clinical situations and with due considerations to new developments. Authors, editors, and the publisher cannot be held responsible for any typographical or other errors found in this book.

Cover art is a computer simulation of the patellofemoral joint. It was created at the Columbia University Orthopaedic Research Laboratory and is reprinted with permission from RP Grelsamer, WW Colman, and VC Mow, Anatomy and Mechanics of the Patellofemoral Joint, *Sports Medicine and Arthroscopy Review*, Vol 2, p 185, © 1994, Lippincott–Raven Publishers.

Library of Congress Cataloging-in-Publication Data

Grelsamer, Ronald P.
The patella: a team approach/
Ronald P. Grelsamer, Jenny McConnell.
p. cm.
Includes bibliographical references and index.
ISBN 0-8342-0753-2 (hardcover)
1. Patella—Diseases. 2. Patella—Surgery.
3. Patella—Wounds and injuries—Physical Therapy.
I. McConnell, Jenny. II. Title.
[DNLM: 1. Patella—physiopathology.
2. Pain—therapy. 3. Physical Therapy.
WE 870 G825p 1998]
RD561.G74 1998
617,5′82—dc21
DNLM/DLC
for Library of Congress
97-46654
CIP

Copyright © 1998 by Aspen Publishers, Inc.
All rights reserved.

Aspen Publishers, Inc., grants permission for photocopying for limited personal or internal use. This consent does not extend to other kinds of copying, such as copying for general distribution, for advertising or promotional purposes, for creating new collective works, or for resale. For information, address Aspen Publishers, Inc., Permissions Department, 200 Orchard Ridge Drive, Suite 200, Gaithersburg, Maryland 20878.

Orders: (800) 638-8437
Customer Service: (800) 234-1660

About Aspen Publishers • For more than 35 years, Aspen has been a leading professional publisher in a variety of disciplines. Aspen's vast information resources are available in both print and electronic formats. We are committed to providing the highest quality information available in the most appropriate format for our customers. Visit Aspen's Internet site for more information resources, directories, articles, and a searchable version of Aspen's full catalog, including the most recent publications: **http://www.aspenpub.com**
Aspen Publishers, Inc. • The hallmark of quality in publishing
Member of the worldwide Wolters Kluwer group.

Editorial Services: Jane Colilla

Library of Congress Catalog Card Number: 97-46654
ISBN: 0-8342-0753-2

Printed in the United States of America
1 2 3 4 5

EASTERN WASHINGTON
UNIVERSITY LIBRARIES
CHENEY, WA 99004

To my wife and best friend Sharon who gave up many an evening and weekend while I sifted through references, sat at the computer, or padded our long-distance phone bill.
To my children Dominique and Marc from whom I constantly learn and to my parents who made my education possible!

Table of Contents

Contributors

Ronald P. Grelsamer, MD
Chief
Hip and Knee Reconstruction
Maimonides Medical Center
Brooklyn, New York
Staff Orthopaedic Surgeon
The Hospital for Joint Diseases
Beth Israel Medical Center
New York, New York
Member of the International Patellofemoral
    Study Group

Glenn S. Kasman, MS, PT
Physical Medicine and Rehabilitation
Virginia Mason Medical Center
Seattle, Washington

Jenny McConnell, PT, GDMT, MBiomedE
Director
McConnell & Clements Physiotherapy
Sydney, Australia
Director
McConnell Institute
Marina del Rey, California

John E. McNerney, DPM
Chief of Podiatric Surgery
Pascack Valley Hospital
Westwood, New Jersey
Consultant/Team Podiatrist
New York Football Giants
New Jersey Nets Basketball Team
New Jersey Devils Hockey Team
New Jersey MetroStars Soccer Team
Kean College of New Jersey
Union, New Jersey

Preface

Twenty years ago when Ficat and Hungerford published a book on disorders of the patella, the question was "why an entire book on the patella?" Today the question could be "why another book on the patella?" Indeed, since the publication of Ficat and Hungerford's seminal book, there have been two English-language books on the subject and two further editions of the original work.

The Patella: A Team Approach represents the collaborative editorial efforts of an orthopaedic surgeon and a physical therapist, and the chapters have been written by an orthopaedic surgeon, two physical therapists, and a podiatrist. This reflects the well-accepted opinion that most patellofemoral problems can be addressed by an appropriate nonoperative program.

This book is designed to help the health professional deal with the patient who presents with what is often referred to as "patellar pain." There are no chapters on patella fractures or quadriceps or patellar tendon ruptures; nor is there a chapter on the patella in total knee replacement surgery. These subjects are very well covered in other texts. On the other hand, this book addresses topics not addressed in other books on the patella. Chapters on controversies (Chapter 1), classification of patellofemoral disorders (Chapter 9), the foot and orthotics (Chapter 13), taping (Chapter 12), and the failed patella (Chapter 15) all contribute to making this work significantly different.

Medical texts fall into two categories: multiauthor and single-author works. Each approach has its pros and cons. Multiauthor texts provide varying points of view, but the information presented may be contradictory. Single-author texts provide a more unified approach, but they reflect the author's bias. Although this book is technically a multiauthor text, it is conceptually a single-author text; all chapters have been written by or under the umbrella of the two senior authors. Although we have tried to separate fact from opinion and to present different points of view, our biases surely shine through.

It is our hope that health professionals who read this book will gain an appreciation of the fundamental concepts and the numerous controversies surrounding the patella.

Ronald P. Grelsamer, MD
Jenny McConnell, PT, GDMT, MBiomedE

Acknowledgments

I thank my friend and colleague Jean-Pierre Farcy, MD, for introducing me to the world of the patella by suggesting that I visit Philippe Cartier, MD, in Paris. Philippe, in turn, exposed me to surgical and philosophical approaches I had never dreamed of.

John Fulkerson, MD, and Alan Merchant, MD, further broadened my horizons and have shown me that nice guys can indeed finish first.

The dedicated members of the International Patellofemoral Study Group have all indirectly contributed to this text by tempering some of my heretofore unshakable beliefs.

Van Mow, PhD, Gerard Ateshian, PhD, Daniel Kwak, PhD, Tom Gardner, ME, and the entire team at the Columbia University Orthopaedic Research Laboratory have put in countless hours to fine-tune, carry out, carry out again, analyze, and re-analyze some of the findings reported on in Chapter 3 (not to mention putting up with my incessant queries).

Jenny McConnell, PT, GDMT, MBiomedE, from Australia, has made terrific contributions to the treatment of patellar disorders. It has been a privilege to have her as a coeditor (my local phone company will be sorry to see this project come to its conclusion). I thank Lloyd Hines, PT, for introducing us.

I thank Douglas Hertford, MD, Steven Shankman, MD, and the Radiology Department at the Columbia-Presbyterian Medical Center in New York for their ongoing radiological guidance and their photographic contributions to this text.

My long-time friend Georges Dremeaux has demonstrated terrific patience and has contributed the beautiful illustrations in Chapter 2.

My department chairman Allan Strongwater, MD, and my colleagues Jeffrey Klein, MD, and Hershel Samuels, MD, in addition to taking the Orthopaedic Department at the Maimonides Medical Center to ever greater heights, have allowed me to take the time to complete this work.

My earliest mentor Howard Kiernan, MD, was the first to point out to me that patella malalignment is underdiagnosed and over-operated. Nas Eftekhar, MD, has always stressed the importance of careful preoperative screening in orthopaedic surgery.

My colleagues and residents at the Maimonides Medical Center, the Hospital for Joint Diseases, and the Beth Israel Medical Center in New York have constantly queried and questioned the concepts in this book, and I am grateful for their intellectual stimulation.

Ms. Mary Anne Langdon from Aspen Publishers, Inc, has stood by us as we labored far past the deadline. Without her patience and understanding, this book would never have been possible. Mr. Stephen Zollo from Aspen Publishers, Inc, saw the merits of this combined orthopaedic surgeon/physical therapist collaboration and gave this project the thumbs up. My secretary, Denise Court, orchestrated the shuffling of manuscripts; for this I am eternally grateful. Final thanks to Ms. Jane Colilla and her team for putting it all together.

On behalf of patients who will be helped by this book, to all of you I say thank you!

Ronald P. Grelsamer, MD

CHAPTER 1

What Causes Pain? and Other Fundamental Controversies

NOMENCLATURE: THE TOWER OF BABEL

Health professionals use certain terms with the assumption that listeners and readers will attach the same meaning to those terms as they do. When it comes to common terms pertaining to the patella, nothing could be further from the truth. Reviewing articles in the scientific literature is next to impossible when the authors have not defined terms such as *subluxation* and *instability*. Unfortunately editors have not demanded this of their authors.

Reading through a definition of terms is a dry, tedious process. But, it is absolutely necessary to do this at the outset if we are to understand one another.[1]

Subluxation

Entire papers have been written about the results of surgery for patellar subluxation without a clear explanation of what the authors mean by *subluxation*. At a recent meeting of the International Patellofemoral Study Group, 20 participants with a particular interest in the patella were asked to define subluxation. Not only were there nearly as many definitions as there were participants, but the group could not reach consensus until its third meeting. Possible definitions include the following:

- a clinical sensation of giving way attributable to patellar "instability" (see below for discussion of this term)
- a sign on the physical examination
- a radiological finding whereby the patella is medially or laterally displaced with partial loss of normal contact between the articulating surfaces
- a combination of clinical and radiological signs and symptoms
- any form of clinical or radiological malalignment (Under this definition, even patellar tilt is considered a subluxation.)

Within each of these definitions there is still room for disagreement. For example, giving way can be the result of patellar pain with secondary muscle atrophy. Would this still be subluxation? Perhaps the patient has to specifically feel the patella move. But patients are not always accurate in their impressions. As for a radiological definition, picking a reference point or points against which to determine the medial-lateral displacement of the patella is difficult (see Chapter 5). Moreover, excessive lateral displacement of the patella may only be apparent when imaging is carried out in a certain manner, which may vary from patient to patient.

My personal preference has been to reserve the term *subluxation* for the clinical situation where the orthopaedist (or other health professional) believes that the patella slips out of the trochlea in such a way as to be noticed by the patient.

However, the consensus at the October 1996 meeting of the International Patellofemoral Study Group was to reserve the term *subluxation* for objective studies where abnormal medial-lateral displacement could be documented via imaging or instrumentation. If the patient notes giving way, this would simply be referred to as *giving way* or *functional (symptomatic) subluxation*.

Instability

Instability is more clearly a clinical (rather than radiological) term. It encompasses giving way (as a result of the patella partially slipping out of the trochlea) and dislocation (complete displacement of the patella out of the trochlea, which requires manual repositioning). Instability need not be symptomatic; when it is symptomatic, investigators are urged to say so (eg, "50 patients with symptomatic instability were assessed").

Malalignment

To some people, malalignment is synonymous with subluxation. However, as noted above, this means many things to many people. The patella is aligned with respect to three axes (six degrees of freedom); any abnormality of translation or rotation with respect to any of these three axes represents malalignment. As such, medial-lateral translation, patella alta and patella infera, tilt, and rotation all represent malalignment. In my opinion, some form of malalignment is present in the vast majority of patients with pain pertaining to the patella (with the exception of young teenagers and patients who have sustained blunt trauma to the knee). Although excessive athleticism or poor training can cause pain about the patella, those individuals who develop pain often have an underlying malalignment. I believe that "overuse pain" without malalignment is rare, and "idiopathic"

patellar pain is even more rare. Not everyone shares this opinion.

Anterior Knee Pain

Some people use the term *anterior knee pain* in reference to pain pertaining to the patella. This term replaces the term *chondromalacia*, which was used for many years to indicate the same thing. I do not favor the term *anterior knee pain* because pain from patella malalignment need not be anterior (see Chapter 4).

Normal

"What is normal?" is a question often heard in reference to the patella. One does find such questions in reference to the anterior cruciate ligament or the menisci because there is a narrow range of anatomic variation, and deviations from this range most commonly cause symptoms sooner or later. With respect to the patella, not all abnormalities are symptomatic. In addition, a number of abnormalities are common, which leads to the question of whether an abnormality that is common can truly be called an abnormality (see Additional Readings).

Part of the confusion comes from the fact that the word *normal* can be used in two ways: (1) the lay or statistical definition, whereby normal means "common," and (2) the medical definition, which will not be found in any dictionary (a medically normal condition is one that will not lead to pain or disability). Is it normal to have diabetes, cancer, or heart disease? In the first sense of the word, yes it is normal. A significant percentage of the population has one of these conditions. In the medical sense, it is obviously not normal to have diabetes, cancer, or heart disease.

This same discussion applies to the patella. Patella malalignment is common, and therefore many signs of malalignment are normal (or "common"). The clinical expression of patellar malalignment is variable, and it can be difficult to determine whether a given sign is medically abnormal. The issue of whether it is normal for a patella to be laterally positioned on routine magnetic resonance imaging (MRI) scanning is a good example of this discrepancy between statistical normality and medical normality (see Chapter 5). Tilting of the patella on the physical and radiological examination is also subject to this kind of semantic confusion.

Stress/Force

The terms *stress* and *force* are often used interchangeably. This is a serious error because, although these terms are related, they are quite different. Think of the confusion that would be created by using the words "cloud" and "rain" interchangeably.

A *force*, which is often expressed in pounds or kilograms, can be thought of as a weight. *Stress*, on the other hand, is force divided by area. Although the force exerted on part of a joint is of some importance, it is the stress that is of critical importance. The force exerted on the patellar cartilage may be significant during a certain portion of a given activity; however, if it is distributed over a large area, the stress may be well within tolerable limits. Conversely, an ordinary force concentrated on a small area can be excruciating (see Chapter 3).

There are several types of stress. *Compressive stress* is most closely related to the general concept of pressure. But there is also *tensile stress* (as when pulling on a material) and *shear (tangential) stress* (as when running a hand on a table top). The term *shear stress* is commonly used in a completely unsubstantiated manner—most commonly in discussion pertaining to the patella (as in "performing a particular exercise causes high shear stresses on the patella").

As an example of the confusion caused by these terms, it has been reported that the joint reaction force at the patellofemoral joint is three times the body weight with deep-knee bends to 90 degrees.[2] This information would be far more useful if the contact area were factored in. The joint reaction force may be great, but the stress may not be.

Glide

Glide is a term used to describe the medial-lateral position and movement of the patella. It is a term used mostly by physical therapists. Orthopaedists and engineers are more likely to use the term *translation* or (medial/lateral) *displacement*. Unlike the terms *stress* and *force*, there is no right or wrong here—simply convention.

Arthritis/Arthrosis

To some, the terms *arthritis* and *arthrosis* are synonymous. To others, *arthritis* denotes an inflammatory condition such as rheumatoid arthritis whereas *arthrosis* represents a breakdown of articular cartilage from anything but an inflammatory condition. In this text, the terms are used interchangeably and *inflammatory arthritis* is specified when this is what is meant.

Patellar Realignment

To some, this term refers to "open," inpatient procedures—as opposed to lateral retinacular releases, which are outpatient procedures involving at most a relatively small incision (see Chapter 14). The distinction is made to differentiate major procedures from less major procedures. I believe that any procedure carried out to alter the tracking of the patella qualifies as a realignment procedure. There is no such thing as minor surgery—only minor surgeons.

Patellar Height

A patella that lies too proximally or too distally within the trochlea is said to exhibit abnormal patellar height. There is agreement with respect to the nomenclature of the "high-riding" (excessively proximal) patella—*patella alta*. But a "low-riding" patella (one that lies too distally) is called *patella baja* by some and *patella infera* by others (*baja* is Spanish and *infera* is Latin).

WHAT CAUSES PATELLAR PAIN?

Remarkably, the answer to this question is not completely clear. In patients with symptomatic instability, the pain can be readily attributed to stretching or tearing of the soft tissues. In frank dislocations, osteochondral fractures—which, naturally, are painful—can occur in addition to the tearing of the soft tissues.

The cause of pain is more complicated in patients who have no obvious instability. A number of theories have been advanced, and it is possible that the etiology of the pain is not the same for all patients.

The theory that was advanced earlier in this century (see section on chondromalacia below) is that chondral lesions are painful. Until recently, all investigators agreed that these lesions were likely due to trauma. But because everyone falls on the knee at some point, why doesn't everyone have patellar pain?

In 1941 Wiberg correlated patella shapes (as seen in axial roentgenographic projections) with chondral lesions (chondromalacia) and accordingly developed his classification of normal and abnormal (bony) patellar shapes (see Chapter 5). In the Wiberg type I patella, the (bony) medial facet is equal in size to the lateral facet (this type is rare). The Wiberg type II patella features a medial facet that is smaller than the lateral facet (this type is most common). In the Wiberg type III patella, the medial facet is much smaller than the lateral facet and is convex (Wiberg did not specifically mention this feature).[3,4]

Much more recently, Buard et al found a correlation between the morphology of the trochlea and the incidence of cartilage lesions.[5] These authors found that steep trochleas (smaller than normal sulcus angle—see Chapter 5) have a high incidence of lesions. Specifically, they found that although only 19% of knees in their study were steep, they accounted for 40% of the lesions.

Arnoldi put forth another theory, whereby pain is secondary to increased venous pressure.[6] Using techniques similar to those used by Ficat in assessing osteonecrosis of the hip, Arnoldi determined that patients with patellar pain have higher patellar venous pressure than patients without pain. Osteotomies of the patella in which the patella was wedged open with a longitudinal cut provided short-term relief in a number of patients. Dye noted (during experimentation on himself) that introduction of fluid into the bony patella leads to "sharp lancinating pain."[7]

The most commonly accepted theory is Ficat's theory of excessive lateral pressure[3,4] (also termed lateral patellar compression). According to this theory, the malaligned patella places excessive stress on the lateral facet, and this translates to pain (the subchondral bone is richly innervated[8]). The patella is not laterally displaced, but it is tilted (lateral side down). In my opinion, this is the most common form of patella malalignment. It is readily diagnosed on the physical examination and can usually be confirmed on plain radiographs. This condition can coexist with lateral translation of the patella. Putz et al,[9] who found that bone is more dense laterally in patellae with lateral lesions, give credence to Ficat's hypothesis.

Reducing the tilt can improve the patient's symptoms. However, this reduction is effected by a release (division) of the lateral retinaculum, which leads to the theory of denervation. Fulkerson has found that patients with patellar pain exhibit fibrosis of the nerves within the lateral retinaculum.[10] Division of the retinaculum with its fibrosed nerves could conceivably improve pain, regardless of its effect on patellar tilt. Because the sensory innervation of the patella comes in large part from its superomedial aspect via branches of the saphenous nerve, some people have postulated that when operations on the medial side of the patella work (imbrications, advancements of the vastus medialis obliquus), they do so simply by further denervating the patella.

Pain can occur medially due to altered stresses in the medial subchondral bone and/or from stretching of the medial soft tissues when the patella subluxates.[8]

Outerbridge[8] popularized the concept of an osteochondral ridge as the source of chondromalacia and pain in patients with normally aligned knees. He described this as a horizontal ridge of bone covered with cartilage at the junction of the anterior femur and medial femoral condyle—present to a certain degree in all knees. Those in whom it is particularly prominent are at risk for (true) chondromalacia and pain.

Martinez-Moreno[11] has noted an increased distance from the tibial plateau to the insertion of the semitendinosus in patients with patellar pain and chondral lesions. Distal insertions increase the flexion moment of the pes muscles but decrease the internal rotation moment (the tibia becomes thinner distal to the tibial tuberosity). He has postulated that this decreased internal rotation moment of the tibial internal rotators can contribute to patellar pain via external rotation of the tibia.

The fat pad is quite sensitive to pain, and some have considered this to be the initiating agent.[12,13]

Localized osteoporosis with secondary cartilage changes has been proposed as the cause of lesions and pain.[14]

Varus knees have been associated with increased patellar pain,[15–18] possibly as a result of lateralization of the tibial tuberosity occasionally associated with this morphology (external rotation of the upper tibia associated with genu varum). Likewise, increased tibial torsion has been noted in patellofemoral "instability."[19]

Lateral displacement of the patella is a well-known phenomenon. In addition, some investigators believe that even in the nonsurgical patient medial subluxation/displacement rarely can be a source of pain.[20]

Patients with patellar pain commonly have pain with prolonged knee flexion ("movie theater sign"), and it is unclear whether this is due to vascular congestion or persistent traction on irritated nerves.

Chondral lesions of the odd facet may be due to friction from a plica (J. Hart, MD, personal communication). Isolated erosion of the central trochlea is referred to as a *lunge lesion* in reference to the deceleration noted in fencing-like activities.

A number of other conditions can cause pain about the patella for reasons completely unrelated to malalignment. In such cases, one would not expect great success from physical therapy or surgical protocols designed to address malalignment. Accordingly, it is particularly important to differentiate malalignment pain from "patellar" pain resulting from overuse, inflammatory conditions (eg, rheumatoid arthritis), neuroma, neuropathy, plica, tumor (benign or malignant), a dorsal defect, an osteochondritis dissecans lesion,[21] osteonecrosis,[22] femorotibial arthritis, iliotibial band (ITB) tendinitis, posttraumatic patellofemoral arthritis, infrapatellar contracture syndrome posterior cruciate ligament tear, bipartite patella, loose bodies, meniscal tears, reflex sympathetic dystrophy (RSD), or RSD-like conditions (see Chapters 8 and 15). Unfortunately, these conditions can coexist with patellar malalignment, and sorting out the source(s) of pain can be quite difficult. (Note to orthopaedists: In the United States you need not spend much time thinking about this as you are not recognized as being in a "cognitive" branch of medicine.)

WHY AREN'T ALL MALALIGNED PATELLAE PAINFUL? WHY DOES ONLY ONE KNEE HURT?

The two above questions are obviously related. Why do some malaligned patellae hurt and not others? The same could be asked of flat feet. The answer lies in the concept articulated by Dupont that patellar malalignment is a clinical condition of variable penetration (personal communication). Stated differently, malalignment is a necessary but not sufficient condition for pain to develop.

For some patients, a combination of malalignment and trauma is required to initiate long-lasting patellar pain. A typical scenario for such a patient is one where the malaligned knee is completely asymptomatic until the patient sustains blunt trauma to the front of the knee[23–25] (such as by falling onto the front of the knee or hitting the knee against a dashboard). I have termed this combination of circumstances the "double-crush syndrome" (a term first used in the upper extremity to describe a combination of cervical radiculopathy and carpal tunnel syndrome). Patients who are treated only for the blunt trauma to the knee may be labeled malingerers when symptoms persist (after the obligatory arthroscopy, naturally). These patients will not get better until the patella malalignment is recognized and treated appropriately.

I tell my patients that people with malaligned knees are akin to someone riding a bicycle on the edge of a cliff. All is well until a strong wind blows them off the cliff—which may or may not ever happen.

HOW ARE PAIN AND INSTABILITY RELATED?

One can have pain without instability and vice versa. Instability, though, can cause pain in a number of ways: the medial soft tissues can be stretched, cartilage can be damaged, or an osteochondral fracture can be created.

WHAT WILL REPLACE THE TERM *CHONDROMALACIA*?

From the 1930s until about a decade ago, the term *chondromalacia patellae* was synonymous with pain pertaining to the patella. It is a rather dated term, and most people in the field have abandoned it. However, it still deserves discussion because no term has been universally accepted as a replacement for chondromalacia and it still has a recognized insurance diagnosis code in the United States (717.7).

The concept that cartilage changes are pathological and potentially painful is hardly new. In the 1700s Hunter warned that from Hippocrates to the present age it is universally allowed that ulcerated cartilage is a troublesome thing and that when once destroyed it is not repaired. Konig and Aleman were two of the first to use the term *chondromalacia*, but Aleman himself apparently referred back to a 1906 text when using the term.[17,26–30] They noted softening (malacia) of the cartilage (chondro) and extrapolated a correlation with patellar pain. All of these inves-

tigators attributed the cartilage lesions to trauma. The concept that articular lesions could be secondary to malalignment is relatively recent.[17,19]

The term *chondromalacia* has gone through five stages:

- *Era 1.* From roughly the mid-1920s to the mid-1930s, *chondromalacia* was the term given to lesions of the patella.
- *Era 2.* In the mid- to late 1930s, the term *chondromalacia patellae* (chondromalacia of the patella) became synonymous with patellar pain associated with cartilage lesions.[31–33]
- *Era 3. Chondromalacia patellae* was used to describe patellar pain with or without the presence of cartilage lesions.[14]
- *Era 4.* By the mid-1970s it had become increasingly clear that the patella can be painful in the absence of any chondromalacic lesions and that chondromalacic lesions need not be painful.[8,34–37] Ficat and Hungerford asserted that the following 1908 comment from Büdinger could be applied to chondromalacia: "'Internal derangement' will simply not disappear from the surgical literature. It is the symbol of our helplessness in regards to a diagnosis and our ignorance of the pathology."[38]
- *Era 5.* Today, the term *chondromalacia* has fallen completely out of favor to the point that its use (other than to describe a specific pathological entity) reflects poorly on the user.

The term *chondromalacia*, despite its significant drawbacks, served a purpose. Everyone knew roughly what was meant. Everyone now agrees that it is a poor term, but no one has agreed on a new term. Replacement candidates have included *anterior knee pain* (but, as noted, anterior knee pain need not be related to patella malalignment, and the pain from malalignment need not be anterior); *patellar pain* (this term, likewise, need not be related to malalignment, and pain pertaining to patella malalignment may not be over the patella); *extensor mechanism dyspla-*

sia[39]; and *patellar malalignment* (this last term has my vote because, in my opinion, every adult with patellar pain not caused by one of the miscellaneous conditions listed above has some type of malalignment; this term makes it clear what category of conditions one is and is not talking about—namely, neuromas, hemangiomas, overuse, and many other conditions not related to malalignment that can cause pain about the knee).

DOES PATELLA MALALIGNMENT LEAD TO KNEE ARTHRITIS?

When discussing malalignment and knee arthritis, one must distinguish between *patellofemoral arthritis* and *femorotibial arthritis*— both of which arguably can be related to patellofemoral malalignment.

If one believes that malalignment leads to cartilage degeneration on the lateral portion of the patella, then it does not take a great leap of faith to imagine frank arthritis developing about the patellofemoral joint.[7,40,41] Conversely, realignment of a malalignment patella should halt the progression of arthritis.[42] Of course one rarely sees pure patellofemoral arthritis, which means one of two things: (1) malalignment is rarely severe enough to lead to arthritis or (2) patellofemoral arthritis rapidly leads to femorotibial arthritis in that area. The second point is not hard to fathom when one considers that the patella articulates with the femoral condyles. It is recognized that the patellofemoral joint is one of the more problematic areas of total knee replacement surgery, and in my opinion, this is related to the fact that a number of these patients have patella malalignment to begin with. A study from Japan found a correlation between patella malalignment and subsequent patellofemoral and femorotibial arthritis.[41]

CAN THERE BE PAIN IN THE ABSENCE OF CARTILAGE LESIONS?

Although cartilage lesions were once thought to be the *sine qua non* of patellar pain, it has now become clear that patellar pain from malalignment can exist in the absence of visible cartilage lesions. In addition, the absence of lesions visible to the naked eye does not preclude the presence of abnormalities within the cartilage. For example, blunt trauma can cause damage to the deeper layers of cartilage. Visual examination of the articular surface does not constitute a full examination of the articular cartilage.

ARE THERE DIFFERENCES BETWEEN ADULTS AND ADOLESCENTS WITH KNEE PAIN?

Adolescents are different from adults when it comes to pain about the patella. Some adolescents can be told with confidence that they will grow out of their condition. Indeed, a number of adolescents have pain in the absence of any clinical or radiological malalignment, which eventually resolves. They are not really "malalignment" patients. Perhaps the vastus medialis obliquus lags in development relative to other muscles about the knee and the patient has a transient muscle imbalance.[2]

In the case of adults, no such statement can be made. In the first place, if a patient has pain that is not caused by one of the miscellaneous causes listed above, I can almost always detect an element of malalignment. Second, my experience tells me that adults with symptomatic malalignment generally do not get better from simply waiting things out. Those who get better from waiting things out usually do not go to the doctor. Perhaps adolescents go to the doctor more quickly than adults because their parents are anxious and are not going to wait things out without clearance from the doctor. Regardless of the reason, some adolescents need no treatment other than simple analgesics and can be told to wait it out. This is never good advice for adults.

Some health professionals believe that patellar pain in adolescents can be a sign of psychological problems. Anybody at any age can somatize, or seek attention through suffering, yet I would be exceedingly leery of suggesting this to parents. When I am convinced that there is no malalignment, no mechanical problems, and none of the miscellaneous conditions listed above, I advise the patient and the parents that the condition will resolve on its own and that I will be glad to follow the patient on a regular basis, as needed.

Figure 1–1 is my personal algorithm for the workup and treatment of "patella" pain.

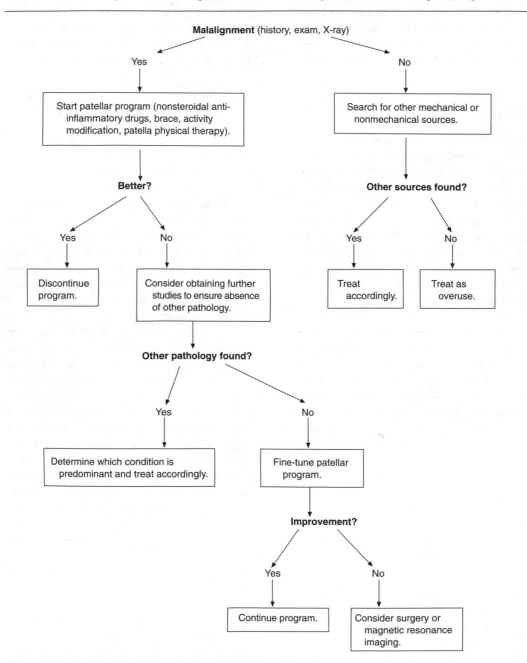

Figure 1–1 An Algorithm for the Workup of "Patella Pain"

REFERENCES

1. The International Patellofemoral Study Group. Patellofemoral semantics—the tower of Babel. *Am J Knee Surg.* 1997;10:92–95.

2. Grana WA, Krieghauser LA. Scientific basis of extensor mechanism disorders. *Clin Sports Med.* 1985;4:247–256.

3. Fulkerson JP. *Disorders of the Patellofemoral Joint.* 3rd ed. Baltimore: Williams & Wilkins; 1997:125.

4. Ficat P, Ficat C, Bailleux A. Syndrome d'hyperpression externe de la rotule. *Rev Chir Orthop.* 1975;61:39–59.

5. Buard J, Benoit J, Lortat-Jacob A, et al. Les trochlées fémorales creuses. *Rev Chir Orthop.* 1981;67:721.

6. Arnoldi CC. Patellar pain. *Acta Orthop Scand.* 1991; 62(suppl 224).

7. Dye SF, Vaupel GL. The pathophysiology of patellofemoral pain. *Sports Med Arthrosc Rev.* 1994; 2:203–210.

8. Outerbridge RE. The etiology of chondromalacia patellae. *J Bone Joint Surg.* 1961;43B:752.

9. Putz R, Müller-Gerbl M, Eckstein F, et al. Are there any correlations between superficial cartilaginous alterations and subchondral bone density (CT-OAM) in the femoropatellar joint? *Orthop Trans.* 1991;15:497.

10. Fulkerson JP. Anatomy of the knee joint lateral retinaculum. *Clin Orthop.* 1980;153:183.

11. Martinez-Moreno JL. Syndrome douloureux rotulien idiopathique: une hypothèse étiopathogénique. *Rev Chir Orthop.* 1994;80:239–245.

12. McConnell J. Fat pad irritation—a mistaken patellar tendonitis. *Sport Health.* 1991;9(4):7–9.

13. Buckley CK. Patello-femoral syndrome, the initiating agent. *Orthop Trans.* 1991;15:344.

14. Darracott J, Vernon-Roberts B. The bone changes in "chondromalacia patellae." *Rheumatol Phys Med.* 1971; 11:175.

15. Milgrom C, Finestone A, Eldad A. Patellofemoral pain caused by overactivity. *J Bone Joint Surg.* 1991; 73A:1041.

16. Cistac C, Cartier PH. Diagnostic et traitement des déséquilibres rotuliens du sportif. *J Traumatol Sport.* 1986;3:92–97.

17. Ficat P. Lateral fascia release and lateral hyperpressure syndrome. In: Pickett JC, Radin EL, eds. *Chondromalacia of the Patella.* Baltimore: Williams & Wilkins; 1983:95–112.

18. Harrison MM, Cooke TDV, Fisher SB, Griffin MP. Patterns of knee arthrosis and patella subluxation. *Clin Orthop.* 1994;309:56–63.

19. Turner MS. The association between tibial torsion and knee joint pathology. *Clin Orthop.* 1994;302:47–51.

20. Pinar H, Akseki O, Karaoglan O, et al. Kinematic and dynamic axial computed tomography of the patellofemoral joint in patients with anterior knee pain. *Knee Surg Sports Traumatol Arthrosc.* 1994;2:170.

21. Desai SS, Patel MR, Michelli LJ, et al. Osteochondritis dissecans of the patella. *J Bone Joint Surg.* 1987; 69B:320–325.

22. Yamaguchi H, Masuda T, Sasaki T, Nojima T. Steroid-induced osteonecrosis of the patella. *Clin Orthop.* 1988;229:201.

23. Insall JN, Falvo KA, Wise DW. Chondromalacia patellae—a prospective study. *J Bone Joint Surg.* 1976; 58A:1.

24. Armstrong CG, Mow VC, Wirth CR. Biomechanics of impact-induced microdamage to articular cartilage: a possible genesis for chondromalacia patella. In: Finerman G, ed. *American Academy of Orthopaedic Surgeons Symposium on Sports Medicine: The Knee.* St. Louis, MO: CV Mosby Co; 1985:70–84.

25. Atkinson PJ, Haut RC. Subfracture insult to the human cadaver patellofemoral joint produces occult injury. *J Orthop Res.* 1995;13:936–944.

26. Aleman O. Chondromalacia post-traumatica patellae. *Acta Orthop Scand.* 1928;63:194.

27. Fulkerson JP. *Disorders of the Patellofemoral Joint.* 3rd ed. Baltimore: Williams & Wilkins; 1997.

28. Karlson S. Chondromalacia patellae. *Acta Orthop Scand.* 1940;83:347.

29. Mansat CH, Bonnel F, Jaeger JH. *L'Appareil Extenseur du Genou.* Paris: Masson; 1985.

30. Hirsch C. A contribution to the pathogenesis of chondromalacia patella: a physical, histologic, and chemical study. *Acta Orthop Scand.* 1944;90(suppl):83.

31. Chaklin VD. Injuries to the cartilages of the patella and the femoral condyle. *J Bone Joint Surg.* 1939;37:133.

32. Silfverskiold N. Chondromalacia patellae. *Acta Orthop Scand.* 1938;9:214.

33. Slowick FA. Traumatic chondromalacia of the patella. *N Engl J Med.* 1935;213:160–161.

34. Casscells SW. Gross pathological changes in the knee joint of the aged individual. *Clin Orthop.* 1978;132:225.

35. Goodfellow JW, Hungerford DS, Woods C. Patellofemoral mechanics and pathology, II: chondromalacia patellae. *J Bone Joint Surg.* 1976;58B:291.

36. Stougard J. Chondromalacia of the patellae: physical signs in relation to operative findings. *Acta Orthop Scand.* 1975;46:685.

37. Abernathy PJ, Townsend P, Rose R, et al. Is chondroma-
    lacia patella a separate clinical entity? *J Bone Joint
    Surg*. 1978;60B:205.

38. Ficat RP, Hungerford DS. *Disorders of the Patel-
    lofemoral Joint*. 2nd ed. Baltimore: Williams &
    Wilkins; 1977.

39. Insall JN, Bullough PG, Burstein AH. Proximal "tube"
    realignment of the patella for chondromalacia patellae.
    Clin Orthop. 1979;144:63–69.

40. Bentley G, Beecham G. Presentation to the Eighth Com-
    bined Meeting of the Orthopaedic Associations of the
    English Speaking World, 1987.

41 Iwano T, Kurosawa H, Tokuyama H, et al. Roentgeno-
    graphic and clinical findings of patellofemoral osteoar-
    thritis. *Clin Orthop*. 1990;252:190–197.

42. Harrison MHM. The results of a realignment operation
    for recurrent dislocation of the patella. *J Bone Joint
    Surg*. 1955;37B:559.

ADDITIONAL READINGS

Boden BP, Pearsall AW, Garrett WE, Feagin JA Jr. Patellofemoral instability: evaluation and management. *J Am
Acad Orthop Surg*. 1997;5:47.

Grelsamer RP, Newton PM, Staron RB. The medial-lateral
position of the patella on routine MR Imaging: when is
normal not normal? *J Arthrosc*. 1998;14:1–6.

CHAPTER 2

Normal and Abnormal Anatomy of the Extensor Mechanism

The patella functions within a complex web of muscles, tendons, and other soft tissues collectively called the *extensor mechanism*. This chapter is therefore entitled "The Anatomy of the Extensor Mechanism" rather than "The Anatomy of the Patella."

EMBRYOLOGY

The word patella means "little plate" in Latin and, as bones go, it is rather small and rather round. There are a number of embryological features of interest to the clinician. In the human embryo, the patella initially lies proximal to its final position and gradually migrates distally.[1-3] Patella alta (see Chapter 5) can therefore be seen as a developmental arrest—the knee's equivalent of the undescended testicle. (Other studies by the same authors suggest that the patella may actually start in a relatively low position [S. Dye, personal communication; September 1996].) Membranes originally separate the patella from the femur and the tibia from the femur. These membranes disappear to a variable extent, their remnants appearing as fibrous bands called plicae.[4] One membrane completely separates the suprapatellar pouch from the patellofemoral joint and the rest of the knee. In rare cases, this condition persists. Normally, there is just one

ossification center in the patella, which is present by the time a child reaches the age of 3. Ossification is complete in girls by age 10 and in boys by age 13 to 16.[2,3] In some patients there can be more than one ossification center. When one of those centers is superolateral and it fails to fuse with the rest of the patella, the patient is said to have a bipartite patella, which can be symptomatic (see Chapter 7).

NORMAL ANATOMY

Although almost every portion of the human anatomy from the pelvis down (including hips and feet) has an effect on the extensor mechanism, the extensor mechanism proper begins above the hip joint and terminates at the tibial tuberosity. The extensor mechanism includes the four muscles of the quadriceps, the patella, the patellar tendon, all the other soft tissues attaching to the patella, and the tibial tuberosity. The blood supply and innervation are also key parts of the anatomy of the extensor mechanism.

The Skin and Subcutaneous Layers

The skin is quite mobile over the knee, just as it is over the dorsum of the hand, over the proximal interphalangeal (PIP) joints of the fingers, and over the extensor surface of the elbow. This mobility allows the knee to flex more than 120 degrees. Accounting for this mobility is a relative lack of fibrous connections between the skin

Special thanks go to SD Kwak, PhD, and the Columbia University Orthopaedic Research Laboratory for assistance with Figures 2–4 and 2–5.

and the underlying fascia. However, some fibrous connections do exist within the loose areolar tissue between the fascia and the skin, which are critical to the success of patellar taping (see Chapter 11).

Beneath the areolar tissue is the *superficial fascia* or *arciform layer*[2,3] (an extension of the fascia lata[5]), and deep to this is the intermediate oblique layer, which blends in with the patellotibial ligaments and may be absent in some people.[2,3] In performing open procedures about the knee (including patellar realignments), some surgeons begin their medial and lateral flaps prior to dividing the arciform layer and the intermediate oblique layer. This is an error because it does not allow the creation of thick flaps. It is extremely easy to create the flaps once the above-mentioned layers have been divided because they naturally peel off of the next layer— the deep longitudinal layer. This layer represents a continuation of the quadriceps tendon and is densely adherent to the patella.

Between the skin and the patella are potential spaces called bursae. These are akin to collapsed balloons that make their presence felt when they become inflamed and painful. They assist in lubrication, allowing one layer to slide over the next. There are three bursae (separating the subcutaneous tissue, the arciform layer, the intermediate oblique layer, and the deep longitudinal layer) (S. Dye, personal communication).

Muscles

The quadriceps consists of the rectus femoris, the vastus intermedius, the vastus lateralis, and the vastus medialis. The vastus medialis can be subdivided into the vastus medialis proper (or longus) and the vastus medialis obliquus. Taken as a group, the four muscles act as extensors of the knee when the foot is off the ground (as when a person kicks a ball); more commonly, they act as decelerators when the foot is on the ground, keeping the knee from collapsing when the foot strikes the ground.

The *rectus femoris* originates at the anterior inferior iliac spine, while the other muscles of the quadriceps originate on the femoral shaft.

The rectus femoris is the only one of the four muscles to cross the hip joint. This gives the hip joint considerable importance with respect to the extensor mechanism. Extension of the hip is an integral part of quadriceps stretching. The line of action (direction of pull) of the rectus femoris is not parallel to the femoral shaft, but rather subtends an angle of about 5 degrees with the femoral shaft (this is said to be the insertion angle of the muscle).

The *vastus intermedius* has a line of action similar to that of the rectus femoris but differs in two ways: its origin is on the proximal part of the femur (and therefore does not cross the hip joint), and its line of action is directly in line with the femur (and therefore forms an angle of about 5 degrees with the rectus femoris).

The *vastus lateralis* originates from the vastus ridge at the base of the greater trochanter and from a tough fibrous band at the posterior aspect of the femur called the linea aspera. It inserts anteriorly into the quadriceps tendon and laterally into the lateral retinaculum. It has a line of action of about 20 to 40 degrees to the long axis of the femur in the frontal plane (20 degrees for the upper fibers, up to 40 degrees for the lower fibers). One group of investigators found that the lower fibers of the vastus lateralis are separated from the main body of the muscle by a thin layer of fat and, as such, form an anatomically distinct vastus lateralis obliquus muscle.[6]

The *pennation angle* is the angle formed by the individual muscle fibers with the line of action of the muscle, and it is expressed as an average for the entire muscle. When all fibers are essentially parallel to the line of pull, as with the rectus femoris or vastus intermedius, the pennation angle is 0 degrees. At the other extreme are the pectoralis major and deltoid, which are fan shaped. The pennation angle for the vastus lateralis is 5 degrees.

The *vastus medialis longus* (VML) originates from the medial aspect of the upper femur and inserts anteriorly into the quadriceps tendon. It has a line of action of approximately 18 degrees off the long axis of the femur in the frontal plane (see Appendix 2–A). The pennation angle has been estimated to be about 5 degrees.[7]

The *vastus medialis obliquus* (VMO) is distinct from the VML.[8] It originates from the distal medial femur and adductor tubercle and inserts into the medial retinaculum and superomedial portion of the patella. Normally, the VMO comes as far distal as the upper third or half of the patella, and its lowermost fibers can be nearly horizontal.[9] Its tendinous portion is short, broad, and blends in with the medial retinaculum. It is usually not easy to see where the VML ends and where the VMO begins. In some patients, a thin layer of fat can be seen separating the two muscles. The VMO has a line of action of about 50 to 65 degrees off the long axis of the femur in the frontal plane, which is quite a bit less vertical than the bulk of the quadriceps[10] (Figure 2–1).

The *physiological cross-section* is an estimate of a muscle's maximum force-generating capacity and factors in the volume of the muscle, the length of the muscle fibers, and the pennation angle. The physiological cross-section is proportional to the overall volume of the muscle and inversely proportional to the length of the individual muscle fibers. It is also proportional to the cosine of the pennation angle. When the pennation angle is low, as with all the muscles of the quadriceps including the VMO, it is a negligible factor because its cosine is close to 1. My colleagues and I have recently analyzed the physiological cross-section of the VMO and found it to be approximately 30% of the entire vastus medialis complex (see Appendix 2–A). The above features contribute to making the VMO a critical dynamic medializing force.

All the muscles of the quadriceps are innervated by the femoral nerve, which enters the thigh along the medial border of the iliopsoas and fans out to the different muscles. The VMO may have a dual innervation (femoral and saphenous), and some believe that it has its own branch of the femoral nerve, further justifying its distinction from the rest of the vastus medialis.[11]

The *articularis genu* is a small, highly variable muscle that originates from the anterior surface of the distal femur just proximal to the patella and inserts into the suprapatellar pouch. It is flat and wispy and ranges in width from 1.5 to 3

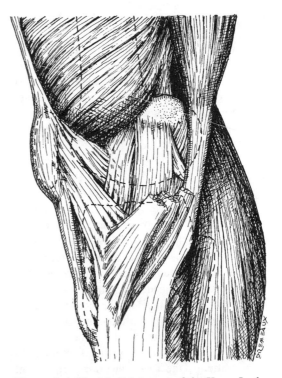

Figure 2–1 The Medial Aspect of the Knee. In the normal knee, the VMO reaches the upper third to upper half of the patella, and the fibers are 50 to 65 degrees off the vertical. Courtesy of Georges Dremeaux, Mt. Kisco, New York.

cm.[5] Its exact role is unclear, but at least one group has attributed patella baja (infera) following knee trauma to a dysfunction of this muscle.[12] Others have said that this muscle retracts the suprapatellar pouch and maintains the pouch's proper position during knee flexion and extension.[10]

The Quadriceps Tendon

The quadriceps tendon represents the confluence of all four muscles tendon units, and it inserts at the anterior aspect of the superior pole of the patella. The tendon has three layers or laminae[13]: the most superficial comes from the rectus femoris, the vastus lateralis and vastus medialis contribute to the intermediate lamina, and the deep lamina comes from the vastus intermedius. The three laminae merge approximately

2 cm from the patella. The tendon tends to be thicker medially, which can be of clinical significance when this tendon is harvested for anterior cruciate ligament reconstructions.[14] It articulates with the trochlea as the knee flexes past 90 degrees and absorbs some of the stresses associated with deep-knee flexion (see Chapter 3). It is prone to degenerate rupture in patients in their 50s and 60s.

The Patellar Tendon

Semantic controversy exists among purists with respect to the name of this structure. The question is whether it is a tendon or a ligament. Because it connects two bones (patella and tibia), it is a ligament; because it represents the attachment of the quadriceps unit to the tibia, it is a tendon. I call it the *patellar tendon*. It originates at the inferior (nonarticulating) pole of the patella and inserts onto the tibial tuberosity. It is approximately 5 to 6 cm long and 3 cm wide. In some patients, the fibers are not parallel but rather fan out from distal to proximal (this can have an effect on the technique used for harvesting a portion of the patellar tendon for anterior cruciate ligament reconstructions, as parallel blades may not always be appropriate). The tendon is invested in a paratenon, a loose fibrillar structure, which is identified and divided in open knee surgery about the patella. The vascular supply is from the underlying fat pad in the proximal third, while the distal third is more directly supplied by branches of the inferior medial and lateral geniculate vessels.[14,15] The tendon contains sensory nerves (wherefore injury is painful) along with mechanoreceptors (Golgi), and Golgi-Mazzoni, Ruffini, and Pacini corpuscles. This tendon rarely ruptures, but when it does it tends to be in people in their teens and 20s.

The Fat Pad

Behind and on either side of the patellar tendon lies the fat pad. It is usually visible and palpable.[16,17] It is richly innervated and sensitive to pain (S. Dye, personal communication). A verti-

cal artery runs medially and laterally, and in most patients a horizontal artery is also present. The foot pad is variable in size; although it is intraarticular, it is extrasynovial.[16] It is limited anteriorly by the patellar tendon, superiorly by the inferior pole of the patella, and posteriorly by the femoral condyles and intercondylar notch. It attaches inferolaterally to the anterior horn of the lateral meniscus and inferomedially to the anterior horn of the medial meniscus.

The Lateral Retinaculum

This thick structure lies along the lateral border of the patella and represents the confluence of many structures including the iliotibial band and lateral patellofemoral ligament.[5,18] The superior genicular artery and vein course in a medial-lateral direction along the ventral surface of the retinaculum near the superior pole of the patella.

The Iliotibial Band

The iliotibial band (ITB), also referred to as iliotibial tract or iliopatellar band,[19] is a remarkable structure (Figure 2–2). It spans two joints, influences three articulations, and is forgotten quite often in the orthopaedic physical exam. It begins as a wide fascia covering the upper lateral pelvis and thigh in continuity with the fascia lata; narrows down to a band along the side of the thigh; remains attached posteriorly to the lateral intermuscular septum; and fans out distally to the patella, the lateral retinaculum, and the tibia (via its attachment to a prominence—Gerdy's tubercle). Terry et al[19] have studied the anatomy of this structure in depth and have termed the portion attaching to the patella the iliopatellar band and the portion attaching to Gerdy's tubercle the iliotibial tract. In the nineteenth century, Gerdy[20] wrote about the insertion of the iliotibial band, and it was Segond[21] who named the tubercle after him. The Belgian anatomist Vesalius was an early reference (1552) for description of the ITB; he considered it to be "the sixth muscle of the tibia," thus em-

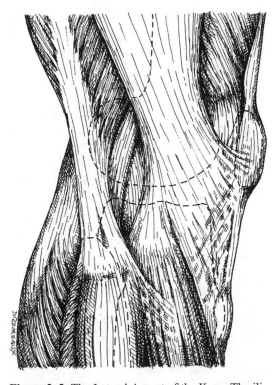

Figure 2–2 The Lateral Aspect of the Knee. The iliotibial band, which is tethered posteriorly, fans out anteriorly into the lateral retinaculum and distally onto Gerdy's tubercle. It is an important dynamic stabilizer of the lateral side of the knee. When excessively tight, it contributes to pulling the patella laterally; it can be the source of "runner's knee" as it rubs against the lateral aspect of the femoral condyle; and it can be a hidden source of anterior knee pain. Courtesy of Georges Dremeaux, Mt. Kisco, New York.

phasizing its distal role.[22] Maissiat studied the ITB extensively,[23] and the ITB has on occasion been called the "band of Maissiat."[22,24]

Proximally, the ITB is indirectly connected to the gluteus medius, the gluteus maximus, the tensor fascia lata, and the vastus lateralis. At that point it is relatively thin (0.2 inch), but it doubles in thickness distally[8] where its strength may compare favorably with that of the anterior cruciate ligament.[19] Because of this connection to the proximal thigh musculature, the ITB can be tensed and can be thought of as a tendon. On the other hand, because of its fixed attachment

posterodistally on the femur, it can also be considered a ligament.[22,24]

The ITB has a number of functions, both static and dynamic. It flexes the hip, and it can flex or extend the knee, depending on the initial position of the knee. With the knee in slight flexion, the ITB is anterior to the axis of rotation and serves to extend the knee. With the knee flexed more than about 30 degrees, the ITB is posterior to the axis of rotation and serves to further flex the knee. Because part of the ITB blends into the lateral retinaculum, it affects patella tracking. During gait, the ITB tenses the lateral side of the thigh and tends to resist the adductor moment about the knee.

Because of its attachments to the lateral retinaculum and to the patella, the ITB has a significant effect on patellar position, patellar tracking (see Chapter 3), and patellar pain—especially when it is excessively tight.

The Medial Retinaculum and Related Structures

The medial retinaculum is far thinner than its lateral counterpart and is not believed to be as significant with respect to patella position and tracking. Beneath the medial retinaculum are patellofemoral, patellomeniscal,[25,26] and patellotibial ligaments.[26] According to some, these are not necessarily visible ligaments but rather are palpable thickenings of the capsule.[5] This accounts in part for the discrepancy in the literature with respect to the presence or absence of these ligaments. Reider et al found that only 6 of 20 specimens had a medial patellofemoral ligament.[5] On the other hand, Conlan et al described a well-defined ligament originating at the adductor tubercle in the same plane as the superficial portion of the medial collateral ligament, and they have provided clear illustrations.[27] They noted that the proximal fibers fan out under the VMO, while the distal fibers attach to the proximal portion of the patella. They noted such a ligament in 23 of 25 specimens. Conlan et al[27] and Fithian et al (personal communication) suggest that the medial patellofemoral ligaments are strong enough to influence patellar tracking and, in fact, are the major (static) medial restraints.

Plicae

A plica is the name given to any fibrous band of tissue that spans part of the knee joint without clear functional role. Vesalius is reported to have first described a knee plica in 1555, specifically the inferior plica about the anterior cruciate ligament (also referred to as *ligamentum mucosum*). It is convenient to think of the plicae as embryological remnants of membranes that at one point separated the compartments. However, this view is somewhat simplistic. Dupont[4] observes that at no point is there a membrane separating the medial from the lateral compartment.

The plica of greatest interest within the context of the extensor mechanism is the medial parapatellar plica, which originates proximal to the patella, courses medial to the patella, and inserts into the fat pad. It is present in a minority of patients, but inflammation of this plica enters into the differential diagnosis of patellar pain. There are many other possible plicae about the knee.[4]

The Tibial Tuberosity

The prominence onto which the patellar tendon attaches is the tibial tuberosity. It usually lies just lateral to the midsagittal plane (midline) of the tibia. In childhood and adolescence, it is separated from the tibial shaft by a growth plate. Because the growth plate does not contribute to the overall length of the bone, it is called an apophyseal rather than an epiphyseal plate.

The Sensory Innervation

Medially, the medial femoral cutaneous nerve ends approximately halfway down the patella after coursing over, through, or under the sartorius.[28] The terminal branch of the nerve to the vastus medialis can also provide sensory fibers to the medial aspect of the patella, and the anterior branch of the obturator nerve can ramify with the subsartorial plexus.[28] The lateral retinacular nerve arising from the sciatic nerve supplies the lateral portion of the patella. In addition to the above-mentioned nerves, the lateral femoral cutaneous nerve can provide sensation to the area just proximal to the patella.[28]

There is considerable variation with respect to the sensory territory covered by each nerve. In some patients, the sensation over the lateral portion of the knee is provided by the medial nerves. In these patients, a medial or midline incision often renders numb the lateral half of the knee. By the same token, some of the pain relief following patella operations on the medial side might in part be due to the simple interruption of sensory nerves (see Chapter 14).

The anterior cruciate ligament has been found to be richly supplied with mechanoreceptors.[29,30] These provide reflex "communication" with the surrounding musculature and belie the concept that ligaments are purely passive. It remains to be determined whether the soft tissues about the patella are equally endowed with mechanoreceptors.

The Vascular Supply about the Patella

The vascular supply to the patella is quite rich. A major vessel enters the patella at the corner of each quadrant in the form of the superior and inferior medial and lateral geniculate arteries (with corresponding veins).[15] Smaller arteries also enter the patella via the inferior and superior pole and help maintain the vascularity to the patella when the genicular arteries have been surgically sacrificed.[31,32] The geniculate vessels fan out into smaller vessels that enter the patella through its dorsal surface via small tunnels that are clearly visible to the naked eye. These give the dorsum of the patella a cribriform (pierced with small holes) appearance.

The vessels are wrapped in a mesh of fine nerves. Thus, any condition affecting the nerves about the knee (eg, reflex sympathetic dystrophy, smoking) will affect the blood supply and therefore the color and temperature of the overlying skin.

The Patella

The patella is often referred to as "a round bone at the front of the knee." If only it were that simple! The patella is nearly as much a piece of cartilage as it is a bone. When viewed dorsally, it is indeed roundish, although the inferior pole in some patients gives it more the appearance of a plump raindrop. Whereas the dorsal surface is all bone, three quarters of the ventral surface is cartilaginous (Figure 2–3). And what cartilage!

The articular cartilage of the patella is the thickest cartilage in the human body. If one believes that form follows function, this cartilage thickness is no accident (see Chapter 3). The patellar cartilage is also unique in that it does not follow the topography of the underlying bone. This can be problematic when one interprets plain X-rays and computed tomography (CT) scans (see Chapter 5). In only 15% of cases does the apex of the bony patella coincide with that of the articular cartilage (when viewed in the axial plane); in 60% of cases, the apex of the articular cartilage is lateral to the apex of the bony patella; in the remaining 25%, it is medial. A matching shift can be appreciated on the trochlear side, where the lowest point of the bony trochlea does not always match the lowest point of the articular cartilage.

The articular surface is oval, with the long axis going in a medial to lateral direction. Thus, when the patella is everted (flipped over) at surgery to expose the articular surface, it always appears that the patella is longer in the medial-lateral direction than in the proximal-distal direction. If the fat just distal to the cartilage is removed, the nonarticulating, non–cartilage-covered inferior pole of the patella is exposed and the patella is once again seen to be roundish.

Patellar cartilage is not one smooth, shield-like surface. Rather, it features a number of facets (Figures 2–4 and 2–5). These facets vary tremendously in size and shape from patient to patient to the point where one could legitimately call them "the fingerprints of the knee." In a given patient, one patella is usually close to be-

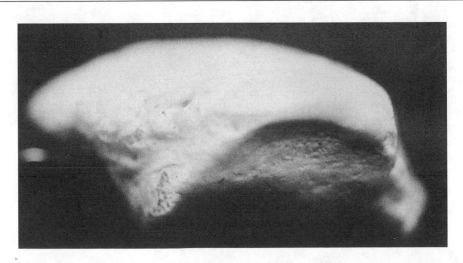

Figure 2–3 The Bony Patella Viewed from the Side. The distal quarter of the patella is nonarticular (has no articular cartilage). Fractures through this portion of the patella are potentially less serious. The ventral aspect of the remainder of the patella is covered with the thickest cartilage in the body. This cartilage does not follow the contour of the underlying bone. Plain radiographs therefore do not give a true measure of the fit between the patella and the underlying trochlea.

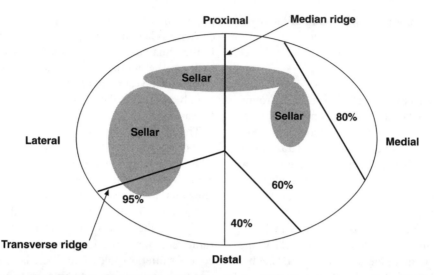

Figure 2–4 Articular Facets: The Fingerprints of the Knee. All patients have a median ridge separating the proximal patella into medial and lateral facets. This ridge goes only halfway down the patella (starting proximally). It veers off in variable fashion toward the medial side and is no longer median. Most patients have a transverse ridge on the lateral side of the patella, but it extends medially in only half of the population. For most patients, the ridges form a λ. The exact pattern is unique to each patient.

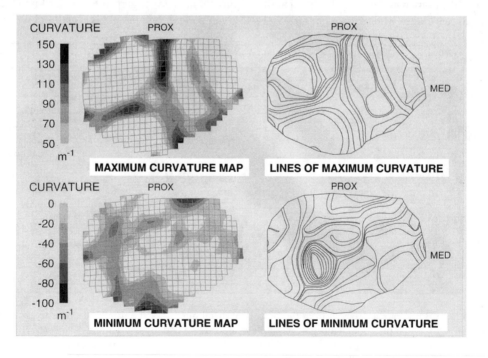

Figure 2–5 Curvature Analysis of a Human Patella

ing a mirror image of the other. In a recent study of unpaired patellae, my colleagues and I found certain common elements to essentially all patellae. Most patients have a median ridge that only goes halfway down the patella (starting proximally), separating the proximal patella into medial and lateral facets. It then veers off in variable fashion toward the medial side and is no longer median (Figure 2–4). Most patients have a transverse ridge on the lateral side of the patella, but it extends medially in about half the population (15 of 39 knees in our study). The median and transverse ridges come together in equally inconstant fashion. The junction may be nearly a right angle; at the other extreme, the two ridges can have no clear junction (in which case, the two ridges are actually one *C*-shaped ridge). In 80% of the patellae, the so-called odd facet was present. This is a smaller facet at the extreme medial portion of the patella, which can be nearly vertical and which articulates with the medial condyle in deep flexion. In addition to the above-mentioned facets, there can be a number of more subtle facets, apparent only with careful scrutiny.

Considering the importance that practitioners assign to cartilage lesions in patellar pain, it is interesting to note that one investigator indicated that the articular cartilage of the patella is insensate (S. Dye, personal communication). This same investigator was surprised to find that probing of the menisci caused pain, as did probing of the trochlea and the femoral condyles.

The articulation between the patella and the trochlea in the axial plane is relatively congruent. That is, as one goes from medial to lateral, there is contact between the patellar cartilage and that of the underlying trochlea. On anatomic sections, there is no contact at the center of the trochlea. During everyday use, it is probable that this space disappears as the patellar cartilage deforms. When the patellofemoral joint is seen from the side, the situation is quite different. Most of the patellar cartilage is not in contact with the trochlea. As such, it can be said that in the sagittal plane the patellofemoral joint is quite incongruent.

One group of investigators found an osteochondral ridge at the most proximal portion of the medial trochlea and postulated that this could be a cause of medial facet chondromalacia.[32] However, other investigators have not found this ridge.[2,33,34]

With the knee in extension, the articular surface of the normal patella lies just proximal to the trochlea. As the knee flexes to about 15 degrees, the articular surface of the patella comes into contact with the trochlea. Part of the patellar surface remains in contact with the trochlea throughout the remainder of the flexion arc (see Chapter 3).

Viewed from the side, the patella is roughly rectangular with a triangular piece tacked on to its distal end (Figure 2–3). This piece is the nonarticulating inferior pole. In normal patients, the longest (diagonal) length of the patella is somewhere between 1.2 and 1.5 times the length of the articular surface. This ratio is important when imaging the patella (see Chapter 5).

Viewed in axial cross-section, the bony patella is V-shaped, the lateral side being longer.

The Trochlea

This is the cartilage-covered, V-shaped groove at the distal end of the anterior femur. The groove consists of the inner walls of the lateral and medial femoral condyles much as a valley flanked by two mountains. In normal knees, the lateral condyle (and therefore the lateral wall of the trochlea) is always higher (protrudes farther anteriorly) than the medial one. This is a characteristic particular to bipedal animals and is a useful sign to anthropologists. It is also useful to us bipedal animals on a day-to-day basis (see Chapter 3).

As noted on X-ray imaging, the so-called sulcus angle of the bony trochlea becomes deeper (steeper) as one progresses distally. However, when one examines the articular surface of the trochlea, it appears that the same sulcus angle is maintained throughout (A. Amis, personal communication). This can be accounted for by a gradual thickening of the articular cartilage as one progresses distally.

The Intercondylar Notch

This is the name given to the vault-like space between the two femoral condyles. The anterior portion of its roof is actually the distal-most portion of the trochlea. The importance of this roof lies in the fact that it is often partially removed during the "notchplasty" portion of an anterior cruciate ligament reconstruction—with unknown long-term effects on the patella. When seen in profile on a lateral X-ray, the roof appears as a line known as Blumensaat's line. This line along with the longitudinal axis of the distal femur subtends at an angle that averages 45 degrees but varies between 25 and 60 degrees.[33]

The Pes Tendons

These tendons are not part of the extensor mechanism. In fact, they flex the knee. But because they can be used for surgery of the extensor mechanism, they warrant a brief description. The pes consists of the sartorius, gracilis, and semitendinosus in that sequence, starting proximally ("Say grace before tea," for those mnemonically inclined). They are innervated by the femoral, obturator, and sciatic nerves, respectively. These muscles originate at the anterior, medial, and posterior portion of the femur, respectively. All three converge just medial and distal to the tibial tuberosity. The sartorius can remain muscular nearly all the way to its insertion. The gracilis and semitendinosus are tendinous about the knee and therefore can be disinserted and used as a ligament substitute.

Hamstring Muscles

These muscles are not part of the extensor mechanism because they flex the knee. However, because they pull the upper tibia posteriorly (and therefore the tibial tuberosity), the hamstrings impart a flexion moment to the patella, pushing the inferior pole of the patella posteriorly into the fat pad. Tightness of the hamstrings has been associated with patellar pain,[35] possibly because of an exaggerated effect on the patella.

ABNORMAL ANATOMY

In patients with malalignment, the anatomy is abnormal in one or more ways. The VMO instead of reaching the upper third or half of the patella may barely reach the patella at all, and its line of pull may be more vertical[36] (Figure 2–6). The combination of these two abnormalities makes the VMO a less effective medial restraint.[37] Electromyography studies suggest that, in patients with malalignment, the electromyographic activity of the VMO is abnormal.[8,12] The entire quadriceps mechanism, including specifically the vastus lateralis, may be abnormal in some patients. Indeed, contraction of the quadriceps in patients with malalignment leads to considerable lateral tilting of the patella (see Chapter 5). This phenomenon is not found in patients with a normal extensor mechanism.[38] Finally, one group of investigators has noted an increase in type 2C muscle fibers in dislocators.[39]

The lateral retinaculum can be excessively tight. In this situation, the patella is laterally tilted (lateral side down) or laterally displaced. There is a chicken and egg situation with respect to whether a tight lateral retinaculum causes a tilted/displaced patella or whether a tilted/displaced patella leads to a tight lateral retinaculum.

The tibial tuberosity can be even more lateral to the midline than usual. This increases the quadriceps angle (see Chapter 3). In adolescence, this tuberosity can become enlarged and painful. When this happens, the patient is said to suffer from Osgood-Schlatter's disease. *Disease* is probably not the correct word here; the condition, although painful, is not serious and is usually self-limited.

The parts or all of the lower extremity can exhibit torsional deformities, with one deformity "attempting" to compensate for another. For example, the hip can be anteverted. The femoral shaft can be internally rotated. The patella can follow the femur and point medially (the "squinting patella") or can remain in its normal position, which then gives it a lateralized appearance ("grasshopper" appearance). A high-riding, lateralized patella can also give this ap-

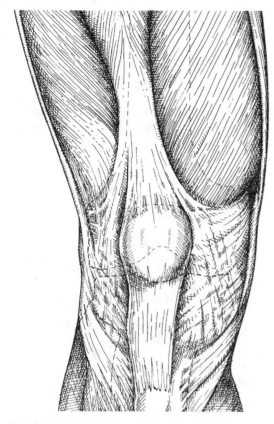

Figure 2–6 Frontal View of the Abnormal Extensor Mechanism. The VMO is dysplastic: it barely reaches the top of the patella, and the line of action of the muscle is about 25 degrees off the vertical rather than the normal 50 degrees. Courtesy of Georges Dremeaux, Mt. Kisco, New York.

pearance, even without internal rotation of the femur. The tibia can exhibit torsion proximally, distally, or both. Proximally, torsion is usually external, which leads to a lateralized tibial tuberosity. These types of complex, top-to-bottom rotational deformities have given rise to the term "miserable malalignment"—referring to the patient's as well as the doctor's feelings.

The patella can have any number of shapes. When viewed from the lateral side, the inferior pole can be long and the articular surface short, giving the patella a long-nosed "Cyrano" appearance. Conversely, the inferior pole can be quite short and the articular surface relatively

long. These unusual shapes can throw off standard interpretations of patellar height (see Chapter 5).

The patella can lie farther proximal than normal with respect to the trochlea. Thus, the so-called height of the patella is greater than normal, a condition called *patella alta*. Brattström[33] refers to Schulthess,[34] who wrote in 1899, as the first to occupy himself with this condition. Conversely, the patella can be too far engaged into the trochlea (too close to the tibial plateau), a condition called *patella infera* or *baja*.

When viewed in a tangential fashion (as if looking at one's own patella), the patella is horizontal when the leg is in neutral rotation. However, it is common in patients with malalignment for the patella to be tilted. Unless the patient has had surgery, tilt is always such that the medial side is elevated and the lateral side depressed (posterior).[26]

When viewed in axial cross-section, the medial bony facet can be excessively small, there may be no separate medial and lateral bony facet, or the patella may look like a hunter's cap (as described by Wiberg[40]) or a pebble.

The trochlea can be shallow, the problem being either excessive thickness of the floor of the trochlea or insufficient height of one or both femoral condyles. One group has found that the medial portion of the trochlea is most variable. Shallow trochleas tend to "point" more medially (ie, the bisector of the sulcus angle points more medially), whereas steeper trochleas point more laterally.[41] This may in part account for increased congruence angles in dislocators (see Chapter 5).

The nerves in the lateral retinaculum can exhibit fibrosis as noted in one study of patella malalignment.[18]

The entire extensor mechanism can be tight. In some cases, this condition is mild and amenable to stretching. In other cases, the tightness is severe and can require a major surgical release (beginning at the hip). Such tightness can be caused by scarring down of the quadriceps (from trauma or injections) or can be congenital (in conjunction with a neuromuscular disease). Patients with permanent dislocation of the patella from childhood have a seriously tight extensor mechanism. This may be either the cause or the result of the chronic dislocation. Either way, when the patella is recentered, these patients lose their knee flexion unless a major soft tissue release is carried out concomitantly.

A plica can become thickened and inflamed (it has been referred to as a "pseudomeniscus").

As the knee flexes, it can catch, pop, and be painful.

A bursa can become inflamed, in which case it fills with fluid and may be painful. This can occur seemingly spontaneously (as with the olecranon bursitis about the elbow), or it can be the result of chronic irritation (eg, from scrubbing the floor). It can fill with blood in cases of trauma, and it can become infected.

REFERENCES

1. Doskocil M. Formation of the femoropatellar part of the human knee joint. *Folia Morphol.* 1985;33:38.

2. Dye SF. An evolutionary perspective of the knee. *J Bone Joint Surg.* 1987;69A:976.

3. Dye SF. Patellofemoral anatomy. In Fox JM, Del Pizzo W, eds. *The Patellofemoral Joint.* New York: McGraw-Hill; 1993:1–12.

4. Dupont JY. Synovial plicae. *Knee.* 1994;1:5–19.

5. Reider B, Marshall JL, Koslin D, et al. The anterior aspect of the knee joint. *J Bone Joint Surg.* 1981; 63A:351–356.

6. Hallisey MJ, Doherty N, Bennett WF, et al. Anatomy of the junction of the vastus lateralis tendon and the patella. *J Bone Joint Surg.* 1987;69A:545.

7. Wickiewicz TL, Roy RR, Powell PL. Muscle architecture of the human lower limb. *Clin Orthop.* 1983; 179:275–283.

8. Lieb FJ, Perry J. Quadriceps function: an anatomical and mechanical study using amputated limbs. *J Bone Joint Surg.* 1968;50A:1535–1548.

9. Bose K, Kanagasuntheram R, Osman MBH. Vastus medialis oblique: an anatomic and physiologic study. *Orthopedics.* 1980;3:880.

10. Hughston J, Walsh WM, Puddu G. *Patellar Subluxation and Dislocation.* Philadelphia: WB Saunders Co; 1984. Saunders Monographs in Clinical Orthopaedics, no. 5.

11. Günal I, Arac S, Sahinoglu K, et al. The innervation of the vastus medialis obliquus. *J Bone Joint Surg.* 1992;74B:624.

12. Mariani P, Caruso I. An electromyographic investigation of subluxation of the patella. *J Bone Joint Surg.* 1979;61B:169–171.

13. Puddu G, Cipolla M, Cerullo G. Tendinitis. In: Fox JM, Del Pizzo W, eds. *The Patellofemoral Joint.* New York: McGraw-Hill; 1993:177–192.

14. Stäubli HU, Schatzmann L, Brunner P, et al. Quadriceps tendon and patellar ligament cryosectional anatomy and structural properties in young adults. *Knee Surg Sports Traumatol Arthrosc.* 1996;4:100–110.

15. Scapinelli R. Blood supply to the human patella: Its relation to ischemic necrosis after fracture. *J Bone Joint Surg.* 1967;49B:563–570.

16. Duri ZAA, Aichroth PM, Dowd G. The fat pad: clinical observations. *Am J Knee Surg.* 1996;9:55–66.

17. Hoffa A. The influence of the adipose tissue with regard to the pathology of the knee joint. *JAMA.* 1904;42:795–796.

18. Fulkerson JP. Anatomy of the knee joint lateral retinaculum. *Clin Orthop.* 1980;153:183.

19. Terry GC, Hughston JC, Norwood LA. The anatomy of the iliopatellar band and iliotibial tract. *Am J Sports Med.* 1986;14:39.

20. Gerdy PN. *Troisième monographe des maladies des organes du mouvement.* Paris: Victor Masson; 1855.

21. Segond P. Recherches cliniques et experimentales sur les e'panchements sanguins du genou par entorse. *Progres Med.* 1879;6:319.

22. Jacob HAC, Huggler AH, Ruttiman B. In-vivo investigations on the mechanical function of the tractus iliotibialis. In: Huiskes R, Van Campen D, De Wijn J, eds. *Biomechanics: Principles and Applications.* The Hague: Martinus Nijhoff; 1982.

23. Maissiat JH. *Etudes de physique animale.* Paris: Bethune et Plon; 1843.

24. Thomsen W. Zur Statik und Mechanik der gesunden und gelahmten Hufte: Ueber die Bedeutung des Tractus iliotibialis (Maissiat). *Z Orthop Chir.* 1934;60:212–231.

25. Andrews JR, Thornberry R. The role of open surgery for patellofemoral joint malalignment. *Orthop Rev.* 1986;15:72.

26. Fulkerson JP, Shea KP. Disorders of patellofemoral alignment: current concepts review. *J Bone Joint Surg.* 1990;72A:1424.

27. Conlan T, Garth WP, Lemons JE. Evaluation of the medial soft-tissue restraints of the extensor mechanism of the knee. *J Bone Joint Surg.* 1993;75A:682–693.

28. Horner G, Dellon L. Innervation of the human knee joint and implications for surgery. *Clin Orthop.* 1994; 301:221–226.

29. Schultz RA, Miller DC, Kerr CS, et al. Mechanoreceptors in human cruciate ligaments. *J Bone Joint Surg.*
1984;66A:1072–1076.

30. Solomonow M, Baratta R, Zhou BH, et al. The synergistic action of the anterior cruciate ligament and thigh
muscles in maintaining joint stability. *Am J Sports Med.*
1987;15:207–213.

31. Björkström S, Goldie IF. A study of the arterial supply
of the patella in the normal state, in chondromalacia patellae and in osteoarthritis. *Acta Orthop Scand.*
1980;51:63–70.

32. Scuderi G, Scharf SC, Meltzer L. Evaluation of patella
viability after disruption of the arterial circulation. *Am J
Sports Med.* 1987;15:490–493.

33. Brattström H. Patella alta in non-dislocating knee joints.
Acta Orthop Scand. 1970;41:578–588.

34. Schulthess W. Zur pathologie und therapie der
spastischen Gliederstarre. *Z Orthop Chir.* 1899;6:1–13.

35. Grana WA, Krieghauser LA. Scientific basis of extensor
mechanism disorders. *Clin Sports Med.* 1985;4:247–
256.

36. Outerbridge RE, Dunlop J. The problem of chondromalacia patellae. *Clin Orthop.* 1975;110:177–193.

37. Boucher JP, King MA, Lefebvre R, et al. Quadriceps
femoris muscle activity in patellofemoral pain syndrome. *Am J Sports Med.* 1992;20:527–532.

38. Nove-Josserand L, Dejour D. Dysplasie du quadriceps
et bascule rotulienne dans l'instabilité rotulienne objective. *Rev Chir Orthop.* 1995;81:497–504.

39. Floyd A, Phillips P, Khan MRH. Recurrent dislocation
of the patella. *J Bone Joint Surg.* 1987;69B:790.

40. Wiberg G. Roentgenographic and anatomic studies on
the femero-patellar joint. *Acta Orthop Scand.* 1941;
12:319–410.

41. Buard J, Benoit J, Lortat-Jacob A, et al. Les trochlées
fémorales creuses. *Rev Chir Orthop.* 1981;67:721.

ADDITIONAL READINGS

Eckhoff DG, Montgomery WK, Stamm ER, Kilcoyne RF.
Location of the femoral sulcus in the osteoarthritic knee.
J Arthroplasty. 1996;11:163–165.

Harris NL, Smith DAB, Lamoreaux L, et al. Central quadri-
ceps tendon for anterior cruciate ligament reconstruction.
Part I: morphometric and biomechanical evaluation. *Am J
Sports Med.* 1997;25:23–28.

Siu D, Rudan J, Wevers HW, Griffiths P. Femoral articular shape and geometry. *J Arthroplasty.* 1996;11:
166–173.

Appendix 2–A

Analysis of Vastus Medialis Longus and Vastus Medialis Obliquus Characteristics

In a recent study (Raimondo, Ahmad, Grelsamer, April, Henry, Patella stabilization: a quantitative evaluation of the vastus medialis obliquus muscle, *Orthopaedics*, 1998) 21 formalin-preserved cadavers (16 female, 5 male, average age 79 years) were dissected to expose the vastus medialis longus (VML) and vastus medialis obliquus (VMO). The insertion angle was assessed to the nearest degree with a goniometer. Muscle fibers extending from the origin to the insertion of the muscle were removed and measured to the nearest millimeter. Volume was determined for the entire muscle by water displacement in a graduated cylinder.

The insertion angle for the VMO was 52 +/– 2 degrees, while the insertion angle of the VML was 18 +/– 2 degrees.

Fiber length was 6.3 +/– 0.4 cm for the VMO and 8.5 +/– 0.3 cm for the VML.

The muscle volume was 20 +/– 8 cc for the VMO and 67 +/– 29 cc for the VML.

The physiological cross-section was calculated to be 3.1 +/– 1.3 cm^2 for the VMO and 7.9 +/– 3.3 cm^2 for the VML.

CHAPTER 3

Applied Mechanics of the Patellofemoral Joint

THE PATELLA—A LEVER OR A PULLEY?

What does the patella do and how does it do it? The patella gives the extensor mechanism a greater mechanical advantage. Depending on what activity a person is engaged in and what stage of the flexion-extension cycle is being analyzed, the patella magnifies either force or displacement—typical functions of levers. The patella also changes the quadriceps' direction of force—a typical pulley function.

The patella increases the moment arm of the quadriceps extensor mechanism,[1-6] and this effect is mostly present at about 20 degrees of flexion.[6] According to one calculation, at 0-degree flexion, the patella accounts for approximately one third of the quadriceps' moment arm about the center of rotation of the knee.[1] Simply put,

This chapter was adapted with permission from RP Grelsamer, WW Colman, and VC Mow, Anatomy and Mechanics of the Patellofemoral Joint, *Sports Medicine and Arthroscopy Review*, Vol 2, pp 178–188, © 1994, Lippincott–Raven Publishers.

I thank the following for their help with the biomechanical analyses: Gerard Ateshian, PhD; S. Daniel Kwak, MS; Thomas R. Gardner, MS; and Rajeev Kelkar, MS. This work was supported by a DePuy Orthopaedic Research and Education Foundation (OREF) Development Award.

Special thanks go to SD Kwak, PhD, and the Columbia University Orthopaedic Research Laboratory for assistance with Figures 3–7 and 3–8.

the presence of the patella allows knee flexion and extension to occur with a lesser amount of quadriceps force (ie, the patella is functioning as a lever). Conversely, without the patella, the extensor mechanism must work harder. In such a situation, a greater force is generated by the quadriceps, and this leads to greater forces and stresses across the femorotibial joint. These stresses, in turn, can lead to degeneration of the joint.[7] (*Clinical implication*: After a patellectomy, a patient may be able to compensate in the short run for the lack of a patella, but the femorotibial forces will be increased, and the patient could be at risk for later femorotibial arthritis.[7] This alone is a good reason for regarding the patellectomy as a procedure of last resort.)

In addition to increasing the lever arm of the quadriceps, the patella redirects the force exerted by the quadriceps. For this reason, the patella could be considered a pulley. However, a pulley, unless used in combination with other pulleys, changes the direction of a force but does not change the magnitude of that force. A rope going around a simple pulley has equal tension on either side of the pulley. This is not the case with the patella. A number of investigators have found through calculations and experimental work that the tension in the quadriceps tendon is generally different from that in the patellar tendon (eg, Kaufer,[1] Ahmed,[2] Hirokawa,[4] Grood,[6] Denham,[7] Huberti,[8] van Eijden,[9] Bishop,[10] Amis,[11] Buff[12]) (Figure 3–1). With flexion greater than approximately 50 degrees, most in-

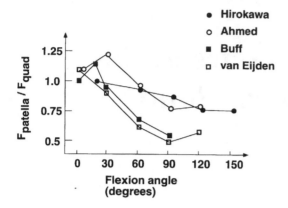

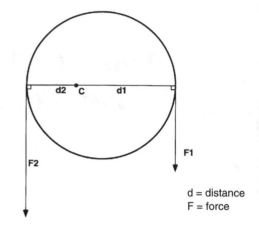

d = distance
F = force

Figure 3–1 Ratio of Quadriceps Tendon Force/Patellar Tendon Force versus Degree of Knee Flexion (as per Four Investigators). *Source:* Reprinted with permission from RP Grelsamer, WW Colman, and VC Mow, Anatomy and Mechanics of the Patellofemoral Joint, *Sports Medicine and Arthroscopy Review*, Vol 2, p 179, © 1994, Lippincott–Raven Publishers.

Figure 3–2 Illustration of an Eccentric Pulley (a Model for the Patella). Because the axis of the pulley is eccentric, the moment arms d1 and d2 are different. Moreover, because in a static situation F2 × d2 = F1 × d1, F1 and F2 are necessarily different also. For similar reasons, the forces in the quadriceps and patellar tendons are different. *Source:* Reprinted with permission from RP Grelsamer, WW Colman, and VC Mow, Anatomy and Mechanics of the Patellofemoral Joint, *Sports Medicine and Arthroscopy Review*, Vol 2, p 179, © 1994, Lippincott–Raven Publishers.

vestigators agree that the force in the patellar tendon is less than the force in the quadriceps tendon. (*Implication*: In this large range, the patella does not amplify the force of the quadriceps.) Regarding flexion from 0 to 50 degrees, there is some disagreement: certain investigators[2,8,12] have found that in this approximate range of flexion, the tension in the patellar tendon is greater than that in the quadriceps (in this range, the patella would function as a classic lever, magnifying the force of the quadriceps). But another investigator[4] reported that this is only true in the narrow range from 0 to 20 degrees, and that from 20 degrees to full flexion the tension in the patellar tendon is less than or equal to that of the quadriceps. Regardless of who is correct about this question, it is clear that the force in the quadriceps tendon is different from that in the patellar tendon. Thus, the patellar mechanism can be considered an eccentric pulley or a cam, as both redirect the force and change its magnitude (Figure 3–2).

Because the fulcrum (patella) is situated between the applied force (quadriceps) and the resistance to be moved (tibia), the lever in question is similar to a type I lever.[13] Most type I levers multiply (ie, increase) the force. This is not the case here because the quadriceps force is greater than the weight of the leg[6] and, in the open-chain mode, this is increasingly true as the knee approaches extension. On the other hand, because the quadriceps force is greater than the weight of the tibia, the displacement of the tibia is greater than displacement of the quadriceps (a lever multiplies either force or displacement). This is a common phenomenon in the human body: strength is sacrificed for displacement (as in the shoulder and elbow). This simple concept arises from the equilibrium moment equation.

Moment = Force × Distance = Constant on either side of a given joint at a given time

The different tensions in the patellar and quadriceps tendons and the complex lever actions of the patella are due to the different mo-ment arms of the two tendons.[6,7,12] In a simpli-fied, two-dimensional equilibrium static analy-sis of the patellofemoral joint (PFJ), assuming frictionless point contact (Figure 3–3), there are at least four moment arms pertaining to the ex-tensor mechanism. The distances d_1 and d_2 are the moment arms of the active quadriceps force and the resisting patellar tendon force, relative to the contact point C, between the patella and the trochlea. The distances d_3 and d_4 are the moment arms of the patellar tendon force and the weight of the leg, respectively, relative to the femo-rotibial contact point C_2. There is a fifth moment arm, which is not measured but a calculated mo-ment arm: the effective moment arm. This is the moment arm the quadriceps would require to carry out flexion-extension if the extensor mechanism were considered to have a single moment arm unit. This effective moment arm derives from the equilibrium moment equations, and thus must take all four moment arms into ac-count and is equal to $(d_1 \times d_3)/d_2$ (see Appendix 3–A for derivation). The moment arms most rel-evant to the patella are d_1 and d_2. As the knee flexes, the point of contact (C_1 in Figure 3–3) moves and leads to changes in d_1 and d_2. These changes, which can be measured from plain ra-diographs, will cause a difference in tension be-tween the patella and quadriceps tendons. The magnitude of this difference will depend on the flexion angle.[2,6,12] (*Clinical implications*: A par-tial patellectomy and patellar resurfacing in knee arthroplasty will affect all the moment arms, d_1, d_2, d_3, and d_4, and will therefore affect the effec-tive moment arm of the extensor mechanism. The extent to which this is true remains to be de-termined for each patient, as is the specific clini-cal consequence.)

If the goal is to minimize the contact force F_1, the quadriceps force F_q, or the patellar tendon force F_p, the forces F_1, F_p, F_q can be calculated as a function of the weight W of the lower leg for various anatomic conditions. This can be done by measuring the distances d_1 to d_4 on a plain ra-diograph view of a PFJ, and by using equations 5 and 6 of Appendix 3–A, along with some el-

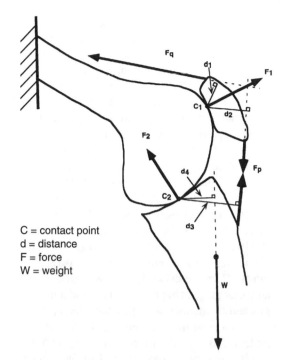

C = contact point
d = distance
F = force
W = weight

Figure 3–3 A Two-Dimensional Force Analysis of the Knee in an Open-Chain Configuration. The model assumes frictionless point contact between the articu-lating surfaces and a quasi-static situation. F_q, F_p, and W are the quadriceps force, the patellar tendon force, and the weight of the leg, respectively; d_1 and d_2 are the moment arms about C_1 for the quadriceps and pa-tellar tendon force, respectively; d_3 and d_4 are the mo-ment arms about C_2 for the patellar tendon force and the weight of the leg, respectively; F_1 and F_2 are the joint reaction forces for the patellofemoral and femo-rotibial joints, respectively. *Source:* Reprinted with permission from RP Grelsamer, WW Colman, and VC Mow, Anatomy and Mechanics of the Patel-lofemoral Joint, *Sports Medicine and Arthroscopy Review*, Vol 2, p 180, © 1994, Lippincott–Raven Pub-lishers.

ementary trigonometric relationships. The force F_2 can also be calculated.

THE QUADRICEPS (Q) ANGLE

When viewed in the frontal plane (straight on) the quadriceps does not function in a straight line. It "rounds a corner." Thus, the quadriceps angle is defined as the angle subtended by the patellar tendon and by a line from the center of the patella to the anterior superior iliac crest. It has been a great source of confusion, misinterpretation, and controversy. It is quite clear, however, that in the knee without surgery, the quadriceps angle is always positive (ie, as the quadriceps contracts, the bowstring effect tends to displace the patella laterally). This may explain why the lateral side wall of the trochlea is higher and more prominent than its medial counterpart. The only muscular restraint to this lateral displacement is the vastus medialis obliquus (VMO). Because of this important function, the VMO deserves special mention. It originates mostly from the distal, tendinous portion of the adductor magnus but also from the adductor longus and the medial intermuscular septum,[14] and it has its own nerve supply.[15] The VMO normally inserts into the superomedial aspect of the patella, as far down as one half of the patellar length.[14] In patients with malalignment, the VMO may barely reach the top of the patella, and the fibers are likely to be more vertical than the normal oblique angle (see Chapter 2). Not surprisingly, the VMO is the major focus of all patellar rehabilitation programs, and the search for VMO-preferential exercises continues. According to some investigators, we may be chasing windmills.[16]

Different values of normal have been reported for the quadriceps (Q) angle, and there is still a question about the different Q angles for men and women. Some believe that, because women have a wider pelvis, the anterior superior iliac spine—the origin of the Q angle—is more lateral, thus giving a somewhat larger Q angle. This has not been proven, and it is not clear that on average women have a significantly greater Q angle. Regardless of this controversy, the practitioner can safely use 10 to 15 degrees as a normal range for the Q angle when the knee is extended or slightly flexed. The Q angle decreases with flexion because of the progressive internal rotation of the tibia relative to the femur. There are many pitfalls in measuring the Q angle: if the patella is subluxed laterally out of the trochlea, the Q angle as measured clinically loses much of its value because the clinician will measure a falsely normal angle. Assessment of the true Q angle requires the patella to be centered. Alternatively, the center of the trochlea can be estimated and used as a reference. This can only be done radiologically (see Chapter 5).

A valgus limb alignment increases the Q angle, because the entire upper tibia including the tibial tuberosity is lateralized. This has led to the notion that high Q angles are a particular problem in women with valgus knees. However, practically speaking, the Q angle is really a measure of the position of the tibial tuberosity relative to the midline of the trochlea.[17] The position of the tibial tuberosity is the major variable in the assessment of the Q angle, and the position of the tibial tuberosity is the major determinant of the Q angle. Varus knees with external torsion of the upper tibia present some of the biggest Q angles.[18,19] In fact, there is a school of thought that patellar malalignment (including tilt) is more prevalent in varus than in valgus knees.[20,21]

PATELLOFEMORAL CONTACT AREA

Distribution

The retropatellar surface has several distinct facets, and the total articulating surface of the patella (10.7 ± 1.6 cm^2) is much smaller than its mating femoral trochlear surface (29.5 ± 1.5 cm^2). A joint is said to be perfectly congruent if there are no gaps of noncontact between the two sides of the joint. The patella can be considered congruent or incongruent, depending on the direction from which it is viewed (see Chapter 2). Normal articular cartilage has excellent lubrication and wear characteristics.[22,23] Even at the very high loads and low sliding speeds normally found in the PFJ,[24] the cartilage provides a low-friction articulation. The normal anatomic features of the PFJ—such as the concavity of the trochlea and convexity of the retropatellar surfaces—along with the various soft connective tissues and muscles, provide the joint with the required stability. The transverse congruency ensures medial-lateral stability, whereas the sagittal incongruency provides an excellent setting with respect to lubrication requirements.

Only part of the patella articulates with the trochlea at any given time. Contact studies, whether done with dye staining,[25] silicone rubber casting,[26] pressure film,[27–30] methylmethacrylate,[31] or stereophotogrammetry,[32–35] have qualitatively given the same results (ie, in the early degrees of flexion, the distal portion of the patella articulates with the proximal trochlea). As the knee flexes, the contact area moves proximally on the patella. At 90 degrees, the superior portion of the patella is in contact with the trochlea. With further flexion, the contact area moves back toward the center of the patella. At full flexion, the medial facet no longer touches the medial trochlea. However, a small, relatively vertical cartilaginous border of the medial facet, which is referred to as the "odd facet" and is present about 80% of the time, often articulates with the inner border of the medial femoral condyle in deep flexion.[35] (*Clinical implications*: Knowing the site of a patellar chondral lesion can influence a rehabilitation program. For example, for patients with a distal patellar lesion, any type of strenuous activity in the early degrees of flexion may be painful and contraindicated. The location of a patellar lesion may influence the results of Maquet- and Fulkerson-type procedures, which seek to unload arthritic lesions. A painful proximal lesion may not be well decompressed by procedures that elevate the tibial tuberosity as they may elevate mostly the distal portion of the patella.)

Magnitude

In full extension and at 0-degree flexion, there is no patellofemoral contact.[25,31] Some investigators, however, have found contact at 0-degree flexion, and they have quantified it.[2,8] This discrepancy may be due to experimental differences, because defining 0 degrees can be harder than it seems. (There is also a the common misuse of the terms *full extension*, *maximal extension*, *neutral extension*, and *0-degree flexion*. *Neutral extension* and *0-degree flexion* are synonymous, and their definition is self-explanatory. *Full extension* and *maximal extension* are also synonymous, but they are not automatically equivalent to neutral extension; in some patients, *full extension* and *maximal extension* actually refer to *hyperextension*. Thus, one cannot put maximal force on the quadriceps and call that *neutral extension* or *0-degree flexion*. If a patient has no ability to hyperextend, then the four terms are synonymous.)

The tibial crest can be considered a straight line, but the anterior aspect of the femur is bowed. The femoral head is not usually present in knee specimens (nor visible on magnetic resonance imaging studies of the knee) and, therefore, a line drawn from the center of the hip to the center of the condyles cannot be used. Simple visual alignment can be used, but it is subject to slight error.

Using visual alignment to define 0-degree flexion, my colleagues and I have found that there is indeed no contact between the articular surface of the patella and that of the trochlea at 0 degrees of flexion. There can, of course, be contact between the articular surface of the patella and the suprapatellar bursa. The first contact between the articular surface of the patella and that of the trochlea varies from patient to patient, but it is usually present by about 15 degrees of flexion.

There is universal agreement that from 0 to 60 degrees of flexion the magnitude of the contact area increases as the knee flexes (see Figure 3–4). Some individuals believe that the area quadruples as the knee flexes from 10 to 60 degrees.[2,27,30] The magnitude of the contact area with flexion greater than 60 degrees is subject to more controversy. According to some investigators, the magnitude of the contact area remains constant between 60 and 90 degrees,[27] whereas others see a continued rise in this range.[8,25,28,31,36]

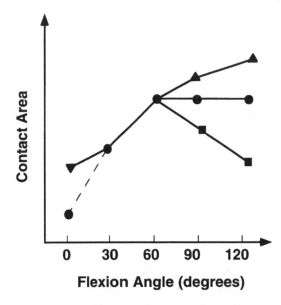

Figure 3–4 Qualitative Graph of Contact Area versus Knee Flexion According to Various Authors. *Source:* Reprinted with permission from RP Grelsamer, WW Colman, and VC Mow, Anatomy and Mechanics of the Patellofemoral Joint, *Sports Medicine and Arthroscopy Review*, Vol 2, p 182, © 1994, Lippincott–Raven Publishers.

Others see a peak at 60 degrees, with diminution from 60 to 90 degrees.[29] Likewise, with flexion greater than 90 degrees certain investigators see a continued rise in contact area,[37] others see leveling off of the contact area,[8] and yet others see a considerable drop-off from 90 to 120 degrees.[2,27,38]

These differences can be accounted for in part by specimen-to-specimen variability, varying techniques of area assessment,[32,33] and variations in time of load application. Differing applied quadriceps forces may also play a role. Some studies have found significant changes in contact area when the quadriceps force increases from 500 N to 2500 N,[37] from 500 N to 2000 N,[39] or from 100 N to 1500 N.[38] However, another study reported that changing the quadriceps force from 700 N to 1500 N changed the contact area very little and did not change the overall contact pattern at all.[2,27]

CONTACT LOAD (JOINT REACTION FORCE) AND PRESSURE

Stress is defined by the following formula:

$$\text{Stress} = \text{Force} \div \text{Area}$$

One needs to know both the contact load (force) and the contact area to calculate the contact stress. A good example of the difference between stress and the force (load) is a person crossing a snowfield with a snowshoe on one foot and a regular shoe on the other. Both shoes exert the same force on the snow, but the stress exerted by each shoe is quite different because of the surface area over which the force acts. Likewise, the force on the patellar articular cartilage must be considered in the context of the contact area over which the force acts.

Pressure is a special state of stress in which the load acting on an area is perpendicular to the area for all planes through the point of interest. Pressure in air or water satisfies this condition. Because normal articular cartilage is nearly frictionless, the load acting on it is nearly perpendicular to the surface. (A frictional component acts tangentially to the surface and thus causes the joint reaction force to act at an oblique angle to the surface.) Thus, the terms *contact stress* and *contact pressure* are often used synonymously in the literature, and this is acceptable. Unfortunately, the terms *force* and *stress* are often used interchangeably, which is a major error.

From a clinical point of view, it is the stress (not the force) within the material that is important. Thus, to calculate the stress acting on the cartilage surface, one must be able to determine both the force and the contact area by measuring them experimentally or calculating them using a theoretical model.

Force, stress, and area can be either measured or calculated. The distinction between the two methods becomes blurred when one realizes that measurements can require considerable calculations pertaining to the measuring instruments.[32] Calculations alone[4,9,40–43] or in combination with measurements[1,2,6,12,27–30,44–48] have been used to assess force and stress. Qualitatively, there has recently been more agreement than disagreement about these techniques.

Closed Kinetic Chain

In a closed-chain activity (when the foot is against a rigid surface, such as during a leg press or squat), the joint reaction force on the PFJ increases as the knee flexes from 0 to 90 degrees (Figure 3–5A). The contact area increases also, but the change is less than that of the force. Therefore, the stress increases from 0 to 90 degrees.

From 90 to 120 degrees, the force levels off or even decreases[28] as the quadriceps tendon comes into contact with the trochlea and begins to account for some of the total joint reaction force and contact area (Figure 3–5B). According to some investigators,[28] the contact area decreases only slightly in this range, and the stress decreases from 90 to 120 degrees.

Other investigators[2] have found a smaller decrease in force and contact area past 90 degrees and have noted considerable specimen-to-specimen variability with respect to pressure.

Open Kinetic Chain

In an open-chain activity (when the foot is not in contact with a surface, such as during leg curls and extensions), the forces across the patella are lowest at 90 degrees of flexion (Figure 3–6). The quadriceps and patellar tendons are nearly at right angles to each other at this point, and the joint reaction force at the PFJ will therefore be a relatively high proportion of the quadriceps force. However, it is a high proportion of a low force at this angle,[49] and the joint reaction force is therefore quite low.

As the knee extends from this flexed position, the quadriceps force increases, the joint reaction force increases (then decreases past 45 degrees), and the contact area progressively decreases. The net result is an increase in contact stress until early flexion, after which the entire patella slides proximal to the trochlea and there is no longer contact between the two cartilaginous

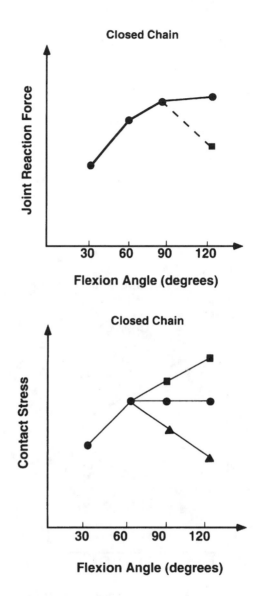

Figure 3–5 Closed-Chain Activity. **(A)** Qualitative graph of joint reaction force versus knee flexion for a closed-chain activity. The dashed line represents the work of investigators who noted significant contact between the quadriceps tendon and the trochlea and accounted for this in their assessment. **(B)** Qualitative graph of joint contact stress (as reported by three different investigators). *Source:* Reprinted with permission from RP Grelsamer, WW Colman, and VC Mow, Anatomy and Mechanics of the Patellofemoral Joint, *Sports Medicine and Arthroscopy Review,* Vol 2, p 183, © 1994, Lippincott–Raven Publishers.

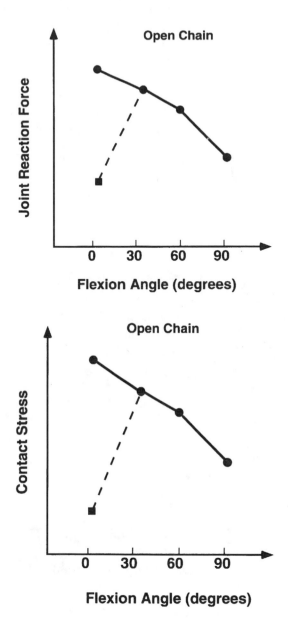

Figure 3–6 Open-Chain Activity. (A) Joint reaction force and (B) stress versus knee flexion for open-chain activity. The dashed line represents current thinking about the force and stress one can expect if there is no contact between the patella and the trochlea at 0 degrees of extension. *Source:* Reprinted with permission from RP Grelsamer, WW Colman, and VC Mow, Anatomy and Mechanics of the Patellofemoral Joint, *Sports Medicine and Arthroscopy Review*, Vol 2, p 184, © 1994, Lippincott–Raven Publishers.

surfaces. At 0 degrees of flexion, the quadriceps force is high, but the joint reaction force is low because the femur and tibia are nearly parallel and because there is no contact between the two cartilaginous surfaces. Likewise, contact stress is low. In hyperextension, the patellar cartilage stress is low because the patella is actually lifted off the distal femur and does not overlap with the trochlea. (*Clinical implications:* Open-chain exercises are most safely carried out from 60 to 90 degrees, especially if there are distal lesions. From a point of view of cartilage stress, straight leg raises with the knee at 0 degrees or hyperextended are equally safe. Closed-chain exercises are safest in the 0- to 45-degree range, especially if there are proximal lesions.)

As more information pertaining to the PFJ becomes available, some of these concepts may be refined or modified.

PATELLA TRACKING

The tracking of the patella as the knee flexes and extends has been the subject of much debate.[3,50,51] Depending on what coordinate system one uses (see below), the patella can be seen to take a relatively wobbly path down the trochlea, with this path varying from patient to patient. Soft-tissue restraints play a role,[52,53] as do the bony and cartilaginous anatomy of the joint. The relative importance of these structures as determinants of patellar kinematics is still under investigation.[2,5,52,53] For example the articular facets are remarkably intricate and variable (see Chapter 2), and their geometry may greatly influence patellar tracking.[2,3,52,53] The main ridges are the (vertical) median ridge in the superior half of the patella, the transverse ridge in the lateral half of the patella, and the disto-medial ridge. These ridges give the undersurface of the patella a vaguely inverted *Y* appearance. In certain patients, the ridges truly form an inverted *Y*, and these patients can be said to have a true inferior facet (Figure 3–7). This inferior facet articulates with the flat, proximal trochlea in early flexion. As the patella enters and seats itself into the trochlea, the (proximal) medial and lateral

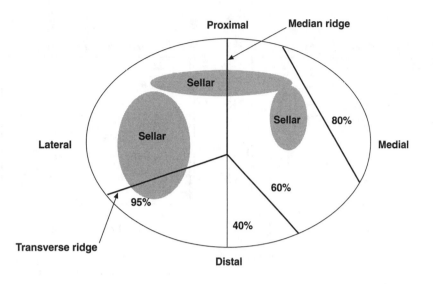

Figure 3–7 Articular Facets (Schematic Representation). Note the constant horizontal ridge laterally and the constant vertical ridge proximally. Thus, the superolateral facet is the only constant facet. One cannot truly talk of a medial and lateral facet when looking at the articular surface (see Chapter 2).

facets articulate with the inner walls of the femoral condyles.[35]

The choice of coordinate systems is a rather arcane subject to most clinicians. Yet it is critical to the interpretation of studies on tracking. For example, in a *global coordinate system*, the patella is deemed to be at the zero position when the knee is extended. All measurements of displacement are made relative to this initial zero position. Equally significant, measurements are made relative to a rigid device such as the rig in which the knee is mounted. When using an *anatomic coordinate system*, the patellar position is given relative to the coordinates centered on the underlying femur. In a situation where the patella might move medially from an initially lateralized position, the global coordinate system gives the patella a "medial" value. But if the patella is still lateralized with respect to the midline, the anatomic coordinate system gives the patella a "lateral" value (as well it should, from the clinician's point of view).

The entire tracking pattern can be affected by the choice of the coordinate system. In a study of

seven cadaveric knee joints, my colleagues and I found that the tracking pattern in the global coordinate system varied greatly from specimen to specimen (L Blankevoort, SD Kwak, CS Ahmad, TS Garder, et al, unpublished data, 1997). In the anatomic coordinate system, however, all patellae started in a slightly lateral position (relative to the center of the femur), all moved medially in the first degrees of flexion, and all patellae then tracked "straight" (ie, without any medial or lateral deviation relative to the chosen longitudinal axis) (see Figure 3–8). For the clinician, the anatomic coordinate system is intuitive, but many biomechanics studies express their results with respect to a global coordinate system.[3,54,55]

One of the difficulties in determining the position of the patella in an anatomic system is defining the center of the coordinates. When one says that the patella is "lateral," the obvious question is "lateral to what?" Figure 3–8 shows the tracking of the patella when the patella is assessed relative to the "center" of the distal femur. Using a least-squares technique, the articular surface of

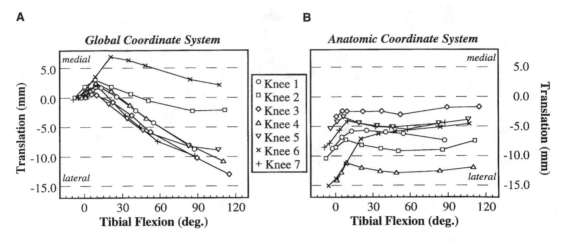

Figure 3–8 Patellar Tracking. (**A**) Patellar tracking relative to a global coordinate system. Each patella appears to have its own particular tracking pattern. (**B**) Patellar tracking relative to an anatomic system. Patellae by and large start slightly lateral to the middle of the femur, move medially, and then track straight down the trochlea. The concept that the patella takes a wobbly, unpredictable path is probably an artifact of the coordinate system.

the posterior condyles is fitted with spheres whose centers are connected (this defines the x axis). The midpoint of this line is the origin of the coordinate system.

The position of the patella can also be assessed relative to the bottom of the trochlea, although the trochlea itself often follows a C-shaped course (apex medial).

In vitro testing has represented a major portion of the tracking studies performed on the patella and, despite the advent of computerized imaging, in vitro testing will most likely continue to be of considerable interest for the foreseeable future. My colleagues and I have noted that a number of investigators omit the iliotibial band (ITB), and we recently studied its in vitro effect on tracking (SD Kwak, CS Ahmad, TR Gardner, H Wu, et al, unpublished data). Not surprisingly, omission of this tendon while maintaining the VMO shifted the contact area medially. Proportionally, the contact area on the patella shifted much more than did the patella as a whole. There was relatively little change in the position of the patella itself (0.3 mm with 90 N pull at the proximal portion of the ITB), most likely as a result of the ITB being tethered to the posterolateral femur and acting more as a liga-

ment than as a tendon with regard to the patella (see Chapter 2).

It is important for the clinician to know what is normal to aid in the interpretation of data from magnetic resonance imaging (MRI) and computed tomography (CT). As a corollary, how does one define the medial-lateral position of the patella? The medial-lateral position can be determined by a "congruence angle" similar to that used on Merchant views,[56] by a line drawn through the apex of the trochlea to the apex of the patella,[57] or by a measure of patellar displacement relative to one or both condyles.[58] The normal patella is centered in the trochlea when the knee is flexed. At 0-degree flexion, using stereophotogrammetry,[32] my colleagues and I have found that the patella is displaced laterally (which is not controversial)—but only by a few millimeters.[59]

One has to be careful in applying these data to the interpretation of MRI results. In a recent investigation, we found that, in 59 of 60 patients without evidence of patellar problems, the patella lay centered over the underlying femur on routine MRI tests prescribed to be in neutral extension (see Chapter 5). Based on a number of factors, we concluded that most patients were positioned with their knee in a few degrees of flexion during routine MRI tests.

MATERIAL PROPERTIES OF PATELLOFEMORAL CARTILAGE

Cartilage can be considered a biphasic material[22,23,60,61]—possessing a freely flowing fluid phase and a porous-permeable, fiber-reinforced solid phase. When cartilage is under compression or tension, water and ions can flow through it—at the expense of great frictional drag. The biphasic interpretation of cartilage physiology readily accounts for the observed phenomena of *cartilage creep* (change in dimensions over time when a constant load is applied) and *stress relaxation* (change in stresses over time when a constant deformation is imposed). It is my opinion that texts and theories referring to cartilage as a one-phase, elastic material are inaccurate and will not stand the test of time. In its simplest form, three material parameters can predict the behavior of articular cartilage in compression: (1) the permeability (the ease with which a fluid flows through a porous material), (2) compressive aggregate modulus (a combination of Young's modulus and Poisson's ratio), and (3) Poisson's ratio (a measure of lateral expansion or contraction with axial compression or tension). Further refinements of the biphasic theory have sought to include the effects of ion-induced swelling and are included in the triphasic theory.[60]

Experiments on the cartilage of the mating surfaces of the PFJ have shown that the cartilage on the patella generally has a lower modulus, higher permeability, and greater thickness than that of the distal femur.[22,62] Advantages may be afforded the patella because of these parameters. For example, because of its relatively low stiffness and high permeability, the stability of the joint may be improved as the patella seats itself more deeply into the trough of the trochlea. This deeper seating will increase the contact area and therefore decrease the contact stress. However, higher permeability and greater deformation lead to high load carriage by the collagen-proteoglycan collagen matrix, which may, in turn, lead to matrix damage and subsequent degeneration.[22] This may explain the prevalence of patellar lesions relative to trochlear lesions.

GAIT ANALYSIS

Gait characteristics of patients with patellofemoral pain have not been extensively studied. Greenwald et al[63] have used a commercial motion analysis system to study knee motion in subjects with and without patellofemoral pain. They noted that, at midstance during stair descent, patients with patellofemoral pain exhibited significantly more knee extension; presumably, this is a protective mechanism (against pain) rather than an intrinsic change in knee dynamics. This may be an area for future research.

IN VITRO TECHNIQUES—PRESENT AND FUTURE*

Stereophotogrammetry (SPG) is a science developed in the nineteenth century and currently used for determining the quantitative anatomy and contact areas of the PFJ. SPG is used to obtain precise three-dimensional measurements of an object through the process of simultaneously photographing the object with two cameras, measuring the two-dimensional images, then combining them with appropriate mathematical computations.[32,33,64] The object points may consist of points on an articular surface, in which case, three-dimensional models of the joint surface can be obtained. A typical layout of a photogrammetry apparatus is modeled in Figure 3–9. The object to be measured is placed within the workspace of a calibration frame[33,65] and fitted with markers (calibration targets) whose three-dimensional coordinates are known *a priori* relative to some fixed laboratory reference frame. The calibration targets are used to

---

*This section has been written with the assistance of Van C Mow, MD, and Gerard A Ateshian, MD, from the Columbia University Orthopaedic Research Laboratory.

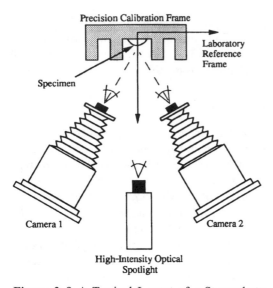

Figure 3–9 A Typical Layout of a Stereophoto-grammetry Apparatus. Two cameras photograph a specimen within the calibration frame. *Source:* Reprinted with permission from RP Grelsamer, WW Colman, and VC Mow, Anatomy and Mechanics of the Patellofemoral Joint, *Sports Medicine and Arthroscopy Review*, Vol 2, p 185, © 1994, Lippincott–Raven Publishers.

calculate the precise position and orientation of the cameras relative to the laboratory reference frame. A fine grid providing discernible object points is optically projected onto the surface.[33,66] The object is simultaneously photographed from two cameras, and two images called stereograms are obtained. The stereograms are then digitized using a high-accuracy digitizer and stored in a computer. The three-dimensional coordinates of all object grid points are calculated using the known positions of the calibration targets. The joint surface model can be visualized, scaled, and rotated using computer graphics software. Characteristics of the surface such as surface area or curvature may be calculated and displayed. In close-range SPG, measurement accuracy has been reported in the range of 0.02 mm to 0.20 mm.[33,65–71]

An example of a computer graphics model for the PFJ produced using the SPG technique can be seen in Figure 3–10. Note the congruence of the articular surfaces of the PFJ in the horizontal plane. Precise geometries, like those obtained by SPG, are essential for accurate biomechanical models of the PFJ.[33] In assessing malalignment and congruency, one must remember that the contours obtained from plain radiographs are those of the subchondral bone, not of the articulating cartilage surfaces. Because it is the cartilage surfaces that bear the load, it is essential to quantify the geometric characteristics of these surfaces. Plain radiographs or CT scans cannot do this. MRIs will most likely be able to do this in the future.

INTERACTIVE MANIPULATION OF JOINT SURFACE MODELS

An advantage of obtaining three-dimensional computer models of articular surfaces is that they can be manipulated interactively on a computer screen. Different configurations can be generated so that they simulate physiological conditions. For example, a Merchant view of the articular cartilage surface can be simulated and visualized, as shown in Figure 3–10. Furthermore, at any particular position of the articular surfaces, it is possible to estimate the regions of

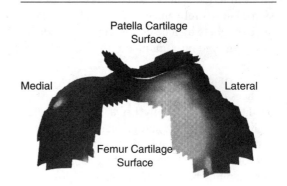

Figure 3–10 Computer Model Generated by Stereophotogrammetry. *Source:* Reprinted with permission from RP Grelsamer, WW Colman, and VC Mow, Anatomy and Mechanics of the Patellofemoral Joint, *Sports Medicine and Arthroscopy Review*, Vol 2, p 185, © 1994, Lippincott–Raven Publishers.

contact in the joint by assessing the overlap of the surfaces (Figure 3–11), where the patellar and femoral regions of contact are shown at 30 degrees of flexion. To simulate patellar malalignment or assess realignment procedures, the patellar surface can be translated and rotated on the computer. The resulting areas of overlap can be displayed (Figure 3–11B), demonstrating a dramatic reduction in the size of the contact area.[34] The ability to predict the change in con-tact from a computer model may be useful as a clinical tool for predicting the outcome of a surgical procedure such as lateral release, medial plication, or tibial tubercle osteotomy. With such techniques, computer-assisted orthopaedic surgery, in which the patient's articular surface topography is initially quantified noninvasively using MRI and then analyzed by the orthopaedic surgeon, may soon become a reality.

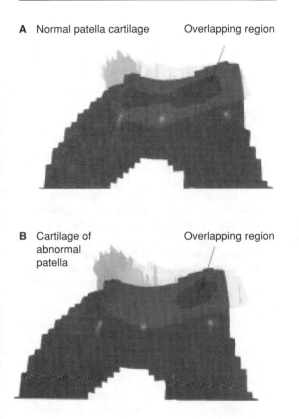

Figure 3–11 Computer Simulation of Different Physiological Conditions. (**A**) Normal and (**B**) abnormal patella alignment is simulated. As the patella is lateralized, the contact area is seen to shift and to diminish. *Source:* Reprinted with permission from RP Grelsamer, WW Colman, and VC Mow, Anatomy and Mechanics of the Patellofemoral Joint, *Sports Medicine and Arthroscopy Review*, Vol 2, p 186, © 1994, Lippincott–Raven Publishers.

FUTURE DIRECTIONS

With regard to the nonoperative treatment of the patella, it remains to be seen whether or not short-arc, open-chain exercises are beneficial. The answer to this question depends on anatomic factors dictating contact areas and stresses and ability of cartilage to sustain the normally high loads found in the PFJ. My colleagues and I hope to use current developing techniques in our laboratory[72] to help provide deeper insights into how contact areas are related to PFJ anatomy, how PFJ reaction force and patellar tracking vary with joint anatomy, and how different surgical procedures affect anatomic and biomechanical characteristics of the PFJ. Keeping in mind other investigators' work in this area, we plan to assess contact area before and after realignment procedures to determine the significance of this parameter and to document some basic rationales for some of the commonly used surgical techniques.

"Hamstring facilitation" is a concept more recently introduced in the physical therapy world. As more information is obtained, I will explain and discuss this concept in a subsequent edition.

To better interpret routine MRIs, the normal medial-lateral position of the patella (ie, relative to the articulating surfaces) in extension needs to be established, taking into account the difference between 0 degrees and full extension.

Finally, an understanding of the pathophysiologic processes at the cellular and extracellular matrix level early in the degenerative process may ultimately help practitioners prevent and treat patellar pain.

REFERENCES

1. Kaufer H. Mechanical function of the patella. *J Bone Joint Surg.* 1971;53A:1551–1560.

2. Ahmed AM, Burke DL, Hyder A. Force analysis of the patellar mechanism. *J Orthop Res.* 1987;5:69–85.

3. van Kampen A, Huiskes R. The three-dimensional tracking pattern of the human patella. *J Orthop Res.* 1990;8:372–382.

4. Hirokawa S. Three-dimensional mathematical model analysis of the patellofemoral joint. *J Biomech.* 1991; 24:659–671.

5. Heegaard J, Leyvraz PF, van Kampen A, Rakotomanana L, et al. Patellar stability as a function of joint anatomy. *J Bone Joint Surg.* 1993;75B(suppl):140–141.

6. Grood ES, Suntay WJ, Noyes FR, Butler DL. Biomechanics of the knee-extension exercise. *J Bone Joint Surg.* 1984;66A:725–734.

7. Denham RA, Bishop RED. Mechanics of the knee and problems in reconstructive surgery. *J Bone Joint Surg.* 1978;60B:345–351.

8. Huberti HH, Hayes WC, Stone JL, Shybut GT. Force ratios in the quadriceps tendon and ligamentum patellae. *J Orthop Res.* 1984;2:49–54.

9. van Eijden TMGJ, Kouwenhoven E, Verburg J, Weijs WA. A mathematical model of the patellofemoral joint. *J Biomech.* 1986;19:219–229.

10. Bishop RED, Denham RA. A note on the ratio between tensions in the quadriceps tendon and infrapatellar ligament. *Eng Med.* 1977;6:53–54.

11. Amis AA, Farahmand F. Biomechanics of the knee extensor mechanism. *Knee.* 1996;3:73–80. Abstract.

12. Buff HU, Jones LC, Hungerford DS. Determination of forces transmitted through the patellofemoral joint. *J Biomech.* 1988;21:17.

13. Cochran GVB. *A Primer of Orthopaedic Biomechanics.* New York: Churchill Livingstone; 1982.

14. Bose K, Kanagasuntheram R, Osman MBH. Vastus medialis oblique: an anatomic and physiologic study. *Orthopedics.* 1980;3:880–883.

15. Weinstabl R, Scharf W, Firbas W. The extensor apparatus of the knee joint and its peripheral vasti: anatomic investigation and clinical relevance. *Surg Radiol Anat.* 1989;11:17.

16. Grabiner MD, Koh TJ, Draganich LF. Neuromechanics of the patellofemoral joint. *Med Sci Sports Exerc.* 1994;26:10–21.

17. Grana WA, Krieghauser LA. Scientific basis of extensor mechanism disorders. *Clin Sports Med.* 1985;4:247–257.

18. Iseki F, Fujikawa K. Clinical pictures of the osteoarthritis in the knee joint. *J Jpn Orthop Assoc.* 1980; 54:563–574.

19. Fujikawa K, Seedhom BB, Wright V. Biomechanics of the patello-femoral joint. Part II: a study of the effect of simulated femoro-tibial varus deformity on the congruity of the patello-femoral compartment and movement of the patella. *Eng Med.* 1983;12:13–21.

20. Cistac C, Cartier P. Diagnostic et traitment des déséquilibres rotuliens du sportif. *J Traumatol Sport.* 1986;3:92–97.

21. Milgrom C, Kerem E, Finestone A, Eldad A, et al. Patellofemoral pain caused by overactivity. *J Bone Joint Surg.* 1991;73A:1041–1043.

22. Mow VC, Ateshian GA, Ratcliffe A. Anatomic form and biomechanical properties of articular cartilage of the knee joint. In: Finerman GAM, Noyes FR, eds. *Biology and Biomechanics of the Traumatized Synovial Joint: The Knee as a Model.* Rosemont, IL: American Academy of Orthopaedic Surgeons Symposium; 1992:55–81.

23. Mow VC, Ratcliffe A, Poole AR. Cartilage and diarthrodial joints as paradigms for hierarchical materials and structures. *Biomaterials.* 1992;13:67–97.

24. Ozkaya N, Nordin M. *Fundamentals of Biomechanics: Equilibrium Motion and Deformation.* New York: Nostrand Reinhold; 1991.

25. Goodfellow JW, Hungerford DS, Zindel M. Patellofemoral mechanics and pathology. I: functional anatomy of the patello-femoral joint. *J Bone Joint Surg.* 1976;58B:287.

26. Fujikawa K, Seedhom BB, Wright V. Biomechanics of the patello-femoral joint. Part I: a study of the contact and the congruity of the patello-femoral compartment and movement of the patella. *Eng Med.* 1983;12:3–11.

27. Ahmed AM, Burke DL. In vitro measurement of static pressure distribution in synovial joints—part II. Retropatellar surface. *J Biomech Eng.* 1983;105:226–236.

28. Huberti HH, Hayes WC. Patellofemoral contact pressures. *J Bone Joint Surg.* 1984;66A:715–724.

29. D'Agata SD, Pearsall AW, Reider B, Draganich LF. An in vitro analysis of patellofemoral contact areas and pressures following procurement of the central one-third patellar tendon. *Am J Sports Med.* 1993;21:212–218.

30. Retaillaud JL, Darmana R, Devallet P, Mansat M, et al. An experimental biomechanical study of tibial tuberosity advancement. *Rev Chir Orthop.* 1989;75:513–523.

31. Aglietti P, Insall JN, Walker PS, Trent P. A new patella prosthesis. *Clin Orthop.* 1975;107:175–187.

32. Ateshian GA, Kwak SD, Soslowsky LJ, Mow VC. A stereophotogrammetric method for determining in situ contact areas in diarthrodial joints, and a comparison with other methods. *J Biomech.* 1994;27:111–124.

33. Ateshian GA, Soslowsky LJ, Mow VC. Quantitation of articular surface topography and cartilage thickness in knee joints using stereophotogrammetry. *J Biomech.* 1991;24:761–766.

34. Froimson MI, Ateshian GA, Soslowsky LJ, Kelly MA, et al. Quantification of the surfaces and contact areas at the patellofemoral articulation. *Proc Inst Mech Eng.* 1989;5:73–78.

35. Kwak SD, Colman WW, Ateshian GA, Grelsamer RP, et al. Anatomy of the human patellofemoral joint articular cartilage: a surface curvature analysis. *J Orthop Res.* 1997;15:468–472.

36. Seedhom BB, Tsubuku M. A technique for the study of contact between visco-elastic bodies with special reference to the patello-femoral joint. *J Biomech.* 1977; 10:253–260.

37. Hehne HJ. Biomechanics of the patellofemoral joint and its clinical relevance. *Clin Orthop Rel Res.* 1990; 258:73–85.

38. Matthews LS, Sonstegard DA, Hanke JA. Load bearing characteristics of the patello-femoral joint. *Acta Orthop Scand.* 1977;48:511–516.

39. Hille E, Schulitz KP, Henrichs C, Schneider T. Pressure and contact-surface measurements within the femoropatellar joint and their variations following lateral release. *Arch Orthop Trauma Surg.* 1985;104:275–282.

40. Maquet P. *Biomechanics of the Knee.* Berlin: Springer-Verlag; 1976.

41. Mikosz RP, Andriacchi TP, Andersson GBJ. Model analysis of factors influencing the prediction of muscle forces at the knee. *J Orthop Res.* 1988;6:205–214.

42. Yamaguchi GT, Zajac FE. A planar model of the knee joint to characterize the knee extensor mechanism. *J Biomech.* 1989;22:1–10.

43. Steinkamp LA, Dillingham MF, Markel MD, Hill JA, et al. Biomechanical considerations in patellofemoral joint rehabilitation. *Am J Sports Med.* 1993;21:438–444.

44. Huberti HH, Hayes WC. Contact pressures in chondromalacia patellae and the effects of capsular reconstructive procedures. *J Orthop Res.* 1988;6:499–508.

45. Perry J, Antonelli D, Ford W. Analysis of knee joint forces during flexed-knee stance. *J Bone Joint Surg.* 1975;57A:961–967.

46. Ferguson AB, Brown TD, Fu FH, Rutkowski R. Relief of patellofemoral contact stress by anterior displacement of the tibial tubercle. *J Bone Joint Surg.* 1979; 61A:159–166.

47. Haut RC. Contact pressures in the patellofemoral joint during impact loading on the human flexed knee. *J Orthop Res.* 1989;7:272–280.

48. Manouel M, Pearlman HS, Belakhlef A, Brown TD. A miniature piezoelectric polymer transducer for in vitro measurement of the dynamic contact stress distribution. *J Biomech.* 1992;25:627–635.

49. Frankel VH, Nordin M. *Basic Biomechanics of the Skeletal System.* Philadelphia: Lea & Febiger; 1980.

50. Veress SA, Lippert FG, Hou MCY, Takamoto T. Patellar tracking patterns measurement by analytical X-ray photogrammetry. *J Biomech.* 1979;12:639–650.

51. Reider B, Marshall JL, Ring B. Patellar tracking. *Clin Orthop.* 1981;157:143–147.

52. Heegard J, Leyvraz PF, van Kampen A, Rakotomanana L, et al. Influence of soft structures on patellar three-dimensional tracking pattern of the human patella. *Clin Orthop.* 1994;299:235–243.

53. Heegaard J, Leyvraz PF, van Kampen A. Contribution of joint geometry and soft tissue structures on patellar stability. *Trans Orthop Res Soc.* 1994;40:667.

54. Blankevoort L, Huiskes R, de Lange A. The envelope of passive knee motion. *J Biomech.* 1988;21:705–720.

55. Koh TJ, Grabiner MD, De Swart RJ. In vivo tracking of the human patella. *J. Biomech.* 1992;25:637–643.

56. Schutzer SF, Ramsby GR, Fulkerson JP. Computed tomographic classification of patellofemoral pain patients. *Orthop Clin North Am.* 1986;17:235–248.

57. Despontin J, Thomas P. Reflexions sur l'étude de l'articulation femoro-rotulienne par la méthode des tomographies axiales transverses computérisées. *Acta Orthop Belg.* 1978;44:857–870.

58. Laurin CA, Dussault R, Levesque HP. The tangential X-ray investigation of the patellofemoral joint. *Clin Orthop Rel Res.* 1979;144:16.

59. Grelsamer RP, Newton PM, Staron RB. The medial-lateral position of the patella in the "extended" knee. *J Arthrosc.* In press.

60. Mow VC, Hayes WC. *Basic Orthopaedic Biomechanics.* New York: Raven Press; 1991.

61. Mow VC, Newton PM, Grelsamer RP. Biomechanics of articular cartilage and meniscus. In: Fu FH, Harner CD, Vince KG, eds. *Knee Surgery.* Baltimore: Williams & Wilkins; 1994:101–130.

62. Froimson MI, Ratcliffe A, Gardner TR, Mow VC. Differences in patellofemoral joint cartilage material properties and their significance to the etiology of cartilage surface fibrillation. *Osteoarthritis Cartilage.* In press.

63. Greenwald AE, Bagley AM, France EP, et al. A biomechanical and clinical evaluation of a patellofemoral knee brace. *Clin Orthop.* 1996;324:187–195.

64. Ghosh SK. *Analytical Photogrammetry.* Oxford, England: Pergamon Press; 1979:149–156.

65. Ghosh SK. A close-range photogrammetric system for 3-D measurements and perspective diagramming in biomechanics. *J Biomech.* 1983;16:667–674.

66. Huiskes R, Kremers J, de Lange A, Woltring HJ, et al. Analytical stereophotogrammetric determination of three-dimensional knee joint geometry. *J Biomech.* 1985;18:559–570.

67. Selvik G. Roentgen stereophotogrammetry: a method for the study of the kinematics of the skeletal system. *Acta Orthop Scand.* 1974;232(suppl):60.

68. Ateshian GA. B-spline surface-fitting method for articular surfaces of diarthrodial joints. *J Biomech Eng.* 1993;115:366–373.

69. Brown RH, Burstein AH, Nash CL, Schock CC. Spinal analysis using a three-dimensional radiographic technique. *J Biomech.* 1976;9:355–365.

70. Fioretti S, Germani A, Leo T. Stereometry in very close range stereophotogrammetry with nonmetric cameras for human movement analysis. *J Biomech.* 1985; 18:831–842.

71. Stokes I, Greenapple DM. Measurement of surface deformation of soft tissue. *J Biomech.* 1985;1:1–7.

72. Gardner TR, Ateshian GA, Grelsamer RP, Mow VC. A 6 DOF knee testing device to determine patellar tracking and patellofemoral joint contact area via stereophotogrammetry. Proceedings of the ASME Winter meeting, 1994; New York.

ADDITIONAL READINGS

Eckhoff DG, Montgomery WK, Stamm ER, Kilcoyne RF. Location of the femoral sulcus in the osteoarthritic knee. *J Arthroplasty.* 1996;11:163–165.

Sakai N, Luo ZP, Rand J, An KN. Quadriceps forces and patellar motion in the anatomical model of the patellofemoral joint. *Knee.* 1996;3:1–7.

Siu D, Rudan J, Wevers HW, Griffiths P. Femoral articular shape and geometry. *J Arthroplasty.* 1996;11:166–173.

Appendix 3–A

Derivation of Effective Moment Arm

Please refer to Figure 3–3. Assume frictionless point contact and a quasi-static situation.

Summing moments for C_1 and C_2:
For C_1:

$$F_q \cdot d_1 - F_p \cdot d_2 + F_1 \cdot 0 = 0 \qquad (1)$$

For C_2:

$$W \cdot d_4 + F_p \cdot d_3 + F_2 \cdot 0 = 0 \qquad (2)$$

Rearrange Eq. 2 to get:

$$W \cdot d_4 = F_p \cdot d_3 \qquad (3)$$

Solve for F_p from Eq. 1 and substitute into Eq. 2:

$$W \cdot d_4 = F_q \cdot (d_1 \cdot d_3)/d_2 \qquad (4)$$

Therefore, because $W \cdot d_4$ represents the moment due to the weight of the leg, the effective moment arm of the quadriceps mechanism is $(d_1 \cdot d_3)/d_2$.

The quadriceps force from this analysis is given by:

$$F_q = W \cdot (d_4 \cdot d_2/d_1 \cdot d_3) \qquad (5)$$

and the patellar tendon force is given by:

$$F_p = W \cdot (d_4/d_3) \qquad (6)$$

CHAPTER 4

The History and Physical Examination: The Orthopaedist's Perspective

At a recent patella course, the faculty were asked what three findings on the physical exam they considered to be the most important with respect to making a diagnosis of patellar malalignment. Each panelist gave a different answer. Such a discrepancy in answers would not be found at an anterior cruciate ligament or meniscus symposium. Many physical findings have been described in connection with patellar pathology, but no single finding has gained uniform approval as being a clear reflection of clinically significant patellar pathology.

There are two reasons for this. (1) Patellar malalignment is common, and therefore patella-related abnormalities are commonly seen. This has led some investigators to consider these common abnormalities to be "normal" (see Chapter 1). (2) Certain signs and symptoms appear to be common to patellar malalignment and other conditions about the knee. It is therefore easy to mistake patellar pathology for another condition and vice versa.

THE MEDICAL HISTORY

The history of a patient with patellar pain is usually dismayingly nonspecific.

Pain Location

Occasionally the pain is directly anterior but most often not. It is commonly medial or lateral to the patella. The pain can be directly over the medial or lateral joint line, in which case it can mimic a torn meniscus.[1-4] Investigators believe that this is related directly or indirectly to the patellomeniscal/patellotibial ligaments.[3] Pain can even be popliteal,[5-7] possibly secondary to hamstring tightness or spasm, and the ever-present Baker's cyst can therefore be falsely blamed for the pain. Pain near the inferior pole of the patella can be confusing. It can be a reflection of patella malalignment, but can also be related to an inflammation of the fat pad or to one form or another of patellar tendinitis/tendinosis[8,9] (see Chapter 8).

Activities Associated with Pain

Patients often complain of anterior knee pain with prolonged sitting, the "movie theater sign." Classic teaching also has it that pain is worse going down stairs, but in my experience pain going up stairs is just as common, if not more common. Others have also noted this.[3] Consistent with this complaint is the patient's difficulty getting out of a low chair. Patients rarely volunteer this information; it has to be elicited.

Giving Way

The patient may describe giving way as the patella slips out and back in to the trochlea, but a torn anterior cruciate ligament can cause similar symptoms (a diagnosis far more appealing to the orthopaedic surgeon). A loose body, a torn meniscus, or simple muscle atrophy can also lead to giving way.

"Swelling"

The term is put in quotation marks because it is extremely common for patients with knee pain (whatever the cause) to consider their knee to be swollen. Although it can indeed be swollen, very often objectively this is not the case. Therefore, when a patient offers that his or her knee has been swollen, the clinician has to take the information with a degree of skepticism. The painful knee may feel heavy, stiff, and irritated, which may translate into an impression of swelling. True swelling can be the result of an effusion (excessive fluid in the knee, which can be synovial or hemorrhagic) or of synovial inflammation (rheumatological, tuberculous, etc). An effusion represents free fluid in the joint, which can be aspirated (tapped). Synovial inflammation leads to a boggy knee, which is akin to a fluid-filled sponge. It is filled with fluid that cannot be aspirated with a needle.

"Heat"

Many patients report heat about the knee. This is not specific to patellar problems. This heat is usually not observed by the examiner. (This is a particular problem when, over the telephone, patients report "heat about the knee" following surgery.) A knee that is truly excessively warm is indicative of an inflammatory or infectious process. There may or may not have been an injury associated with the onset of symptoms.

"Crunching," "Noise"

Noisy knees are common and not necessarily a cause for concern. Noisy knees that hurt are another story. It has not been determined exactly what causes crepitus—that fine, muffled crunching sound akin to autumn leaves being stepped on. Perhaps this is a reflection of visible articular cartilage damage. However, I have a number of patients with crepitus who have visually intact articular cartilage at the time of arthroscopy. I therefore do not subscribe to that tenet. Admittedly, articular changes not visible to the naked eye could be partly responsible. Changes in the synovium and other soft tissues could also be the cause.

Duration of Symptoms

The duration of symptoms prior to the visit to the doctor or therapist is quite variable. Some patients come in for worsening of what had been until then low-grade, chronic pain; others have a relatively rapid onset of symptoms, which usually occurs after a sudden change or increase in physical activity.

Unilateral or Bilateral Symptoms

Symptoms can be unilateral or bilateral. If a patient has long-term pain in both knees, this should increase the clinician's suspicion that the problem is patellar rather than meniscal—even if the pain and tenderness are over the medial or lateral joint line. The major differential in patients with bilateral knee pain is a rheumatological condition. If there is any question, it is relatively inexpensive to test for the sedimentation rate. If a patient has not had a checkup in a while, this can be a good time to suggest a basic medical examination, including routine, inexpensive laboratory testing. Conversely, patients with unilateral symptoms can find it difficult to understand why they would have pain in only one knee when both knees look the same on X-ray and physical exam. It is even more difficult when, on X-ray, the asymptomatic knee looks worse than the painful one (not an uncommon scenario). It is not always clear what leads one knee and not the other to be painful (see Chapter 1).

THE PHYSICAL EXAMINATION

Examination in the Standing Position

The exam requires the patient to be barefoot and in shorts or a gown. It is tempting to allow the patient to keep the outer garments on, but this is usually inadequate.

The patient is often sitting on the exam table when the doctor or therapist walks in, and it is tempting to start the exam with the patient in that position. This is acceptable, as long as the examiner remembers to test the patient standing and walking at the end of the exam. However, I prefer to start with the patient standing and walking.

The patient should face the examiner and stand in his or her natural position. If the feet are rotated outward or inward, ask the patient to stand with the feet pointing forward. Do the patella and the foot line up? When the patella faces forward, is the foot externally rotated? When the foot is forward, does the patella look inward ("squinting patella") (Figure 4–1)? If so, this indicates a complex rotational problem about the knee, sometimes called "miserable malalignment." This term alone should indicate that the clinician and the patient could be in for a difficult time. The patella in this situation is but an innocent bystander in a rotational malalignment that goes from the hip down to the feet. When the patella points inward, the entire soft tissue envelope of the upper leg is rotated—usually in association with femoral neck anteversion (see discussion of hip examination below). The leg has to turn in order to keep the femoral head seated in the acetabulum. On occasion, the rotation of the thigh is incomplete, to the extent that the patella remains relatively straight. With the underlying thigh rotated inward, the patella now has the appearance of being lateralized. Sometimes it actually is lateralized, which gives the knee a grasshopper appearance.

Is the patient knock-kneed or bowlegged? If so, the patient is at increased risk for patellar pain. A valgus knee increases the quadriceps (Q) angle by displacing the tibial tuberosity laterally. Patients with varus knees can also have very high Q angles when the varus is associated with lateral positioning of the tibial tuberosity. Despite the common wisdom that patellofemoral problems are associated with valgus knees, a number of investigators have noted that a varus alignment is commonly found.[10–12] When pa-

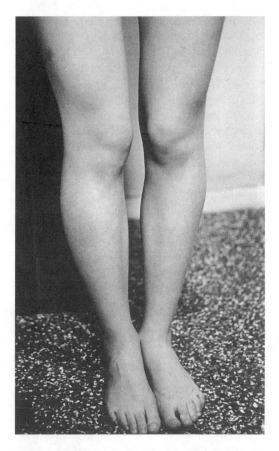

Figure 4–1 Squinting Patellae. The key in diagnosis and treatment is to realize that this is associated with "miserable malalignment," a complex malalignment from the hip down to the feet.

tients approach middle-age and have varus or valgus alignment, medial or lateral femorotibial compartment arthritis may also be part of the differential diagnosis. Of course, patellar pain can coexist with femorotibial arthritis. In such a situation, failure to address both problems can lead to persistence of pain.

When seen from the side, the patient can be assessed for recurvatum. This, along with joint laxity, is not uncommonly associated with patellar problems. One can speculate that the normal internal rotation of the femur that takes place in extension will be exaggerated in recurvatum, and this may have a detrimental effect on the dynamics of the leg. The inferior pole of the patella may be driven posteriorly into the fat pad in such a way as to cause pain.

Don't forget the feet (see Chapter 13). This is easy to do if the patient is still in his or her shoes. High arches and, more commonly, flat feet can alter the mechanics of the knee to the point of causing or contributing to knee pain. The exact biomechanical connection between flat feet and knee pain remains speculative, but the clinical correlation does exist. As the foot pronates, the tibia internally rotates.[3,13] This decreases the Q angle and, thus, one would expect decreased knee pain with flat feet. Clearly then, pain is not necessarily related to a change in the Q angle (unless one assumes that in some patients a decrease in Q angle causes pain simply because for them it is a deviation from normal). The valgus imposed by the flat feet may be a significant factor. When patients with flat feet climb stairs, the center of the knee does not lie over the center of the foot. This is corrected by the proper arch support (see Chapter 13).

Watching the patient's gait gives an indication of how much pain he or she is in. A peg-leg gait (the patient walks with the knee straight as if in a cast) is indicative of pain and/or profound quadriceps weakness. Pain anywhere about the lower extremity can cause this type of gait. An antalgic gait (a relatively quick step on the painful side) is by definition indicative of pain in the leg. Neither the peg-leg nor the antalgic gait are specific for any particular part of the leg, and even a lumbar radiculopathy can cause pain about the thigh, knee, or leg and result in an antalgic gait. If the patient leans to the affected side when walking, this suggests the possibility of pathology about the hip. Pain about the knee can indeed be a reflection of hip pathology. The practitioner should be attuned to this possibility, especially when no tenderness is elicited about the knee itself. In situations where knee pain is actually referred pain from the hip, it is usually medial (presumably via a shared sensory pathway—the obturator nerve and its branches) and lateral when referred from common types of lumbar radiculopathies. Patients are said to have a steppage gait when the hip and knee are flexed more than usual. The patient looks like he or she is climbing a step. This most commonly occurs when the patient has a foot drop, which is usually the result of a peroneal nerve palsy. Pain about the knee in the presence of steppage gait is not likely to be related to patellar malalignment. As the patient walks, watch the feet. The patient may pronate significantly during the so-called foot flat portion of the gait cycle (that is, the feet become flat as the patient rocks forward from the heel onto the ball of the foot). As noted above, this can adversely affect knee mechanics to the point of contributing to the patient's pain.

Examination in the Sitting Position

The patient can now be examined sitting, with the knee bent over the edge of the table. As with the exam of any part of the body, one should look, lightly touch, palpate, and manipulate—in that sequence. There is a natural amount of external tibial torsion as noted on every chairlift (the tips of the skis point outward), and this is the time to check if it is excessive.[14] With the thigh held steady, the foot and leg of some patients can be further rotated externally. If this is the case, and the patient already walks with the leg in some external rotation, one has to be careful with certain types of surgical realignments (see Chapter 14) as the external rotation can be inadvertently exaggerated.

Patellar Height

The articular cartilage of the normal patella begins to make contact with the trochlea in early flexion (approximately 15 degrees). If the patella rides relatively proximally ("high") or distally ("low"), the patient is said to have a patella alta or infera. In either case the mechanics are altered and the possibility of pain exists. Patellar height is difficult to assess clinically. With severe patella alta, the patella points toward the ceiling rather than straight ahead when the patient is sitting. With the leg extended, patella alta leads to the "camelback sign"—two bumps at the front of the knee (the proximal one is the patella, the distal one the fat pad).[15] The patella has to be quite high for these signs to be present.

Skin Color

Is the skin color the same on both sides? Redness or blanching can be associated with sympathetic changes such as those seen in reflex sympathetic dystrophy (RSD) (see Chapter 15).

Patellar Tracking

The patient should be asked to extend the knee. This is the time to assess patellar tracking. Normally, the patella follows a straight line as the knee extends. Although the femur and the (resultant) pull of the quadriceps are about 5 degrees off the vertical in the lateral direction, the patella appears to follow a straight line as the knee goes from flexion to extension. In a small but significant number of patients with patellar malalignment, the patella clearly slips off laterally as the knee approaches extension.[4] This has been called the J sign, a reflection of the path taken by the patella (Figure 4–2). This is a form of subluxation, and a factor to consider in planning surgery. Note that a minority of patients with malalignment do not exhibit a J sign simply because they will not extend the knee (presumably, the phenomenon of the patella slipping laterally is associated with too much discomfort).

Joint Laxity

Joint laxity is associated with patellar pathology, and the patient can be asked to passively push the thumb against the volar aspect of the forearm. Hyperextension of the elbow, recurvatum of the knee, and considerable external rotation of the tibia on the femur can be associated findings (Figure 4–3).

Examination in the Supine Position

With the patient lying supine, the following parameters can be assessed.

Ability To Extend the Knee Fully

Some patients with severe malalignment refuse to extend the knee fully.[16] They know

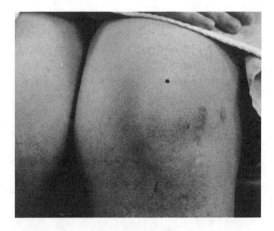

A

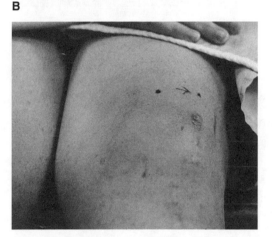

B

Figure 4–2 The J Sign. (**A**) With the knee flexed 90 degrees, the patella is centered. (**B**) As the knee reaches terminal extension, the patella suddenly jumps laterally. This is not common but is quite impressive and is a sign of a rather severe condition.

from experience that as the knee nears full extension, the patella will uncomfortably slip laterally (see J sign above). This is not the locked knee of a torn meniscus or of a loose body.

Hamstring/Achilles Tightness

Tightness of the hamstrings or Achilles tendon has been associated with patellar pain, presumably because of compensatory mechanisms

A

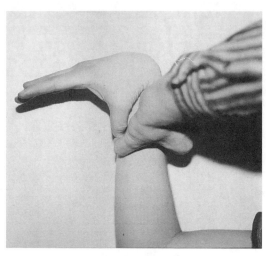

B

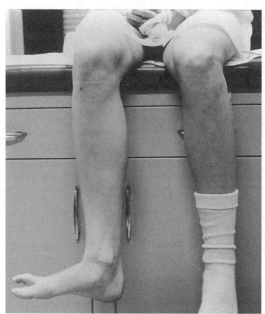

Figure 4–3 Joint Laxity. This is exemplified by (**A**) bringing the thumb to the forearm and (**B**) rotating the tibia externally on the femur to a considerable extent.

in the extensor mechanism. Many investigators have noted that correction of hamstring tightness is correlated with improvements in patellar pain.

VMO Dysplasia

The normal vastus medialis obliquus (VMO) is quite visible and prominent at the supero-medial aspect of the patella (Figure 4–4A). The patient with patella malalignment often has a dysplastic VMO that is barely visible and barely palpable (Figure 4–4B). One of the goals of physical therapy is to strengthen this muscle be-cause it provides the only dynamic medial force on the patella.

The Quadriceps (Q) Angle

Maligned, misunderstood, and misused, the Q angle almost deserves a chapter of its own. First described by Cruveilher in 1840,[17] the Q angle is the angle subtended by a line from the anterior superior iliac spine (ASIS) to the center of the patella and a line from the center of the patella to the center of the tibial tuberosity (Figure 4–5). Investigators have determined that normal is ap-proximately 15 degrees in both men and women (women have a wider pelvis, but this may not significantly affect the ASIS). Some investiga-tors have noted ever so slightly higher values in women and slightly higher values when the Q angle is tested in the standing (versus supine) patient.[18] The Q angle is a measure of the patella's tendency to move laterally when the quadriceps muscles are contracted. The greater the angle, the greater this tendency. The Q angle is not easy to measure and interpret. Rotating the foot outward while holding the thigh obviously increases the Q angle by moving the tibial tuber-osity laterally. The examiner must make an ef-fort to keep the patient's leg in neutral rotation. This is easier said than done in patients with femoral and/or tibial torsion. The examiner must also remember that the Q angle decreases with knee flexion (the tibia internally rotates). When normal values for the Q angle are reported, it is with the knee extended or slightly flexed (5 to 30 degrees). If, unbeknownst to the examiner, the patella is laterally positioned, a falsely normal Q angle will be recorded. Every effort must be made to maintain the patella centered in the trochlea when measuring the Q angle. In any case, beware of the falsely normal Q angle. With

A

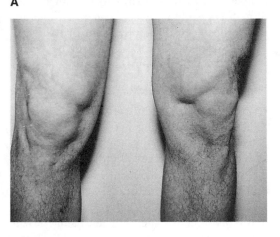

B

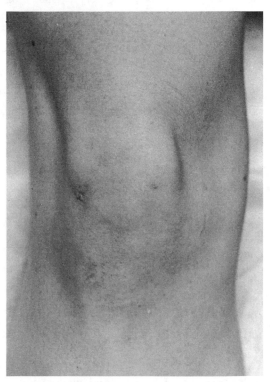

Figure 4–4 VMO Dysplasia. (**A**) The patient demonstrates a normal VMO, clearly visible at the superomedial aspect of the patella. (**B**) The patient demonstrates a dysplastic VMO that does not stand out, and when palpated feels very soft (even as the patient tries to tense the muscle).

the knee flexed 90 degrees, the tibial tuberosity should be in the midline. This is another way of assessing the Q angle at 90 degrees. It does not replace the traditional assessment of the Q angle because the tuberosity can be positioned normally at 90 degrees of flexion but be abnormally lateralized near extension.

Clinical tip: The proximal limb of the Q angle is relatively constant: a line from the anterior superior iliac crest to the middle of the (centered) patella is approximately 5 degrees off from the vertical (for men and women). It is the line from the middle of the patella to the tibial tuberosity that varies from patient to patient. If this line is no more than 10 degrees off the vertical, this means that the Q angle is no greater than 15 degrees (ie, normal). I recommend simply looking at the patellar tendon and determining how far off the vertical it is. If it is 10 degrees or less, it is normal; between 10 and 15 degrees is borderline; more than 15 degrees is abnormal. This method of assessing the Q angle is particularly valuable during surgery when the thigh and pelvis are draped off.

The A Angle

Arno[19] has described the A angle, an angle subtended by the longitudinal axis of the patella and an imaginary line drawn from the inferior pole of the patella to the tibial tuberosity (presumably assessed with the patient supine). It is a measure of patellar rotation in the frontal plane. Arno's premise was that excessive rotation (inferior patella pointing laterally) could be a source of pain. He documented the case of one patient whose symptoms resolved with diminution of the A angle through physical therapy—in particular, taping. This case study made no mention of normal values for the A angle; however, if Arno's work is substantiated by other studies it may be worth including this measurement in the patellar exam. To date, I have not been successful in detecting abnormal A angles.

Swelling

The patient may comment that the knee is swollen. The knee can now be examined for the presence of an effusion ("water on the knee") or

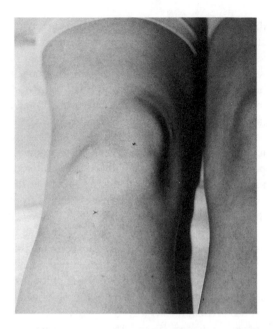

Figure 4–5 The Quadriceps (Q) Angle. The Q angle is the angle subtended by a line from the anterior superior iliac spine (ASIS) to the center of the patella and a line from the center of the patella to the center of the tibial tuberosity. Because the line from the ASIS to the center of the patella is a relatively constant 5 degrees off the vertical (as one notes in performing knee replacement surgery), clinically it is much quicker simply to check the position of the tibial tuberosity. If it is lateralized, the patient has a high Q angle perhaps masked by lateral displacement of the patella itself. (With the knee slightly flexed, the patellar tendon should be off the vertical by no more than 10 degrees. Note that if one then adds the 5 degrees mentioned above, this leads to the normal Q angle of 15 degrees.)

of a boggy synovitis. With effusion, the knee feels like a water balloon to the examiner, and with boggy synovitis it feels doughy or spongy. An effusion can be associated with almost any knee condition. If the effusion is significant enough, it can be tapped and the fluid sent for analysis.

Skin Color and Temperature

If skin color has not been noted yet, this is the time to do so. It is important to determine skin temperature as it compares to the other knee. Skin that is particularly cool can be a sign of reflex sympathetic dystrophy. Skin that is warm can also be a sign of reflex sympathetic dystrophy or of an inflammatory or infectious process.

Palpation for Tenderness

The knee is palpated for areas of tenderness. I prefer to start palpating parts of the knee suspected of being pain-free so as to keep the patient at ease. Tenderness of either joint line can indicate a collateral ligament strain if there has been an injury, a meniscal tear, femorotibial arthritis, or—most significantly for the purposes of this discussion—patella-related pain. The reason for joint-line tenderness in patella malalignment is not agreed upon and probably multifactorial. Interestingly, the very existence of joint-line tenderness as a sign of patellar pathology is unknown to many orthopaedists. I see this on a regular basis during second opinions. This finding was not taught to me during my formal training, and I suspect that it was not taught to these doctors either. I have not seen it written in any common textbook, nor have I seen it described in the other texts on the patella. Yet Karlson recognized this finding at least as far back as 1940, as evidenced by the following statement: "The diagnosis is difficult to make and the differential diagnosis injury to the meniscus . . . causes special difficulties, as in both these ailments [meniscal and patellar pathology] there is a pressure tenderness over the medial joint space."[1] This finding has been confirmed by others,[1–4] and in my own practice I have found this to be absolutely correct. Likewise the McMurray maneuver, traditionally associated with meniscal pathology, can cause medial-lateral displacement of the patella and be painful on that basis alone.[4]

As the distal portion of the iliotibial band (ITB) crosses the lateral femoral condyle, it can be tender. This is probably what is commonly called ITB tendinitis or runner's knee. This is a condition in which a tight ITB rubs against the lateral femoral condyle and becomes irritated with repetitive motion such as seen in running or cycling. I have found that ITB tendinitis coexists quite commonly with patellar tilt, presumably because the ITB is in continuity with the lateral retinaculum.

Very localized tenderness at the medial aspect of the knee away from the joint line can be the sign of a neuroma, especially in a situation where there has been blunt trauma (eg, a fall onto the knee or a car accident). In my opinion, neuromas are quite frequently missed. Eliciting pain from gently squeezing the skin should greatly heighten one's suspicion that a neuroma is contributing to the patient's symptoms. A subcutaneous injection of lidocaine can help confirm the diagnosis.

Tenderness at the anterior aspect of the medial femoral condyle in association with a snapping sensation as the knee is flexed can reflect a symptomatic plica. The plica is a band of fibrous tissue that is variable in its location and presence. In the human embryo, the knee begins as a joint made of separate compartments. The plica may or may not be an embryological remnant (see Chapter 2). The plica usually begins at the medial aspect of the patella and inserts into the fat pad. It is not present in every patient, and its exact points of origin and insertion vary. The diagnosis of a painful plica was quite in vogue in the late 1980s, and many unnecessary plica removals were carried out. There has been at least one report of a patella dislocating following plica removal. This is understandable, because the plica can function as a passive medial restraint. On the other hand, it is certainly possible for a plica to be symptomatic.

Palpation at the tip (inferior pole) of the patella can elicit considerable tenderness and can reflect patellar tendinitis (jumper's knee). This condition can simply be due to overuse or can itself be a reflection of malalignment. Either way, it can be a very stubborn condition.[20] At the other end of the tendon, tenderness over the tibial tuberosity is rare in adults but common in teenagers who suffer from Osgood-Schlatter's disease ("Osgoodschlitis," as far as many patients are concerned). The tibial tuberosity is an apophysis (ie, it has a growth plate that does not contribute to the axial growth of the bone), and it can become enlarged or painful. This condition seems to occur more frequently in patients with an underlying extensor mechanism malalignment (eg, patella alta) but can be idiopathic.

On either side of and directly behind the patellar tendon lies the fat pad. In the orthopaedic literature and in the traditional orthopaedic exam, this structure receives relatively little attention. As is the case with its counterpart just proximal to the trochlea, the fat pad is likely to provide some cushioning (see Chapter 2). It can become inflamed and thus a source of pain. Palpation is easy because the fat pad is readily visible under the skin of most patients. In extreme cases, the fat pad can be sclerotic and painful; in such cases the patient is said to suffer from Hoffa's condition. There is still some controversy as to whether this condition truly exists. The differential diagnosis would include pigmented villonodular synovitis.

Because a major differential diagnosis of knee instability is a rupture of the anterior cruciate ligament, the examiner should perform a Lachman, anterior drawer, and pivot shift test for any patient complaining of giving way. Far less common, but equally significant is the posterior cruciate ligament (PCL) deficiency. The PCL and the extensor mechanism are synergistic to the extent that both resist forward subluxation of the femur (eg, when going down steps). In a situation where the PCL is deficient, the patella will experience larger forces and stresses than normal. The posterior drawer, drop-back, and other PCL-related tests should be performed if there is any question of a PCL tear.

Examination of the Patella Proper

This portion of the exam can begin with the simplest test of all: assessment of tilt. The medial and lateral borders of the patella are lightly palpated (if the examiner's nails blanch, he or she is pressing too hard) (Figure 4–6). If the leg is in neutral rotation, an imaginary line between the fingertips should be horizontal, parallel to the ground. When the patella is tilted, the medial border is higher than the lateral border.

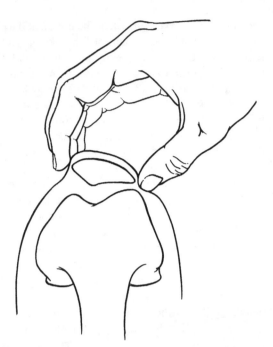

Figure 4–6 Patellar Tilt. The thumb and index lightly palpate the borders of the patella. The normal patella is horizontal. Tilted patellae may be easily reducible, and this correlates with the severity of the malalignment. This is a very sensitive test of malalignment— perhaps the most sensitive test. Of course, patella malalignment (tilt) is common and not necessarily symptomatic. Tilt can therefore be noted in patients without knee pain and in patients with knee pain secondary to nonpatellar conditions.

Practical tip: If the examiner has trouble finding the lateral border of the patella, this is because the patella is tilted. The lateral border has blended in with the lateral condyle.

Note that in patients who have not had surgery, the patella is never tilted the other way (the lateral border is never higher than the medial border). Tilt can be graded from mild to severe in a way that is clearly subjective. Patients with tilt can also be divided into those whose tilt is easily reducible and those whose tilt persists despite the examiner's attempt to correct it. Such reducibility is also subjective. Certain investigators have taken a slightly different tack, suggesting that the patella is abnormal if the lateral border cannot be raised 15 degrees. If such a

measurement could be reliable it would provide an objective measure of reducibility. However, I have difficulty judging 15 degrees. Naysayers will quickly point out that tilt is common. This may be true, but tilt is not normal. Again, the reader is referred to Chapter 1 for a discussion of "common" versus "normal."

Facet Tenderness

When the patella is pushed to one side and then the other, it is possible to curl the fingers around the borders of the patella and to palpate the medial and lateral "facets" (Figure 4–7). With moderate pressure, this should not be painful. When the malaligned patella is the source of the patient's pain, however, it is extremely common for one or both facets to be tender. In teenagers and patients in their early 20s, it is usually the medial facet that is tender; in patients over 25, it is almost always the lateral facet that is tender. I would go so far as to say that if there is no tenderness with this maneuver I would look elsewhere for the source of patient's pain (assuming, of course, that pain is the chief complaint).

What exactly is being tested with this maneuver? After all, between the examiner's fingers and the patella lie the retinaculum, the capsule, and synovium. Tenderness of any of these structures could lead to a positive test. However, it is my impression that if any of these structures is the source of pain, it will be tender to direct palpation (ie, the examiner should be able to elicit tenderness without having to curl his or her fingers under the patella). On the other hand, perhaps by curling fingers under the patella the examiner stretches the soft tissues enough to elicit pain. Regardless, in my opinion, pain from this maneuver is very highly correlated with patellar malalignment.

Assuming that it is the patella that is tender and not the retinaculum, what is it about the patella that makes it tender? Articular cartilage itself cannot be the source of pain because it lacks sensory nerves. However, in a laterally tilted patella, the subchondral bone on the lateral side of the patella can indeed be tender; in the athletically active patient over the age of 30, I believe

A

B

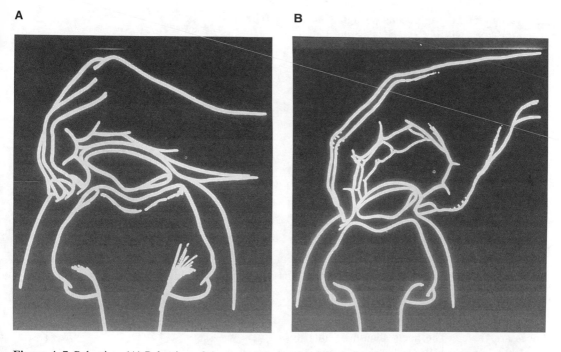

Figure 4–7 Palpation. (**A**) Palpation of the medial facet. This facet is not normally tender. (**B**) Palpation of the lateral facet. This is usually tender in patients over the age of 25 with symptomatic malalignment (except for the small minority who are dislocators and who are pain-free between dislocations).

that this is the source of pain. This still leaves unexplained the source of the medial tenderness in younger patients. If one believes the hypo-hyper pressure theory of malalignment, why should the medial subchondral bone be tender? The reader is referred to Chapter 1 for further discussion of this subject.

The medial-lateral play (glide) of the patella is often mentioned as part of the exam. If the lateral retinaculum is tighter than normal, it will restrict both medial and lateral displacement. I have difficulty interpreting and assessing the medial-lateral displacement of the patella and prefer to assess tilt (another manifestation of relative tightness on the lateral side). Clearly though, medial-lateral play is worth checking because a patient with clinical instability (giving way), patella alta, and extensive medial-lateral play is pathophysiologically different from a patient with pain, severe tilt, and limited medial-lateral play. This will almost certainly affect the

choice of procedures should the patient come to surgery.

The Apprehension (Fairbanks) Sign

For this test, the patient's knee starts in the flexed position (at least 30 degrees). The patient is asked to extend the knee while the examiner pushes the patella laterally. In patients who do not have severe instability, this maneuver causes no pain or apprehension. However, in patients who dislocate or severely sublux their patella, this maneuver leads to the patient's apprehension as evidenced by the patient's grabbing of the examiner's tie, arm (or other part of the anatomy) or by withdrawal of the leg. This is a very specific test (a positive apprehension sign is a sure sign of patellar instability), but overall it is not a sensitive sign of malalignment. The apprehension sign is uniformly negative in patients who have tilt and pain but who do not experience subluxation (giving way) or dislocation.

A variation on the apprehension sign is noted when the knee will not extend, despite the absence of pain or any mechanical block. The patient refuses to have the knee straightened for fear of painful subluxation in extension (see J sign above).

Examination in the Decubitus Position

With the patient on his or her side, tightness of the ITB can be assessed (Ober test) (Figure 4–8). This condition is critical because the ITB is in continuity with the lateral retinaculum. Via this connection, a tight ITB will have a detrimental effect on the patella, and conversely, stretching of the ITB can reduce patellar pain.

Examination in the Prone Position

With the patient lying on the stomach, the knees are flexed. The heels should be able to touch the buttocks. If not, the extensor mechanism is tight. This can be expected to cause undue pressure on the patella when the knee is flexed.

The popliteal space should be evaluated for the presence of masses. Note that a soft, mushy mass toward the medial side of the popliteal space is probably a Baker's cyst, an outpouching of the capsule. It is not serious and usually not painful.

Hip rotation should be assessed. Increased internal rotation is associated with increased femoral neck anteversion, itself associated with patellar pain.[21]

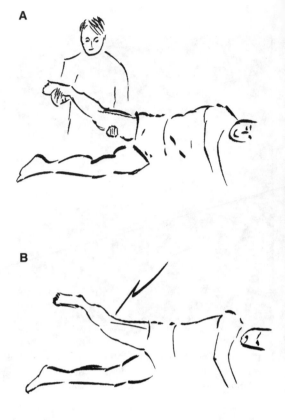

A

B

Figure 4–8 The Ober Test. A most underused test, this part of the examination tests the iliotibial band. (**A**) With the hip extended and the knee slightly flexed, the iliotibial band is at its tightest. Normally, with the leg in this position the knee should be able to touch the exam table. (**B**) In a severely abnormal situation, the leg remains suspended in the air. Tight lateral structures can be a source of chronic (anterior) knee pain.

REFERENCES

1. Karlson S. Chondromalacia patellae. *Acta Orthop Scand.* 1940;83:347.

2. Bentley G, Dowd G. Current concepts of etiology and treatment of chondromalacia patella. *Clin Orthop.* 1984;189:209.

3. Carson WG. Diagnosis of extensor mechanism disorders. *Clin Sports Med.* 1985;4:231–246.

4. Outerbridge RE, Dunlop J. The problem of chondromalacia patellae. *Clin Orthop.* 1975;110:177–193.

5. Arnoldi CC. Patellar pain. *Acta Orthop Scand.* 1991;62(suppl 224).

6. Insall JN, Falvo KA, Wise DW. Chondromalacia patellae—a prospective study. *J Bone Joint Surg.* 1976; 58A:1.

7. Scuderi G, Cuomo F, Scott WN. Lateral release and proximal realignment for patellar subluxation and dislocation. *J Bone Joint Surg.* 1988;70A:856.

8. Duri ZAA, Aichroth PM, Dowd G. The fat pad: clinical observations. *Am J Knee Surg.* 1996;9:55–66.

9. McConnell J. Fat pad irritation—a mistaken patellar tendonitis. *Sport Health.* 1991;9(4):7–9.

10. Ficat P. Lateral fascia release and lateral hyperpressure syndrome. In: Pickett JC, Radin EL, eds. *Chondromalacia of the Patella.* Baltimore: Williams & Wilkins; 1983:95–112.

11. Cistac C, Cartier PH. Diagnostic et traitement des déséquilibres rotuliens du sportif. *J Traumatol Sport.* 1986:3:92–97.

12. Harrison MM, Cooke TDV, Fisher SB, Griffin MP. Patterns of knee arthrosis and patella subluxation. *Clin Orthop.* 1994;309:56–63.

13. Pedowitz WJ, Kovatis P. Flatfoot in the adult. *J Am Acad Orthop Surg.* 1995;3:293–302.

14. Turner MS. The association between tibial torsion and knee joint pathology. *Clin Orthop.* 1994;302:47–51.

15. Hughston J, Walsh WM, Puddu G. *Patellar Subluxation and Dislocation.* Philadelphia: WB Saunders Co; 1984. Saunders Monographs in Clinical Orthopaedics, vol 5.

16. Brattström H. Patella alta in non-dislocating knee joints. *Acta Orthop Scand.* 1970;41:578–588.

17. Ellison AE, Boland AL Jr, DeHaven KE, et al. *Athletic Training and Sports Medicine.* Chicago: American Academy of Orthopaedic Surgeons; 1984:272–273.

18. Woodland LH, Francis RS. Parameters and comparisons of the quadriceps angle of college-aged men and women in the supine and standing positions. *Am J Sports Med.* 1992;20:208.

19. Arno S. The A angle: a quantitative measurement of patella alignment and realignment. *J Sport Phys Ther.* 1990;12:237–242.

20. Fritschy D, de Gautard R. Jumper's knee and ultrasonography. *Am J Sports Med.* 1988;16:637–640.

21. Eckhoff DG, Montgomery WK, Kilcoyne RF. Femoral morphometry and anterior knee pain. *Clin Orthop.* 1994;302:64–68.

CHAPTER 5

Patellofemoral Imaging

Theoretically, practitioners can make the diagnosis of patellar malalignment in a patient presenting with knee pain or instability after taking the history and performing the physical examination. Nevertheless, imaging serves several adjunctive functions:

- It can confirm the diagnosis of malalignment.
- It can qualify the pathology (eg, tilt, height, dysplasia).
- It can quantify the pathology.

All of these can be important with respect to prognosis, surgical planning, and informed consent.

The term *malalignment* has traditionally referred to the medial-lateral position of the patella. However, the patella has a three-dimensional tracking pattern and can be malaligned in several different planes: it can be translated superiorly or inferiorly, and it can be flexed or extended when viewed from the lateral (sagittal) direction.[1,2] It can be tilted or medial-laterally displaced when viewed from an axial direction, and it can be rotated when viewed from a frontal direction.[3] These all qualify as forms of malalignment.

Settegast[4] in 1921 described the first roentgenographic technique for visualizing the patellofemoral joint, and several modifications and

new techniques have since been developed. Although radiographs remain the mainstay of patellar imaging on an everyday basis, more sophisticated modalities including nuclear technetium scanning, computed tomography (CT), and magnetic resonance imaging (MRI) can all be very useful. With the high costs of these newer imaging techniques, it is a challenge to use them in the most cost-effective manner possible.

PLAIN RADIOGRAPHS

For the large majority of patients with malalignment, plain radiographs are the only imaging modality the clinician will need to make the diagnosis. The most important views for determining patellar alignment are the lateral and the axial views.

The Lateral View

Technique

On the ideal lateral X-ray, the posterior condyles overlap perfectly. This is particularly important if one wishes to assess the depth of the trochlea or even patellar tilt (which one should do in any patient with patella malalignment). Most of the time, the specific degree of flexion is immaterial. Occasionally, when patellar height is an issue, it can be useful to view an image of the knee in extension.

Special thanks go to Dr Philippe Cartier for assistance with Figure 5–15.

Patellar Height

A patella alta lies cephalad to its normal position in the trochlea, whereas a patella infera (patella baja) represents the reverse. Even though there is no firm consensus regarding the treatment of these conditions, there is no question about the usefulness of detecting them. Patella infera is usually a postsurgical condition that, when associated with a painful knee, can be a signal to the surgeon to approach with caution.[5,6] Patella alta, in contrast, is usually a congenital or developmental condition that is often associated with other anatomic anomalies such as trochlear and condylar dysplasia. A high-riding patella can be associated with pain and/or instability.

Numerous investigators have created a measuring system for determining patellar height. When a specific location on the femur is used as a reference, the degree of knee flexion must be specified (because the patella moves with respect to the femur when the knee is flexed). When the proximal tibia is used as a reference, the measurement is relatively independent of knee flexion (because the patellar tendon maintains the patella at a constant distance from the tibia).

Blumensaat[7] was one of the first to look for an objective radiographic sign of patella alta. He determined that when the knee is flexed 30 degrees, the inferior pole of the patella should not be cephalad to an anterior prolongation of the intercondylar notch. There are two drawbacks to this technique. (1) The knee must be specifically flexed at 30 degrees. (2) The angle between Blumensaat's line and the longitudinal axis is usually about 45 degrees, but it ranges between 27 and 60 degrees as determined by Brattström[8] in a study of 100 randomly measured patients. If the slope of the intercondylar notch is particularly steep, one could read a falsely positive patella alta. Conversely, if the slope of the intercondylar notch is particularly shallow, one could miss a patella alta.

Labelle and Laurin[9] determined that when the knee is flexed 90 degrees, the superior pole of the patella should just intersect an imaginary prolongation of the anterior cortex. This technique is a natural extension of the physical examination; however its drawback is that the knee must be imaged while flexed at a right angle.

With the leg near extension, the inferior pole of the patella should be entering the trochlea. Exactly how far proximal to the trochlea it can lie before being judged high has not been determined. Norman et al[10] found that with the knee "maximally" extended and the quadriceps contracted, the distance from the distal aspect of the patellar articular surface to the subchondral bone of the femoral condyles was a relatively constant percentage of patient height (approximately 2%). The authors did not specifically define what they considered to be patella alta.

The most commonly used measure in the United States (if its near-universal appearance in US publications is any indication) is the one described by Insall and Salvati in 1971[11] (Figure 5–1). These authors devised a simple, easily remembered parameter that is relatively independent of knee flexion. In their study, they found that the length of the patellar tendon should be approximately equal to the length (diagonal) of the patella. Despite its popularity, the Insall-Salvati ratio has some disadvantages: the tuberosity may be misshapen (eg, from trauma or prior surgery) and the tibial tuberosity may be difficult to visualize because of an over-penetrated radiograph. These points are minor, however, because the posterior aspect of the patellar tendon can be assumed to insert approximately 2 cm from the tibial plateau unless the tuberosity has been displaced. Allowances can be made for the size of the patient. The major disadvantage of this parameter, in my opinion, is the reliance on the inferior pole of the patella as a landmark. It has long been known that patellar morphology in the coronal plane is variable (see the discussion of Wiberg classification below). More recently, investigators have learned that patellar morphology can also be variable in the sagittal plane.[12–15] Of greatest concern with the Insall-Salvati ratio is the fact that a long inferior pole can "fool" the ratio. For example, a long-nosed "Cyrano" patella with its articular surface sitting in an abnormally high-riding position could yield a normal ratio (Figure 5–2). In a 1992 study of 100 patients with patellar pathol-

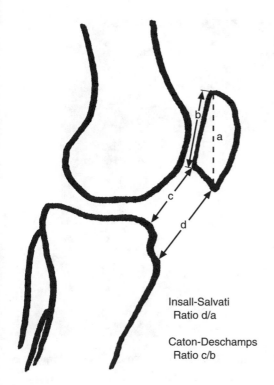

Insall-Salvati
Ratio d/a

Caton-Deschamps
Ratio c/b

Figure 5–1 The Insall-Salvati and the Caton-Deschamps ratios. With the Insall-Salvati ratio, the diagonal length of the patella (**d**) should be equal to the length of the patellar tendon (**a**) ± (20%). This ratio can be applied regardless of the degree of knee flexion. The Caton-Deschamps ratio is the distance from the anterior border of the tibia to the most distal articular surface of the patella (**c**) divided by the length of the patellar subchondral bone (**b**). This ratio should equal approximately 1. *Source:* Reprinted with permission from RP Grelsamer et al, Evaluation of Patellar Shape in the Sagittal Plane—A Clinical Analysis, *American Journal of Sports Medicine*, Vol 22, pp 61–66, © 1994, American Orthopaedic Society for Sports Medicine.

ogy, it was reported that a number of patients with patella alta went undetected by the Insall-Salvati ratio.[12–14]

The Modified Insall-Salvati ratio represents an attempt to circumvent the inferior pole of the patella as a landmark while maintaining the familiar tibial tuberosity.[16] It is often preferable to the original (it does not take much time to look at both ratios). With the Modified Insall-Salvati ra-

tio, the distance from the tibial tuberosity to the most distal point of the patellar articular surface should be less than twice the length of the articular surface (Figure 5–3).

The Blackburne-Peel,[17] de Carvalho,[18] and Caton-Deschamps[5,19] ratios (from Great Britain, Denmark, and France, respectively) are similar. All three use the upper tibia, the distal-most portion of the patellar articular surface, and the length of the patellar articular surface as landmarks; they can all be used, regardless of the degree of knee flexion. The difference between them lies in the upper tibial landmark: Blackburne and Peel draw a line along the tibial plateau (Figure 5–4), de Carvalho et al use the upper border of the tibia, and Caton et al use the anterosuperior corner of the tibia. The normal value for these three ratios is approximately 1 (1.2 for the Caton-Deschamps ratio). They are all easy to apply; however, because they use the length of the articular surface, they are inaccurate in certain patellar morphotypes with a short articular surface. Moreover, the slope of the tibial plateau varies from patient to patient, making any line drawn along it (Blackburne and Peel) a somewhat fickle landmark for patellar height. The anterosuperior angle of the tibia (Caton-Deschamps) is not always present, in which case the Caton-Deschamps ratio reverts to that of de Carvalho. Note that there is a drawback to all the ratios that use the length of the articular surface: this length is not exactly the same in all patients of a given height.[12–14]

Using MRI, Deutsch et al[20] considered a patella to be of normal height when its inferior pole is no more proximal than the superior aspect of the trochlea with the knee extended. Intuitively, this appears to be true, and this theory merits a special study. This measure has the particular advantage of truly being physiological because it assesses the position of the patella with respect to the trochlea. For example, the MRI of a patient with a normally positioned patella but a dysplastic trochlea that begins too distally would be read as patella alta. This is a correct diagnosis because, functionally, the patient would have a patella alta.

Given the multitude of measurement techniques, there appears to be no ideal parameter of

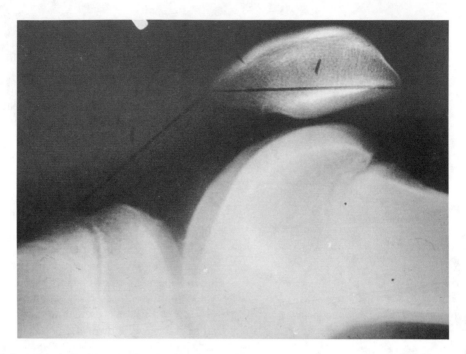

Figure 5–2 A Falsely Positive Insall-Salvati Ratio as a Result of a "Cyrano" (Long-Nosed) Patella Morphology

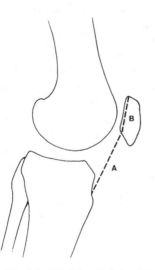

Figure 5–3 The Modified Insall-Salvati Ratio. The distance from the tibial tuberosity to the inferior pole of the patella (**A**) should be less than twice the length of the articular surface (**B**). *Source:* Reprinted with permission from RP Grelsamer and S Meadows, The Modified Insall-Salvati Ratio for Assessment of Patellar Height, *Clinical Orthopaedics and Related Research*, Vol 282, p 173, © 1992, Lippincott-Raven Publishers.

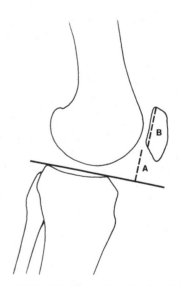

Figure 5–4 The Blackburne-Peel Ratio. The distance from the plateau to the inferior pole (**A**) should equal the length of the articular surface (**B**). *Source:* Reprinted with permission from RP Grelsamer and S Meadows, The Modified Insall-Salvati Ratio for Assessment of Patellar Height, *Clinical Orthopaedics and Related Research*, Vol 282, pp 170–176, © 1992, Lippincott-Raven Publishers.

patellar height. Practitioners are interested in the position of the patellar articular surface with respect to the femur (the patella should engage the trochlea in early flexion). However, any such assessment requires a specific angle of flexion. Any parameter independent of knee flexion requires a fixed point of the upper tibia, and none of the landmarks is foolproof. Finally, if a measurement is going to be independent of the patient's body height, the denominator must be proportional to this height. Neither the length of the patella nor the articular surface of the patella fully satisfies this requirement.

Despite these criticisms, the ratios have their advantages. They are all easy to remember and apply. They can be quickly assessed and, if the practitioner uses these ratios in conjunction with one another, he or she should readily detect clinically significant patella alta or infera. If patella alta or infera is noted on only one of the measurements, one of the above-mentioned anatomic variations of the patella is probably the cause.

Trochlear Dysplasia

Analysis of the femoral trochlea is usually associated with a Merchant-type (axial) view on plain radiograph. Valuable information can also be obtained from the lateral view (Figure 5–5). The subchondral bone of the trochlea is seen as a thin, dense, white line that parallels the lateral femoral condyle and is continuous with the intercondylar notch. This is easily verified by placing a fine wire over the trochlea and over the femoral condyles.[21] The distance between this line and the line representing the subchondral bone of the lateral femoral condyle is, at any given point, a measure of the depth of the trochlea at that point.[21–24] Severe, global dysplasia may be manifest by an overlap of the two lines. An intersection would represent a completely flat, bony trochlea at that point (with a possible area of cartilaginous convexity not necessarily detectable on a Merchant view). I have called such intersections or overlaps the "lateral trochlear sign."[21] Dejour et al called this *croisement*,[24] referred to in the English literature as "crossing," although "overlap" might be better

(the lines do not cross as in an *X* but merge or overlap as in a *Y*). Dejour et al documented that the normal trochlear depth averages 4 mm and that patients with patellar instability can have a trochlear depth of 0 mm at its shallowest. These authors further defined three types of dysplasia: in type I, the overlap of the lines occurs at the proximal trochlea; in type II, there are two areas of overlap—one proximal and one distal; in type III, the overlap is distal, indicating that the trochlea is severely dysplastic over most of its length.

Note that measurements of trochlear dysplasia are predicated on obtaining a perfect lateral X-ray (ie, the posterior condyles overlap precisely on the X-ray picture). In order to obtain this view, it is sometimes necessary to rotate the leg in one direction or the other. Also, excessive external rotation of the leg diminishes the apparent depth of the trochlea and can even lead to a false-positive lateral trochlear (crossing or overlap) sign.[21]

Patellar Morphology

Wiberg noted in 1941 that, when viewed in axial cross-section, the patella can exhibit a variety of shapes[25] (Figure 5–6). He noted further that on autopsy specimens, certain shapes were associated with "chondromalacia." Although the correlation between true chondromalacia and clinical pain is debatable (see Chapter 1), it does seem that certain shapes (eg, Hunter's cap) are associated with clinical problems. My colleagues and I have found that when viewed in a sagittal plane, certain patellar morphologies (both long-nosed "Cyrano" and short-nosed patellae) are associated with painful patella syndromes.[12–14] Specifically, we have looked at a morphology ratio based on the "length" of the patella (à la Insall-Salvati) and the length of the articular surface (Figure 5–7). Most patellae exhibit a ratio between 1.2 and 1.5. Those with a ratio greater than 1.5 give the appearance of having a "long nose" (in fact a relatively long, nonarticulating inferior pole), and those with a ratio less than 1.2 have a "short nose" (Figure 5–8). In my experience, both long- and short-nose patellae are associ-

A

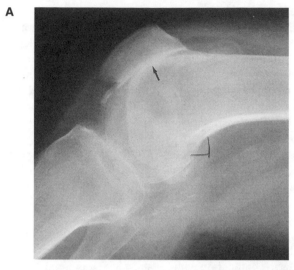

B

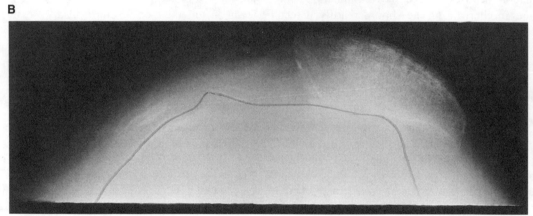

Figure 5–5 The Lateral Trochlear (Crossing) Sign. (**A**) Lateral radiograph of a patient with trochlear dysplasia. The subchondral bone of the trochlea intersects that of the lateral femoral condyle (30 degree external rotation of the leg can also produce such an artifact). (**B**) Axial view confirming the severe dysplasia.

ated with disorders of the extensor mechanism. As noted previously, both of these morphologies have the potential for distorting the classic Insall-Salvati ratio.

The Axial View

Technique

The technique has gradually evolved since 1921 when Settegast described placing the patient prone on the X-ray table and flexing the knee past 90 degrees.[4,26] There are two disadvantages to this approach:

1. the significant (hyper)flexion of the knee (one is most interested in the early degrees of flexion where lateral displacement will be most obvious)
2. the artifact caused by the weight of the patient's leg as it applies pressure to the patella

Jaroschy[27] described a supine technique, which he then modified back to a prone method.

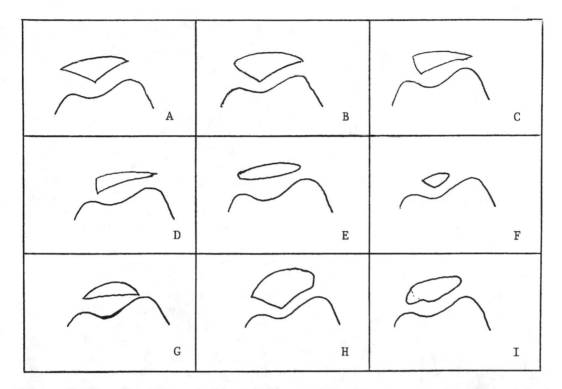

Figure 5–6 Wiberg's Classification of Patellar Morphology in the Axial Plane. (**A**) Type I. (**B**) Type II. (**C**) Type III. There has been some controversy as to which shapes—if any—are actually pathological. Other shapes considered to be potentially pathological include (**D**) Hunter's cap, (**E**) pebble, (**F**) parva, (**G**) half moon, (**H**) magna, (**I**) Baumgartl.

The knee was flexed to no more than 50 to 60 degrees. The beam struck the X-ray plate at an angle of about 45 degrees. Although the lesser degree of flexion was an improvement, there was still the possible artifact from the pressure applied to the patella, not to mention the distortion of the beam striking the plate at a 45-degree angle.[26] Wiberg[25] and Knuttson[28] described a supine technique where the beam was perpendicular to the X-ray cassette. This eliminated the deficiencies of Settegast and Jaroschy's approaches, but by today's standard the knee was still too flexed (greater than 45 degrees). Indeed, the patella had to be higher than the patient's chest or head. Merchant et al[29] created a leg holder that allowed the knee to be flexed over the end of the table, and this allowed the knee to be flexed to a lesser degree.[29] This is the technique currently used. Although Merchant described a knee flexion angle of 45 degrees, the knee can commonly be flexed as little as 30 degrees (Figure 5–9). The limiting factor is the size of the patient's chest (the smaller the flexion angle, the closer the X-ray collimator is to the chest if the beam is to remain perpendicular to the cassette).

Laurin and colleagues[30] described a similar patient position but had the patient hold the cassette and had the beam come from the direction of the feet. This allows extension to about 20 degrees of flexion but perhaps exposes the patient to unnecessary radiation and relies on the patient's appropriate holding of the cassette. It requires a modicum of extra work for the technician to bring the X-ray machine to the foot of the patient.

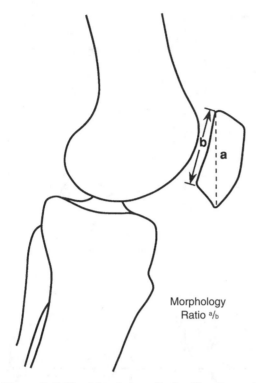

Morphology
Ratio ᵃ/ᵇ

Figure 5–7 The Morphology Ratio. The diagonal length of the patella (**a**) is divided by the length of the articular surface (**b**). A ratio of >1.5 indicated a long-nosed "Cyrano" patella, and a ratio <1.2 indicates a particularly short-nosed patella. *Source:* Reprinted with permission from RP Grelsamer et al, Evaluation of Patellar Shape in the Sagittal Plane—A Clinical Analysis, *American Journal of Sports Medicine*, Vol 22, pp 61–66, © 1994, American Orthopaedic Society for Sports Medicine.

Malghem and Maldague[31] have modified Laurin's technique by collimating the beam to obtain the smallest field size that still includes both patellae and by propping the cassette on the patient's thighs with the help of foam blocks. These authors have also described external rotation of the lower leg during imaging. This is obtained by "firm pulling of the forefoot laterally" while "manual pressure on the lateral side of the upper leg" is maintained to avoid concomitant external rotation of the thigh. Using this approach, they doubled their yield of abnormal images in patients with patella malalignment.[31]

The Sulcus Angle

The sulcus angle is the angle of the bony trochlea (the angle formed by the inner face of both condyles). The sulcus angle does not take into account the articular cartilage. With the knee flexed at 30 to 45 degrees, the normal sulcus angle has been found to be approximately 140 degrees.[32] This measure varies with the angle of knee flexion. When the knee is imaged relatively close to extension, the proximal, shallower portion of the trochlea is assessed; as the knee flexes, the more distal, steeper portion is evaluated. This brings up one of the limitations of standard axial imaging: it only assesses one portion of the trochlea. An area of abnormality can be missed if it is not in the portion of the patella being imaged. Most commonly this problem occurs with areas of dysplasia in the very proximal portion of the trochlea.

One group of investigators found an increased incidence of patellar pain in patients with a steeper trochlea.[33] Patellar instability has traditionally been associated with a more shallow trochlea.[30,33] In severe cases, the trochlea can be flat or even convex.

The Medial-Lateral Position

The treatment of medial-lateral patellar instability has long been debated. Patellar subluxation and dislocation have been shown to correlate with a lateralized resting position of the patella.[34] Merchant[29] in 1974 coined the term *congruence angle*, an objective imaging measurement he devised to demonstrate the medial-lateral position of the patella (Figure 5–10). This measurement was a major breakthrough, because it is independent of leg rotation. This angle uses the apex (posterior-most aspect) of the bony patella as a landmark. It is occasionally tedious to measure, as when double and triple shadows make the apex of the patella difficult to determine. Merchant noted that the average angle was –6 degrees (SD 11 degrees) when all patients except dislocators were assessed, and Aglietti et al[35] found it to be –8 degrees (SD 6 degrees)

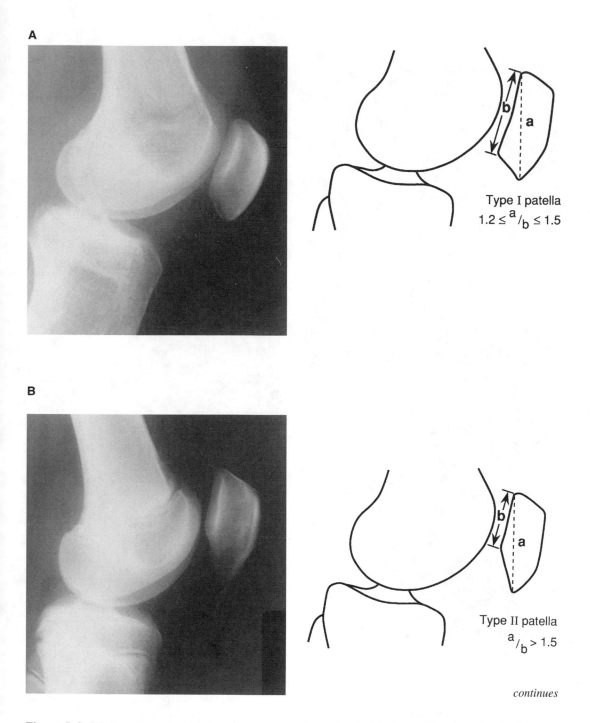

Type I patella
$1.2 \leq \,^a/_b \leq 1.5$

Type II patella
$^a/_b > 1.5$

continues

Figure 5–8 (**A**) Type I Patella; (**B**) Type II "Cyrano" (Long-Nosed) Patella; (**C**) Type III "Dolphin" (Short-Nosed) Patella. *Source:* Reprinted with permission from RP Grelsamer et al, Evaluation of Patellar Shape in the Sagittal Plane—A Clinical Analysis, *American Journal of Sports Medicine*, Vol 22, pp 61–66, © 1994, American Orthopaedic Society for Sports Medicine.

Figure 5–8 continued

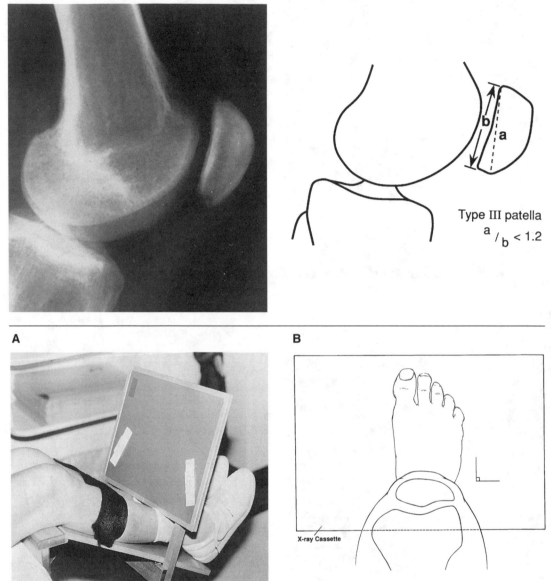

Type III patella
$$a\,/\,b < 1.2$$

Figure 5–9 Technique for Obtaining Merchant (Axial) View. (**A**) The knee should be flexed over the end of the imaging table, and the lower leg should rest on a device that controls the degree of knee flexion. The knee should be extended as much as possible (usually 30 degrees). For a very large person, 45 degrees may be the limit of extension. The position of the collimator is the limiting factor: the more extended the knee, the closer the collimator comes to the patient's chest. (**B**) The foot should be pointing toward the ceiling, and the lower border of the cassette should be parallel to the ground. If the patient exhibits external tibial torsion, the natural foot position can be maintained instead. *Source:* Reprinted with permission from RP Grelsamer, AN Bazos, and CS Proctor, Radiographic Analysis of Patellar Tilt, *Journal of Bone and Joint Surgery*, Vol 75B, pp B22–B24, British Editorial Society of Bone and Joint Surgery.

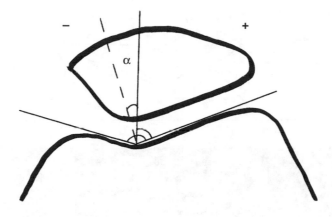

Figure 5–10 The Congruence Angle. This is a measure of the medial-lateral displacement of the patella. It is independent of leg rotation.

when only normal patients were assessed (ie, patients with absence of any knee pathology). Viewed differently, Aglietti's results suggest that the congruence angle should never be positive. The congruence angle does have the undisputedly significant advantage of being relatively independent of leg rotation.

When the practitioner knows that the patella has been imaged with the leg close to neutral rotation, he or she can assess the medial-lateral position of the patella without measuring any angle; the medial and lateral borders of the midpatella are usually level with a line drawn through the apex of the femoral condyles.[36–38] Displacement in any direction is readily noted.

Teitge et al[39] have noted that instrumented medial/lateral pressure applied to the patella can unmask abnormal mobility. Because the patients in Teitge's 1996 study already had a positive apprehension (Fairbank) sign on examination, it is not clear that instrumented displacement of the patella adds much to the average radiographic examination. However, such instrumentation can be useful in situations where objective documentation is necessary.

Patellar Tilt

Abnormal tilt in the axial plane can be detected a majority of the time using the plain Merchant view. Using this technique, Laurin et al[30] and Sasaki et al[40] described different measures of tilt. Both groups of investigators sought to do what Insall and Salvati did for patellar height[11] and Merchant[29] did for medial-lateral displacement: develop a measure of tilt that would be independent of leg position—in this case, leg rotation. Laurin's method uses the subchondral bone of the lateral facet to determine tilt, whereas Sasaki's uses a line connecting the medial and lateral borders of the patella. Both investigators used a line connecting the anterior condyles as a reference landmark. Patients with patella malalignment, however, are the ones most likely to have a form of trochlea/condylar dysplasia. Therefore it has been my position that the anterior condyles are not a reliable reference landmark in those very patients for whom tilt is sought.

As the reference landmark, I prefer to use any horizontal line drawn on the radiograph (Figure 5–11). For this to be an accurate and repeatable landmark, the radiograph must be taken with the foot vertical and the cassette maintained parallel to the ground. This is readily done with a commercially available cassette holder or with a simple leveler placed on top of the cassette (Figure 5–9). If the patient exhibits external tibial torsion, the natural rotation of the feet is maintained. We position the patient, X-ray beam, and cassette

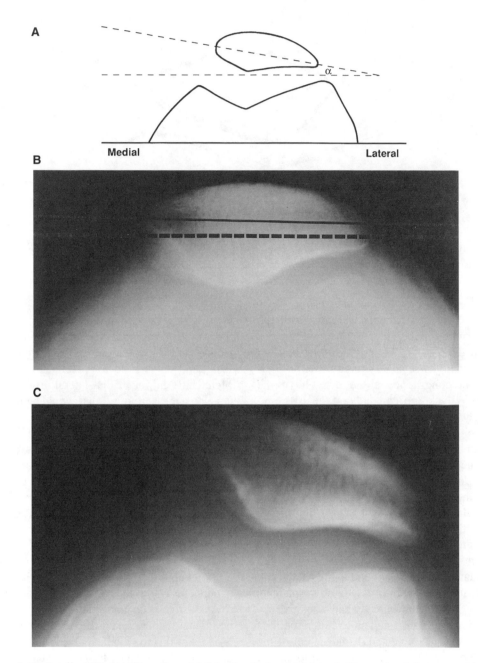

Figure 5–11 Patellar Tilt. (**A**) When the axial (Merchant) view is obtained, tilt can simply be assessed by drawing two lines (the first line comes across the patella from one border to the other; the second can be any horizontal line). The angle (α) subtended by these two lines is the *tilt angle*. This is the radiographic equivalent of the tilt assessed clinically. As the tilt increases clinically, so does the radiographic tilt. Tilt angles >5 degrees are abnormal, and angles >10 degrees correlate highly with clinically significant patella malalignment. (**B**) Normal patellar tilt. (**C**) Clearly abnormal patellar tilt. *Source:* Adapted with permission from RP Grelsamer, AN Bazos, and CS Proctor, Radiographic Analysis of Patellar Tilt, *Journal of Bone and Joint Surgery*, Vol 75B, pp 822–824, British Editorial Society of Bone and Joint Surgery.

as recommended by Merchant, except that we use a knee flexion angle of 30 degrees rather than 45 degrees whenever possible. This method of assessing tilt is less accurate when the radiograph has been taken in an unspecified manner (eg, when it has been taken at another facility). The disadvantages, however, are far outweighed by the advantages of this simple method.

If one considers the tilt angle to be formed by a line joining the corners of the patella and any horizontal line,[41] a tilt angle between 0 and 5 degrees is normal, an angle of 5 to 10 degrees is borderline, and an angle greater than 10 degrees is frankly abnormal (Figure 5–11). This method is so simple and straightforward that abnormal tilt can be readily detected even without the use of an instrument. In a study designed to assess this tilt angle, my colleagues and I found that abnormal tilt was detected in 85% of patients suffering from malalignment pain. The 15% of patients whose malalignment was not detected exhibited either abnormal tilt that became normal at 30 degrees of flexion or malalignment not related to tilt (ie, patella alta or lateral displacement). The false-positive rate was 8% and the accuracy 89%. Relatively few of the patients in this study had tilt with lateral displacement (only 25% had an abnormal congruence angle). It has become our impression that most patients with malalignment have tilt and pain rather than lateral displacement and symptomatic instability.[41]

Miscellaneous X-Ray Parameters

Other X-ray measurements described in the literature include the patella index of Cross and Waldrop,[42] Laurin's patellofemoral index, and Laurin's lateral patellar displacement[30] (Figure 5–12).

Cross and Waldrop[42] from the Hughston clinic describe a patellar index that assesses the relative length of the medial and lateral bony facets as seen on axial imaging. In their 1975 study, these authors found that dislocators have a relatively small medial bony facet.

The patellofemoral index is a ratio of the medial patellofemoral space divided by the lateral patellofemoral space. Normally it is less than or equal to 1.6. Laurin found that patients who were unstable have a ratio greater than 1.6.[30] This is simply an indication that the patella is tilted laterally (the medial space opens up), and the (easier) assessment of tilt supplants this patellofemoral index.

Laurin's lateral patellar displacement is a measure of the medial-lateral displacement of the patella. A line is drawn across the anterior border of the condyles. A perpendicular line is drawn through the center of the medial femoral condyle. If the medial border of the patella is "well away," this represents abnormal lateral positioning.[30]

TECHNETIUM SCANNING

An abnormal bone scan of the patella reflects increased bone turnover, and Dye and Boll[43] found increased incidence of abnormal scans in patients with patellar pathology.[43] These investigators found that improvement in the scans paralleled the clinical course for some patients. The pathophysiological connection between an abnormal scan and patellar pain has not been established other than to show a disturbance of homeostasis. At the present time, it remains an interesting radiological-clinical correlation, and I would not routinely recommend technetium scanning to diagnose patellar malalignment. However, a bone scan could potentially pick up nonmalalignment causes of anterior knee pain such as infections and tumors. It can also be used to detect reflex sympathetic dystrophy (RSD), although it is currently controversial to use it in this way. Not all tumors lead to a positive scan. Saglik et al[44] recently reported on a patient with a painful unicameral bone cyst whose technetium scan was negative. A positive scan can also be useful medico-legally if there is any suspicion of malingering.

COMPUTED TOMOGRAPHY AND MAGNETIC RESONANCE IMAGING

CT and MRI scanning have several advantages over plain radiography in that they have the ability to do the following:

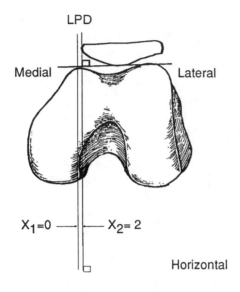

LPD

Medial   Lateral

$X_1=0$ ———|——— $X_2= 2$

Horizontal

Figure 5–12 Laurin Technique of Assessing Medial-Lateral Displacement. A line is drawn through the medial femoral condyle. The horizontal distance to the medial border of the patella is assessed. When applied to MRIs, this technique yields a negative value to a centered patella, which is counterintuitive.

- display axial images of the patella in the range of full extension to 60 degrees flexion (currently CT only)
- visualize the posterior condyles
- image soft tissues such as cartilage
- superimpose images

Their main disadvantages are inconvenience, cost (especially MRI), and radiation (CT).

In obtaining either of these two studies, the orthopaedist is looking for proof or suggestion of patellar malalignment, the presence or absence of cartilage lesions, and/or unrelated knee lesions.

Chondral Lesions

MRI scanning is uniquely capable of assessing the state of articular cartilage. However, a number of parameters affect the detection of articular cartilage lesions: the size of the lesion (breadth and depth), the experience of the radiologist, the strength of the magnetic field, the presence of specialized coils, the choice of imaging sequences, and the presence of a joint effusion.[45,46] As the equipment has continued to improve, so has the MRI's ability to detect smaller lesions. There has been a remarkable flurry of activity in this area throughout the past decade.[47–56]

To date, the most common way to assess the MRI's ability has been to compare the findings from MRI with arthroscopic findings in the same patient. The difficulty has lain in the different rating systems used by surgeons and radiologists. Vallotton et al have recently reported on a radiological rating and correlated it with Noyes' arthroscopic grading system.[46] In a study of 33 knees, they found a perfect correlation between MRI and arthroscopy in three quarters of the cases. In the remaining 25%, MRI tended to underestimate lesions, but this was not uniformly true: on two occasions MRI indicated a deeper lesion than what was appreciated at surgery.

Malalignment

More than a century ago, Roux[57] noted that, unless a patient has an unusual form of malalignment in which the patella subluxates or dislocates in flexion (eg, a short extensor mechanism), the patella usually becomes unstable as it nears extension. A lateralized patella may therefore not be detected by a Merchant view, because this technique requires the knee be flexed to at least 30 degrees. If the Merchant view does not demonstrate malalignment, but the surgeon still suspects lateral or medial deviation (and needs to prove or quantify it), CT or MRI scanning may provide the necessary information.

Measurements of patellar malalignment using CT or MRI should be done by taking mid-transverse cuts of the patella, in the manner described by Fulkerson et al.[58] With respect to leg rotation, the limb can be positioned with the feet pointing up or in the patient's normal walking alignment. Placing the patient in the CT gantry in the lateral decubitus position can facilitate imaging.[58]

Fulkerson et al[26,58] developed a classification scheme based on CT imaging whereby tilt and subluxation are clearly separated, defined, and measured. A patient with malalignment can have either tilt or subluxation (lateral displacement) or have tilt together with subluxation. They determined *tilt* using the angle formed by the slope of the lateral facet and a line drawn across the posterior condyles. Images were taken with the knee at 15 degrees of flexion. Normal tilt is considered to be greater than 7 degrees and is usually greater than 12 degrees. *Subluxation* is assessed as is the congruence angle on a Merchant view. In 10 asymptomatic volunteers, Fulkerson found that the patella is centered as soon as the knee is slightly flexed. The normal congruence angle at this position is 0 degrees. A positive congruence angle indicates lateral subluxation. This is different from the subluxation criteria established by Merchant[29] and then by Aglietti[35] on plain film. (For further discussion of the patellar position at 0 degrees, see the section on controversies later in this chapter).

Guzzanti et al[60] in Italy noted that contraction of the quadriceps during CT scanning could have a significant effect on the position and tilt of the patella. Specifically, lateral tilting of the patella was accentuated as was the lateral displacement (there is still some controversy with respect to the normal medial-lateral position of the patella on routine MRI scanning). Dejour and his team[61] carried out a similar study with respect to quadriceps contraction but also carried it out in normals. They noted that quadriceps contraction only had a significant effect on the patients with malalignment (severe malalignment in their study group consisted of patients with "instability" severe enough to warrant surgery). Dejour et al deemed 20 degrees to be a reasonable cutoff between normal and abnormal tilt, and they measured tilt in the manner that Fulkerson et al described. The degree of knee flexion was not specified.

Laurin's lateral patellar displacement[30] mentioned above is applicable to CT scanning (see Figure 5–12). Kujala[36,37] in Finland quantified this parameter on CT scans (near extension) and determined that normally the medial border of the patella overhangs the vertical line by 3 mm. Thus, the normal lateral patellar displacement index on CT or MRI is –3 mm, and a value of 0 actually corresponds to a laterally positioned patella. I am not fond of numbers that are counterintuitive and would rather see a lateral displacement of 0 as normal. My colleagues and I[38] have therefore further modified Laurin's technique to include a vertical line through the lateral femoral condyle in addition to that through the medial femoral condyle. In the normal patella, the overhang is equal on both sides. Lateral overhang is given a positive number and medial overhang a negative number. When the two are added and divided by two, this gives a measure of medial or lateral displacement (MLD). *Example 1*: When there is equal overhang on both sides, the two numbers cancel out (+2 mm + -2 mm = 0) and the MLD is indeed zero (Figure 5–13). *Example 2*: If this same patella is displaced laterally 2 mm, there will be 4 mm of lateral overhang and 0 mm of medial overhang (+4 mm + 0 mm/2 = 2 mm). *Example 3*: If on this same knee one notes +6 mm of displacement relative to the lateral line and +2 mm of displacement relative to the medial line, this reflects a displacement of +6 mm + +2 mm/2 = 4 mm. (*Note*: These measures of lateral displacement are for investigational use only. Clinically, one needs no measurement to determine that the patella is laterally displaced.)

Although the patella is known to be slightly displaced laterally in extension, my colleagues and I have found that the normal patella is centered on routine MRI scans (Figure 5–14).[38] This is most likely due to slight flexion of the knee (relaxed quadriceps, coil configuration, knee pain, and so forth). Thus, a lateralized patella on MRI scans should not be summarily dismissed as normal. (On the other hand, a lateralized patella is not automatically symptomatic and may

A   **Centered Patella**   B   **Patella Displaced 2 mm Laterally**

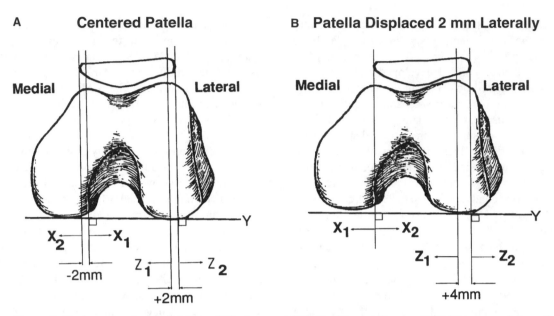

Figure 5–13 Assessing the Medial-Lateral Displacement (MLD) of the patella on an MRI. This is a variation of the Laurin-Kujala technique. A vertical line is drawn through the center of each condyle. Lateral overlap is assigned a positive value and medial overlap a negative value. The medial and lateral overlap are added and divided by two to give the MLD. (**A**) Using this technique, a centered patella will have an MLD of 0, which is an intuitive displacement number for a centered patella. (**B**) If the patella is displaced 2 mm laterally, there will now be 4 mm of lateral overhang and no overhang medially. The MLD will be (4 – 0)/2 = 2 mm, which is an intuitive number for a displacement of 2 mm. *Source:* Reprinted with permission from RP Grelsamer and PM Newton, Imaging of the Patello-Femoral Joint, *Sports Medicine and Arthroscopy Review*, Vol 2, pp 226–236, © 1994, Lippincott–Raven Publishers.

not be the immediate source of a patient's symptoms.)

In addition to detecting malalignment, the effective quadriceps (Q) angle can also be assessed using CT or MRI.[62] The major determinant of the Q angle is not the width of the pelvis or the amount of varus/valgus of the limb but the position of the tibial tuberosity relative to the midline. The center of the trochlea can serve as a reference for the midline. A CT or MRI cut through the trochlea can be superimposed on a cut through the tibial tuberosity, thereby assessing the lateral placement of the tibial tuberosity (trochlear groove-tibial tuberosity [TG-TT] distance (Figure 5–15). The normal TG-TT is approximately 15 mm in maximal knee extension and 9 mm in 30 degrees of flexion.[62] With this

TG-TT measurement, it can be difficult to pick the precise point at the center of the tibial tuberosity.

Computed Tomography/Magnetic Resonance Imaging—Controversies and Future Directions

The Medial-Lateral Position of the Patella on Routine Computerized Imaging

Tracking of the normal patella is recognized to be complex and can vary from patient to patient. The normal patella is, to a variable extent, slightly laterally positioned at extension and is centered in the trochlea in the early degrees of

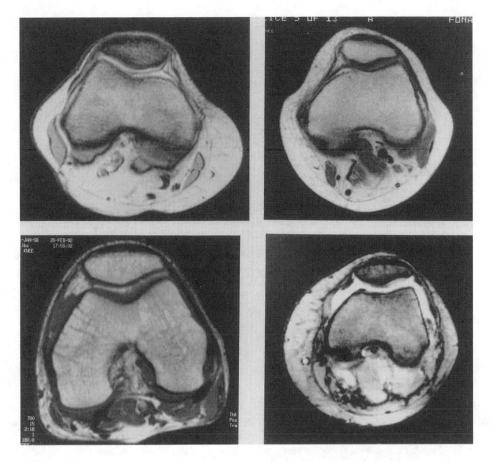

Figure 5–14 Normal Patella. The normal patella is centered over the underlying femur on routine MRI scans. This is most likely due to slight flexion of the knee.

flexion[63,64] (see Chapter 3). This has led some investigators to skip patellar evaluation in extension (0 degrees flexion) and to begin at 5 to 15 degrees of flexion.[20,26] Still not completely accepted is what the normal medial-lateral position of the patella is during routine computerized imaging when the knee is not specifically controlled for flexion. In a recent study involving 60 normal patients (without any demonstrable malalignment on physical or plain radiographic examination), my colleagues and I found that essentially every patient (59/60) exhibited a perfectly centered patella.[38] This was most likely due to (1) a strict definition of "normal" and (2) the slightly flexed position of most knees during

routine imaging. Accordingly, it is our opinion that a patella seen to be laterally positioned on a routine MRI should not be summarily dismissed as normal.

Chondromalacia

In theory, the MRI is ideally suited to detect alterations in cartilage consistency (ie, true chondromalacia). However, the average MRI that is currently available to the clinician cannot detect anything but the largest and deepest of articular cartilage lesions. This continues to be a major source of disappointment and surprise to some patients as they recover from their arthroscopies. Fortunately, the technology for

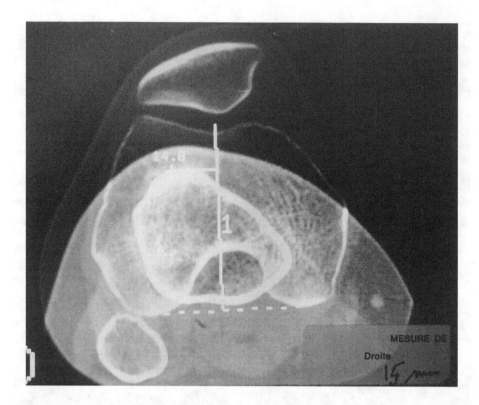

Figure 5–15 Trochlear Groove-Tibial Tuberosity (TG-TT) Distance. Superimposing a cut across the sulcus and another across the tibial tuberosity gives an objective measure of medial-lateral position of the tibial tuberosity. The normal TG-TT is approximately 15 mm in maximal knee extension and 9 mm in 30 degrees of flexion. In effect, the TG-TT is a radiographic way of assessing the effective Q angle (note the abnormal patellar tilt).

---

improved cartilage imaging has been developed, and one can only hope for its rapid dissemination.

Motion Studies

Both CT and MRI allow imaging within a limited range of motion, typically from hyperextension to approximately 30 degrees of flexion, depending on the size of the patient. Sequential cuts are obtained as the knee is brought through the range of motion. These can be displayed as simulated real-time images in a high-tech version of the "bumblebee in flight" card game.

Ultrafast Magnetic Resonance Imaging

Shellock et al[65] demonstrated that MRI scans can now be obtained with sufficient rapidity that a subject might be able to put his knee through a range of motion without having to stop every few degrees for imaging. This technique is indeed more physiological than the previously mentioned technique, although its practical benefits remain to be specifically determined. One problem with this approach is the fact that the patient is supine with the quadriceps relaxed. The availability of standing MRI units may change this.

AN ALGORITHM

The history and physical examination still remain the primary mode for making an accurate diagnosis of a patellofemoral joint disorder. It is my opinion that expensive imaging is overused and is really not required on most patients. Conversely, when ordering plain films, the practice of obtaining only anteroposterior and lateral views should be strongly discouraged when there is a possibility of patellar pathology. For all such cases, the axial view should be routine.

For the anteroposterior view, I recommend that the patient be standing. If the patella is far from the joint or laterally/medially positioned, it already suggests a patellar problem. For the lateral radiograph, the knee can be flexed to any degree. If the knee is scanned in extension, the quadriceps can be contracted to take out the slack. Severe trochlear dysplasia and patella alta or infera can readily be detected on this view. The Caton-Deschamps/de Carvalho/Blackburne ratios are extremely easy to apply and can rapidly suggest abnormal height. If there is any question about patella alta, the Modified Insall-Salvati ratio can also be used. Because of the way the cutoff number of 2 was chosen, this ratio is slightly less sensitive and slightly more specific than the Caton-Deschamps ratio. If the Modified Insall-Salvati ratio also indicates patella alta, chances are very good that the patella is truly high. If the patella is of the long-nosed Cyrano variety, the Caton-Deschamps and the Modified Insall-Salvati ratios tend to slightly overestimate patella alta.

For the axial view, I use a position and setup similar to that described by Merchant et al[29] ex-cept that the knee is flexed 30 degrees rather than 45 degrees. Some subluxation can be detected at 30 degrees that could be otherwise missed at 45 degrees. At 30 degrees, the X-ray tube is very close to the patient's chest, thereby precluding further straightening of the knee. Care must be taken to keep the foot pointing vertically and the cassette horizontal (parallel to the ground). At little cost and radiation to the patient, the surgeon can document tilt, lateral subluxation, and trochlear dysplasia with this view. If radiographs are taken by an unknown person in an unspecified way, and a relatively objective, reproducible measure of displacement is required (for example, for a publication), the congruence angle remains the method of choice. If the leg is close to neutral rotation and displacement is being determined for clinical purposes only, the position of the patella is simply assessed relative to the femoral condyles.

Most patients require no further imaging studies. However, if surgery is contemplated, an MRI or CT scan should be used when subluxation is suspected but not seen on the plain radiographs. This would indeed influence the choice of surgical procedures.[66] The presence and magnitude of an increased Q angle, as explained previously, can be substantiated easily using CT or MRI. If a nonarthroscopic surgical realignment is planned, an MRI may obviate the need for a concomitant arthroscopy.

REFERENCES

1. Fujikawa K, Seedholm BB, Wright V. Biomechanics of the patellofemoral joint. Part 1. *Eng Med.* 1983;12:3–11.

2. van Kampen A, Huiskes R. The three-dimensional tracking pattern of the human patella. *J Orthop Res.* 1992;8:372–382.

3. Reider B, Marshall JL, Ring B. Patellar tracking. *Clin Orthop Rel Res.* 1981;157:143–148.

4. Settegast A. Typische Roentgenbilder von normalen Menschen. *Lehmanns Med Atlanten.* 1921;5:211.

5. Noyes FR, Wojtys EM, Marshall MT. The early diagnosis and treatment of developmental patella infera syndrome. *Clin Orthop.* 1991;265:241–252.

6. Paulos LE, Rosenberg TD, Drawbert J, et al. Infrapatellar contracture syndrome, an unrecognized cause of knee stiffness with patella entrapment and patella infera. *Am J Sports Med.* 1981;15:331–341.

7. Blumensaat C. Die Lageabweichungen und Verrenkungen der Kniescheibe. *Ergeb Chir Orthop.* 1938; 31;149–223.

8. Brattström H. Patella alta in non-dislocating knee joints. *Acta Orthop Scand.* 1970;41:578–588.

9. Labelle H, Laurin CA. Radiological investigation of normal and abnormal patellae. *J Bone Joint Surg.* 1975;57B:530.

10. Norman O, Egund N, Ekelund L, Runow A. The vertical position of the normal patella. *Acta Orthop Scand.* 1983;54:908–913.

11. Insall JN, Salvati E. Patella position in the normal knee joint. *Radiology.* 1971;101:101–104.

12. Grelsamer RP. Patellar morphology in the sagittal plane. *Am J Sports Med.* 1989;17:725. Abstract.

13. Grelsamer RP, Proctor CS, Bazos AN. Patellar morphology in the sagittal plane. *Orthop Trans.* 1990; 14:617.

14. Grelsamer RP, Proctor CS, Bazos AN. Evaluation of patellar shape in the sagittal plane—a clinical analysis. *Am J Sports Med.* 1994;22:61–66.

15. Scuderi GR. The congenital patella nose. *Am J Knee Surg.* 1993;6:159–162.

16. Grelsamer RP, Meadows S. The Modified Insall-Salvati ratio for patellar height. *Clin Orthop.* 1992;282:170–176.

17. Blackburne JS, Peel TE. A new method of measuring patellar height. *J Bone Joint Surg.* 1977;59B:241–242.

18. de Carvalho A, Andersen AH, Topp S, Jurik AG. A method for assessing the height of the patella. *Int Orthop.* 1985;9:195.

19. Caton J, Deschamps G, Chambat P, Lerat JL, et al. Les rotules basses: a propos de 128 observations. *Rev Chir Orthop.* 1982;68:317–325.

20. Deutsch AL, Shellock FG, Mink JH. Imaging of the patellofemoral joint: emphasis on advanced techniques. In: Fox JM, DelPizzo W, eds. *The Patellofemoral Joint.* New York: McGraw-Hill; 1993:89.

21. Grelsamer RP, Tedder JL. The lateral trochlear sign: femoral trochlear dysplasia as seen on a lateral view roentgenograph. *Clin Orthop.* 1992;281:159–162.

22. Maldague B, Malghem J. Apport du cliché de profil du genou dans le dépistage des instabilités rotuliennes. Rapport préliminaire. *Rev Chir Orthop.* 1985;71(suppl II):5.

23. Malghem J, Maldague B. Depth insufficiency of the proximal trochlear groove on lateral radiographs of the knee: relation to patellar dislocation. *Radiology.* 1989;170:507–510.

24. Dejour H, Walsh G, Neyret PH, Adeleine P. La dysplasie de la trochlée fémorale. *Rev Chir Orthop.* 1990;76:45–54.

25. Wiberg G. Roentgenographic and anatomic studies on the femoro-patellar joint. *Acta Orthop Scand.* 1941; 12:319–410.

26. Fulkerson JP. Disorders of the Patellofemoral Joint. 3rd ed. Baltimore: Williams & Wilkins; 1996:83.

27. Jaroschy W. Die diagnostische verwertbarkeit der patellar vernahmen. *Fortschr Geb Roentgenstr.* 1924,31:781.

28. Knuttson F. Über die Roentgenology des Femoro-patellargelenkes sowie eine gute Projecktion für das Kniegelenk. *Acta Radiol.* 1941;22:371.

29. Merchant AC, Mercer RL, Jacobsen RH, Cool CR. Roentgenographic analysis of patellofemoral congruence. *J Bone Joint Surg.* 1974;56A:1391–1396.

30. Laurin CA, Dussault R, Levesque HP. The tangential X-ray investigation of the patellofemoral joint. *Clin Orthop.* 1979;144:16–26.

31. Malghem J, Maldague B. Patellofemoral joint: 30° axial radiograph with lateral rotation of the leg. *Radiology.* 1989;170:566–567.

32. Brattström H. The picture of the femoro-patellar joint in recurrent dislocation of the patella. *Acta Orthop Scand.* 1963;33:373–375.

33. Buard J, Benoit J, Lortat-Jacob A, Ramadier JO. Les trochlées fémorales creuses. *Rev Chir Orthop.* 1981; 67:721–729.

34. Shellock FG, Mink JH, Deutsch AL, Fox JM. Patellar tracking abnormalities: clinical experience with kinematic MR imaging in 130 patients. *Radiology.* 1989; 72:799–804.

35. Aglietti P, Insall JN, Cerulli G. Patellar pain and incongruence. *Clin Orthop.* 1983;122:217–224.

36. Kujala UM, Oesterman K, Kormano M, Nelimarkka O, et al. Patellofemoral relationships in recurrent patellar dislocations. *J Bone Joint Surg.* 1989;71B:788–792.

37. Koskinen SK, Kujala UM. Patellofemoral relationships and distal insertion of the vastus medialis muscle: a magnetic resonance imaging study in nonsymptomatic subjects and in patients with patellar dislocation. *Arthroscopy.* 1992;8:465–468.

38. Grelsamer RP, Newton PM, Staron R. The medial-lateral position of the patella in the extended knee. *J Arthros.* 1998;14:1–6.

39. Teitge RA, Faerber W, Des Madryl P, et al. Stress radiographs of the patellofemoral joint. *J Bone Joint Surg.* 1996;78A:193–203.

40. Sasaki T, Yagi T. Subluxation of the patella. Investigation by computerized tomography. *Int Orthop.* 1986; 10:115–120.

41. Grelsamer RP, Bazos AN, Proctor CS. A roentgenographic analysis of patellar tilt. *J Bone Joint Surg.* 1993;75B:822–824.

42. Cross MJ, Waldrop J. The patella index as a guide to the understanding and diagnosis of patellofemoral instability. *Clin Orthop.* 1975;110:174–176.

43. Dye SF, Boll DA. Radionuclide imaging of the patellofemoral joint in young adults with anterior knee pain. *Orthop Clin North Am.* 1986;17:249–262.

44. Saglik Y, Ucar DH, Yildiz HY, Dogan M. Unicameral bone cyst of the patella. *Int Orthop.* 1995;19:280–281.

45. Peterfy SG, Majumdar S, Lang P, et al. MR imaging of the arthritic knee: improved discrimination of cartilage, synovium, and effusion with pulsed saturation transfer and fat suppressed T1 weighted sequences. *Radiology.* 1994;191:413–419.

46. Vallotton JA, Meuli RA, Leyvraz PF, et al. Comparison between magnetic resonance imaging and arthroscopy in the diagnosis of patellar lesions. *Knee Surg Sports Traumatol Arthrosc.* 1995;3:157–162.

47. Fox JM, Del Pizzo W. *The Patellofemoral Joint.* New York: McGraw-Hill; 1993.

48. Handelberg F, Shahabpour M, Casteleyn PP. Chondral lesions of the patella evaluated with computed tomography, magnetic resonance imaging, and arthroscopy. *Arthroscopy.* 1990;6:24–29.

49. Hayes CW, Sawyer RW, Conway WF. Patellar cartilage lesions: in vitro detection and staging with MR imaging and pathologic correlation. *Radiology.* 1990;176:479–483.

50. Heron CW, Calvert PT. Three-dimensional gradient-echo images MR imaging of the knee: comparison with arthroscopy in 100 patients. *Radiology.* 1992;183:839–844.

51. McCauley R, Kier R, Lynch KJ, et al. Chondromalacia patellae: diagnosis with MR imaging. *Am J Radiol.* 1992;158:101–105.

52. Nakanishi K, Inoue M, Harada K, et al. Subluxation of the patella: evaluation of patellar articular with MR imaging. *Br J Radiol.* 1992;65:662–667.

53. Ochi PD, Yoshio S, Tsukasa K, et al. The diagnostic value and limitation of magnetic resonance imaging on chondral lesions in the knee joint. *Arthroscopy.* 1994;10:176–183.

54. Recht MP, Kramer J, Marcelis S, et al. Abnormalities of cartilage in the knee: analysis of available MR techniques. *Radiology.* 1993;187:473–478.

55. Speer KP, Spizer CE, Goldner JL, et al. Magnetic resonance imaging of traumatic knee articular injuries. *Am J Sports Med.* 1991;19:396–402.

56. Wojtys E, Wilson M, Buckwalter K, Braunstein E, et al. Magnetic imaging of knee hyaline cartilage and intra-articular pathology. *Am J Sports Med.* 1987;15:455–463.

57. Roux C. The classic: recurrent dislocation of the patella: operative treatment. *Clin Orthop.* 1979;144:4–8.

58. Fulkerson JP, Schutzer SF, Ramsby GR, Bernstein RA. Computerized tomography of the patellofemoral joint before and after lateral release or realignment. *Arthroscopy.* 1987;3:19–24.

59. Schutzer SF, Ramsby GR, Fulkerson JP. Computed tomographic classification of patellofemoral pain patients. *Orthop Clin North Am.* 1986;17:235–248.

60. Guzzanti V, Gigante A, Di Lazzaro A, et al. Patello-femoral malalignment in adolescents: computerized tomographic assessment with or without quadriceps contraction. *Am J Sports Med.* 1994;22:55–60.

61. Nove-Josserand L, Dejour D. Dysplasie du quadriceps et bascule rotulienne dans l'instabilité rotulienne objective. *Rev Chir Orthop.* 1995;81:497–504.

62. Goutallier D, Bernageau J, Lecudonnec B. The measurement of the tibial tuberosity-patella groove distance: technique and results. *Rev Chir Orthop.* 1978;64:423–428.

63. Delgado-Martins H. A study of the position of the patella using computerized tomography. *J Bone Joint Surg.* 1979;61B:443–444.

64. Despontin J, Thomas P. Réflexions sur l'étude de l'articulation fémoro-rotulienne par la méthode des tomographies axiales transverses computerisées. *Acta Orthop Belg.* 1978;44:857–870.

65. Shellock FG. Kinematic magnetic resonance imaging. In: Stoller DW, ed. *Magnetic Resonance Imaging in Orthopaedics and Sports Medicine.* Philadelphia: Lippincott; 1993:829–868.

66. Shea KP, Fulkerson JP. Preoperative computed tomography scanning and arthroscopy in predicting outcome after lateral retinacular release. *Arthroscopy.* 1992;8:327–334.

ADDITIONAL READINGS

Dye Sf, Chew MH: The use of scintigraphy to detect increased osseus metabolic activity about the knee. *J Bone Joint Surg.* 75A; 1993:1388–1406.

Mäenpää H, Lehto M. Patellar dislocation has predisposing factors: a roentgenographic study on lateral and tangential views in patients and healthy controls. *Knee Surg Sports Traumatol Arthrosc.* 1996; 4:212–216.

Picard F, Saragaglia D, Montabaron E, et al. Étude morphométrique de l'articulation fémoro-patellaire à partir de l'incidence radiologique de profil. *Rev Chir Orthop.* 1997;83:104–111.

CHAPTER 6

Patellar Instability

As noted in Chapter 1, the term *instability* has different meanings to different people. Here, the term means abnormal, symptomatic, medial-lateral displacement. Instabilities include subluxations and dislocations, both of which can be traumatic or atraumatic. (When the traumatic dislocation occurs in an otherwise normal knee, it is probably a stretch to refer to it as an instability.)

ATRAUMATIC INSTABILITY

Subluxation

As with the term *instability*, the term *subluxation* has different meanings to different people (see Chapter 1). Here the term *subluxation* is used to denote symptomatic, lateral, or medial displacement of the patella. Tilt alone is not considered a form of subluxation for the purposes of this discussion. Patients with subluxation feel a sense of giving way or abnormal motion. This usually occurs when the foot is planted and the upper body twists. In patients who have not undergone surgery, symptomatic subluxation almost always occurs laterally. Although there have been some reports of radiological medial displacement and one report of arthroscopically observed medial positioning of the patella with knee flexion,[1] subluxation as defined here is a *lateral* phenomenon. Moreover, subluxation occurs in the early degrees of flexion—either as the knee just starts to flex or as the knee comes

toward extension. Once the knee is flexed 30 degrees, the patella is engaged into the trochlea and lateral displacement becomes much more difficult and less likely. Patella alta makes subluxation more likely, because the patella lies above the trochlear groove through a greater arc of flexion.

Dislocation

There are three types of dislocation—fixed, habitual, and episodic (recurrent) dislocation.

Fixed Dislocation

In this situation, the patella has never been normally positioned at any degree of flexion. The trochlea is not developed, and the extensor mechanism is foreshortened (Figure 6–1). This is a congenital condition. It can be associated with a fixed flexion contracture of the knee as the extensor mechanism now acts as a flexor.[2]

Habitual Dislocation

In this rare disorder, the patella slips out laterally with each flexion of the knee. The extensor mechanism is abnormally tight, and the only way for the knee to flex is for the patella to slip out laterally. This condition can be due to a neuromuscular disorder (eg, cerebral palsy) or it can be secondary to scarring of the quadriceps. Such scarring can be due to trauma (eg, fracture of the femur) or to repeated injections into the thigh, especially in the neonatal period.[3] I have also

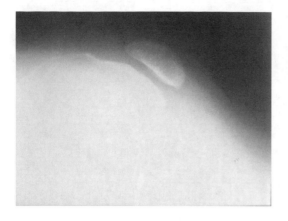

Figure 6–1 Fixed Dislocation. The patella has never been centered, and the trochlea is not developed.

seen such a scenario in a patient with nail-patella syndrome (hereditary onycho-osteodysplasia). Nail-patella syndrome[4] and the related "small patella syndrome"[5,6] are systemic conditions associated with multiple skeletal changes including iliac horns in the former syndrome and ball-and-socket ankle joints in the latter.

When patellar dislocation occurs in patients under the age of 10, one can expect to find any number of associated abnormalities (eg, Marfan's syndrome, dislocation of the hip, excessive valgus deformity, Turner's syndrome).[2]

In both habitual and fixed dislocation, surgery must address the tightness of the extensor mechanism.[7] This involves releasing the quadriceps from the hip joint on down. This procedure can require an incision centered over the patella going up the lateral side of the thigh and back toward the anterior aspect of the hip.

Episodic (Recurrent) Dislocation

Episodic dislocation occurs occasionally and unpredictably. It can be traumatic or atraumatic.

According to Brattström,[8] Meyer and Daunegger suggested in the late nineteenth century that the patella dislocates in extension. However, by the early years of the twentieth century, Wiemuth and Böhler recognized that the patella dislocates in the early degrees (10 to 20 degrees) of flexion. As noted by Brattström,

"The lateral-pulling powers are greater than the medial-pulling…and the patella has not yet completely run into the sulcus."[8] Although there has been some question as to whether the knee is flexing or extending at the time of the dislocation, it matters little.

Recreational dancing is, in my experience, a very common setting for an atraumatic dislocation. The foot is planted, the person twists the upper body and leg, and the knee is only slightly flexed so that the patella is not engaged in the trochlea. With the right anatomic predisposition, the patella slips out laterally. In a person who has never had surgery, it never dislocates medially.

TRAUMATIC DISRUPTIONS OF THE EXTENSOR MECHANISM

Acute disruptions of the extensor mechanism differ from other types of patellar pain insofar as the orthopaedist and patient are dealing with a single, sudden event. These acute disruptions are often related to underlying malalignment, and treatment can be controversial.

Acute Patellar Dislocation

In this situation, the patella has slipped off laterally to the point where the patella is lateral to the lateral femoral condyle, and there is no contact between the patella and the trochlea (Figure 6–2). Manual reduction is required. Dislocations can result from severe trauma or can be relatively atraumatic. In the latter case, the patient is very likely to have some form of patella malalignment with some anatomical abnormalities such as patella alta, increased ligamentous laxity, high quadriceps (Q) angle (see Chapter 3). For example, dancing is not an uncommon cause of dislocation. The foot is planted and the body twists. Simple pivoting during athletics involves similar mechanics (Figure 6–3). In one study, approximately three quarters of dislocations were associated with an athletic injury, while the remaining quarter occurred during activities of daily living (D Fithian, personal com-

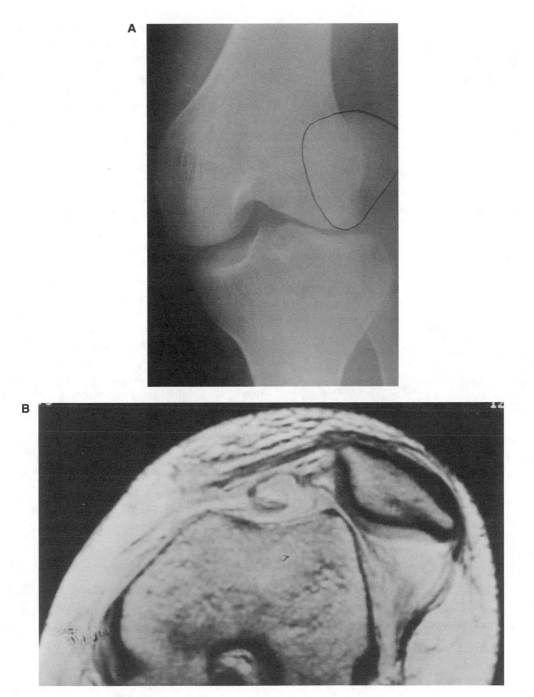

Figure 6–2 Acute Dislocation. (**A**) Anteroposterior radiograph of an acute dislocation. (**B**) Magnetic resonance imaging of a patellar dislocation. Note that the disruption of the medial structures took place at their origin rather than at their patellar insertion. Special studies should not be necessary to diagnose this condition, and sending a patient for a magnetic resonance imaging study prior to reducing the dislocation is cruel and unnecessary. Courtesy of Steven Shankman, MD, New York, New York.

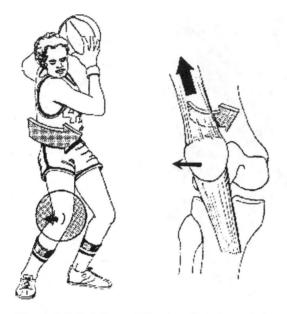

Figure 6–3 Twisting and Pivoting. Twisting and pivoting activities where the foot is planted and the body twists are common causes of relatively atraumatic dislocations. *Source:* Adapted with permission from JC Hughston, WM Walsh, and G Puddu, *Patellar Subluxation and Dislocation*, p 131, © 1984, WB Saunders.

with the articular surface facing away from the femur (Figure 6–4). This requires special maneuvers to reduce the patella and can even require a surgical procedure.

Having reduced the patella, the orthopaedist is now faced with a remarkable array of diagnostic and treatment options (and controversies): these include simple symptomatic treatment and rehabilitation (bracing, physical therapy), magnetic resonance imaging (MRI), arthroscopy, and surgical repair of torn structures with realignment of the patella.

In deciding which option(s) to choose, the surgeon has to consider both the short and long run. In the short run, the surgeon does not want to miss clinically significant acute pathology that might be missed on the physical exam or plain X-rays. The operative term here is *clinically significant*. An MRI study or arthroscopy nearly always reveals some kind of pathology. A loose chondral fragment or osteochondral fracture would be considered significant. On the other hand, calcification within the medial retinaculum is commonly seen in recurrent dislocators,

munication). In this study, slightly under 10% of patients with dislocation had a family history for this condition.

Patient Presentation

The patient has considerable knee pain and refuses to bend the knee. There is obvious swelling about the knee, and the patient is tender about the anterior aspect of the knee. The patella can usually be palpated off to the lateral side of the knee.

Workup and Treatment

The first task is to reduce the patella. Usually, the patella slides off in a straightforward manner with the articular surface facing the femur. In this case, slight hyperextension of the knee and gradual manipulation of the patella back onto the anterior surface of the femur is successful. On rare occasion, the patella flips 90–180 degrees along its long axis, and the patella comes to rest

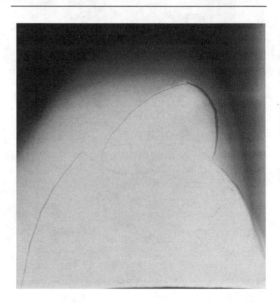

Figure 6–4 The Patella Flipped on Its Longitudinal Axis. The articular surface now points away from the underlying femur. This requires special maneuvers to reduce (reposition) the patella.

does not represent intra-articular pathology, cannot be addressed by an arthroscopy, and does not constitute clinically significant pathology. The odds of finding clinically significant pathology is what remains controversial. One can therefore take one of two approaches: (1) immediate MRI and/or arthroscopy or (2) symptomatic treatment with progression to MRI and/or arthroscopy if pain persists or new symptoms appear. The concept of an informed consumer comes into play. Some patients are particularly upset about having to undergo expensive and time-consuming testing and surgery; others may be more upset about having to undergo these tests after weeks of watchful waiting and time-consuming physical therapy. For some patients, early MRI studies can be a compromise, but these studies will not pick small chondral lesions.

In the long run, the surgeon is thinking about preventing a recurrence of the dislocation. The surgeon therefore needs to know (1) the odds of the patient's suffering further dislocations (ie, the natural history of patellar dislocation) and (2) the long-term effects of the planned procedure (ie, its effects on dislocation and on arthritis and pain). With regard to the first point (recurrent dislocation), patients can be divided into two groups: patients with a normal extensor mechanism and patients with some form of malalignment. In a recent study from Finland, two thirds of patients with recurrent dislocation were in the second group. This is exactly in accordance with the findings of Cash and Hughston.[9] In patients with one or more morphological abnormalities, one can expect a greater rate of recurrence than in patients with a normal extensor mechanism.[9] Therefore, if a patient appears to have had a normal extensor mechanism to begin with (the contralateral knee can be of help in assessing this), the surgeon need not embark on a discussion of the various realignment operations that can be performed (see Chapter 14).

The age of the patient at the time of the initial dislocation is a major factor. The older the patient, the less the chance he or she will experience recurring dislocation. Cash and Hughston[9] reported nearly a linear decrease in dislocation with age, to the point where no patient over the age of 28 at the time of the initial dislocation ever redislocated (the average follow-up was 8 years).

The sex of the patient does not seem to affect the outcome. A number of studies have reported that patella dislocation is a condition seen essentially in women,[10–13] but this is not necessarily the case. For example, in the study by Cash and Hughston, 70% of the patients were men.

Even without having undergone surgery or multiple dislocations, patients who have suffered a patellar dislocation are at risk for developing arthritic lesions. Mäenpää and Lehto reported that patients who only dislocated once had a higher rate of arthritis than patients with recurrent dislocation.[14,15] (*Note*: The two related articles by Mäenpää and Lehto[14,15] feature a wealth of densely presented information that is not adequately reflected by the abstracts. I strongly discourage practitioners from changing their practices without reading these articles in their entirety.) Presumably, it takes greater force to dislocate a normally aligned patella, which results in greater damage to the articular cartilage. This study is consistent with the work of Crosby and Insall,[16] who, based on the follow-up of 26 patients with recurrent dislocation, determined that recurrent dislocation in itself does not lead to arthritis.[16] Crosby and Insall,[16] Marcacci et al,[17] and Trillat et al[18] have noted that dislocations gradually decrease in frequency with time. Surgery usually stops dislocations altogether. In the very long run (30 years), patients with and without surgery function about the same (with surgery consisting of a medialization of the tibial tuberosity in all cases).[17] There is a school of thought (to which I subscribe) that persistent patellar instability can increase the risk of patellofemoral arthritis. This was the conclusion of at least one group who formally studied a cohort of patients suffering from patellofemoral arthritis.[19]

If the patient has some abnormality of the extensor mechanism, the surgeon should consider a procedure to prevent further dislocations. Here the surgeon must weigh the (significant) pain and inconvenience to the patient each time the patella dislocates against some of the long-term side effects of common realignment procedures. Indeed, some of the procedures have been reported to cause painful arthritic lesions years after the operation. The Hauser procedure falls into this category.[20] Even without performing the Hauser procedure, Mäenpää and Lehto[14,15] found a greater rate of arthritis in patients who had surgery versus those who did not. Even though there may have been a selection bias in the study (the patients who were operated on may have been worse off to begin with), the study does suggest that certain types of surgery do not prevent the onset of arthritis and can even hasten it.

Because there are so many procedures for patella realignment, it is hard to make sweeping condemnations of surgery for the dislocating patella. Rather, the surgeon and patient have to be aware of the track record of those of who have come before them and tread carefully into the world of surgical repair for the acute patellar dislocation. In addition to the procedures listed in Chapter 14, inspection of the origin of the vastus medialis obliquus (VMO) and of the medial patellofemoral ligament at the adductor tubercle may be warranted in patients with acute dislocation. Whereas some patients tear their VMO at the insertion on the patella, others can sustain an intrasubstance tear, and others avulse the VMO from the adductor tubercle (Figure 6–2B).

Results

Cash and Hughston[9] reviewed 100 patients (103 knees) who suffered from acute dislocation and were followed an average of 8 years (range 2 to 26 years). They noted that the older the patient at the time of the initial dislocation, the less the chance of redislocation. (This is similar to findings on the shoulder.) Patients did reasonably well with nonoperative treatment, provided that the contralateral knee demonstrated no malalignment.

Crosby and Insall[16] reviewed 81 patients who were treated surgically and 26 patient treated nonsurgically. They noted a "disturbingly high" rate of arthritis in patients who underwent a tibial tuberosity transfer, but no late arthritis in patients who underwent soft-tissue corrections only.

Marcacci et al[17] reviewed 16 patients with bilateral patellar dislocations who had been treated operatively on one side and nonoperatively on the other side. Surgery consisted of a "capsuloplasty by the Roux technique" with a reference to Roux's 1888 article in which he described medial transposition of the tibial tuberosity (see Chapter 14). Follow-up ranged from 20 to 45 years (average 30 years). All but one operated knee ceased to dislocate after surgery. The nonoperated knees continued to dislocate, but the frequency decreased over time. At the time of last follow-up, patients found that both knees functioned equally. They all had arthritic changes, and these did not correlate with their symptoms.

Recommendations

Patients who have sustained a patellar dislocation require the following:

1. *Examination of the other knee to assess underlying malalignment.* If malalignment is found on the contralateral knee, chances are that malalignment is present on the injured side.
2. *Plain radiographs including axial views at the lowest possible angle of knee flexion.* This will further help in assessing alignment, even though X-rays tend to underestimate malalignment (see Chapter 5). A fracture or loose body might be noted.
3. *Further investigation with MRI or arthroscopy.* This will further determine the presence of loose bodies, osteochondral fractures, and other possible damage. I would recommend MRI because it is noninvasive. Although arthroscopic evaluation may provide more information (eg, small articular cartilage lesions not detected on MRI), the added information

will not change the management of the patient. Loose bodies and fractures, which are the main concern, will be noted on the MRI. Equivocal findings can be investigated by arthroscopy.

Patients without underlying malalignment require no further surgical treatment once any acute pathology has been addressed. Patients with underlying malalignment should have the malalignment surgically addressed. Although the dislocations gradually decrease in frequency over time, each dislocation is very painful and requires a trip to the doctor or the emergency department. Reporting on long-term follow-up following surgery invariably involves just one surgical procedure applied to every patient. If a procedure is chosen in such a way as to address the patient's particular pathology—no more, no less—I do not see surgery as increasing that patient's risk of developing arthritis.

Patellar Tendon Rupture

Disruptions of the extensor mechanism move proximally as patients get older. Thus, patella tendon ruptures tend to occur in younger patients (in their teens and 20s). In some patients, the rupture is idiopathic to the extent that no particular cause can be found other than the jumping or deceleration the patient was engaged in at the time of the injury (eg, basketball). Blaming the activity itself is not particularly satisfying because the activity is usually no different from that practiced by other athletes. Yet only a very small minority of athletes rupture their patellar tendon.

A subgroup of patients appear to have a predisposition to this type of injury because their extensor mechanism is abnormal to begin with. Specifically, patella alta appears to be the abnormality most commonly encountered in patients with rupture of the patellar tendon. This obser-

vation is based on personal experience and warrants a formal study. These patients are also prone to having unusually shaped patellae, and the practitioner must assess patella height (alta) very carefully (see Chapter 5). Imaging of the other knee has to be used for this purpose.

Differentiating between the patient whose rupture is idiopathic and the patient with an underlying abnormality of the extensor mechanism is important when it comes to counseling the patient about the future. With the former patient, the rupture could have been caused by an exceptionally violent injury and can possibly be considered an isolated event. With the latter patient, I tell the patient that he or she is at risk for future problems with the extensor mechanism and I review the activities that put the patient at risk.

Treatment of patella tendon ruptures is surgical. On occasion, the tendon can be reapproximated, but often the tendon has been stretched and shredded much like an anterior cruciate ligament. The tendon must therefore be reconstructed. To this end, the semitendinosus and gracilis tendons can be woven through the inferior portion of the patella and through the tibial tuberosity in a figure-of-eight manner. If the tendon has been repaired, the semitendinosus and gracilis tendons can be used in similar fashion to reinforce the repair. Other reinforcement options include placing a cerclage wire around the patella and attaching it to a Steinman pin across the tibial tuberosity. This is applied with the patient's knee in extension. When the knee flexes, the wire shares some of the tension with the repaired or reconstructed tendon.

Patella Fractures and Rupture of the Quadriceps Tendon

These injuries are not usually associated with abnormalities of the extensor mechanism, and the reader is referred to texts on orthopaedic trauma for a discussion of their management.

REFERENCES

1. Dupont JY. Arthroscopic assessment of lateral to medial patellar maltracking: report of seven cases. *Knee.* 1995; 2:47–52.
2. Aichroth P. Patellar dislocation in children. *Knee.* 1996; 3:85–87. Abstract.
3. Bergman NR, Williams PF. Habitual dislocation of the patella in flexion. *J Bone Joint Surg.* 1988;70B:415.
4. Duthie RB, Hecht F. The inheritance and development of the nail-patella syndrome. *J Bone Joint Surg.* 1963; 45B:259–267.
5. Scott JE, Taor WS. The "small patella" syndrome. *J Bone Joint Surg.* 1979;61B:172–175.
6. Dellestable F, Pere P, Blum A, et al. The "small-patella" syndrome. *J Bone Joint Surg.* 1996;78B:63–65.
7. Gao GX, Lee EH, Bose K. Surgical management of congenital and habitual dislocation of the patella. *J Pediatr Orthop.* 1990;10:255–260.
8. Brattström H. Shape of the intercondylar groove normally and in recurrent dislocation of the patella. *Acta Orthop Scand.* 1964;(suppl)68.
9. Cash JD, Hughston JC. Treatment of acute patellar dislocation, *Am J Sports Med.* 1988;16:244.
10. Cofield RH, Bryan RS. Acute dislocation of the patella: results of conservative treatment. *J Trauma.* 1977; 17:526–531.
11. Fondren FB, Goldner JL, Bassett FH. Recurrent dislocation of the patella treated by the modified Roux-Goldthwait procedure. *J Bone Joint Surg.* 1985; 67A:993–1005.
12. Goldthwait JE. Slipping or recurrent dislocation of the patella: with the report of eleven cases. *Boston Med Surg J.* 1904;150:169–174.
13. Rorabeck CH, Bobechko WP. Acute dislocation of the patella with osteochondral fracture: a review of eighteen cases. *J Bone Joint Surg.* 1976;58A:237–240.
14. Mäenpää H, Lehto MUK. Patellar dislocation: the long-term results of nonoperative management in 100 patients. *Am J Sports Med.* 1997;25:213–217.
15. Mäenpää H, Lehto MUK. Patellofemoral osteoarthritis after patellar dislocation. *Clin Orthop.* 1997;339:156–162.
16. Crosby EB, Insall JN. Recurrent dislocation of the patella: relation of treatment to osteoarthritis. *J Bone Joint Surg.* 1976;58A:9.
17. Marcacci M, Zaffagnini S, Iacono F, et al. Results in the treatment of recurrent dislocation of the patella after 30 years' follow-up. *Knee Surg Sports Traumatol Arthrosc.* 1995;3:163–166.
18. Trillat A, Dejour H, Couette A. Diagnostic et traitement des subluxations récidivantes de la rotule. *Rev Chir Orthop.* 1964;50:813–824.
19. Iwano T, Kurosawa H, Tokuyama H, et al. Roentgenographic and clinical findings of patellofemoral osteoarthritis. *Clin Orthop.* 1990;252:190–197.
20. Hampson WGJ, Hill P. Late results of transfer of the tibial tubercle for recurrent dislocation of the patella. *J Bone Joint Surg.* 1975;57B:209–213.

ADDITIONAL READINGS

Arnbjörnsson A, Egund N, Rydling O, et al. The natural history of recurrent dislocation of the patella: long-term results of conservative and operative treatment. *J Bone Joint Surg.* 1992;74B:140–142.

Barbari S, Raugstad TS, Lichtenberg N. The Hauser operation for patellar dislocation: 3–32 year results in 63 knees. *Acta Orthop Scand.* 1990;61:32–35.

Garth WP, Pomphrey M, Merrill K. Functional treatment of patellar dislocation in an athletic population. *Am J Sports Med.* 1996;24:785.

Hawkins RS, Bell RH, Anisatte G. Acute patellar dislocation: the natural history. *Am J Sports Med.* 1986; 14:117–120.

Juliusson R, Markhede G. A modified Hauser procedure for recurrent dislocation of the patella. *Arch Orthop Trauma Surg.* 1990;103:42–46.

MacNab I. Recurrent dislocation of the patella. *J Bone Joint Surg.* 1952;34A:957–967.

CHAPTER 7

Nontraumatic Conditions Related to Malalignment

OSGOOD-SCHLATTER'S CONDITION

In 1903 Robert Osgood[1] and Carl Schlatter,[2] who were a continent apart (United States and Germany, respectively), described a condition that now bears their name—painful swelling of the tibial tuberosity in adolescents. The condition is not related to a specific traumatic event or unusually intense athletic activity, although teenagers with this condition are athletic. It is a condition traditionally associated with boys; however, some believe that girls are increasingly prone to this condition, presumably because of their increased participation in sports.[3] Bilaterality has been noted in 20% to 30% of cases,[4] and siblings of patients with Osgood-Schlatter's have a greater chance of having the condition than the general population. It is self-limited (ie, if left untreated, the pain resolves, although the bump remains). But it can take months or years to resolve, and few parents are willing to wait.

A number of investigators have noted the correlation between Osgood-Schlatter's and patella alta. I have also noted a high incidence of patella alta in patients with this condition, but a chicken-and-egg situation has arisen: does patella alta lead to Osgood-Schlatter's or vice versa?[5,6] It appears to me that the former is most likely. Patella alta diminishes the patella's complex lever action, which leads to a loss of mechanical advantage; this, in turn, leads to greater force requirements by the quadriceps muscles.

This increased force translates to increased tension within the patellar tendon and increased tension on the tibial tuberosity. Hughston et al[5] have also espoused this view.

A number of patients have either persistent or renewed pain into adulthood that is not necessarily only about the tibial tuberosity. Krause et al[7] noted a 60% incidence of symptoms into adulthood. It is my impression that patients whose condition is secondary to malalignment (eg, patella alta) are more likely to have symptoms into adulthood. A separate category of patients with persistent symptoms includes those who form a painful ossicle within the distal portion of the patellar tendon (Figure 7–1). These ossicles can be quite large, and a fracture through an ossicle has been reported.[8] Such patients require removal of the ossicle for pain relief.[4]

Fragmentation of the proximal portion of the patella has been reported in conjunction with Osgood-Schlatter's. When present, this condition is surprisingly asymptomatic.[9]

Classic treatment for Osgood-Schlatter's condition consists of application of cold packs to the area; anti-inflammatory medication[10]; application of a knee immobilizer; consideration of physical therapy for modalities; and a careful explanation of the condition to the patient, parents, coach, and/or counselor. Steroid injections are not indicated for this particular condition. (*Note*: Micheli[11] has specifically noted that anti-inflammatory medications do not work, and he has postulated that the failure is secondary to a

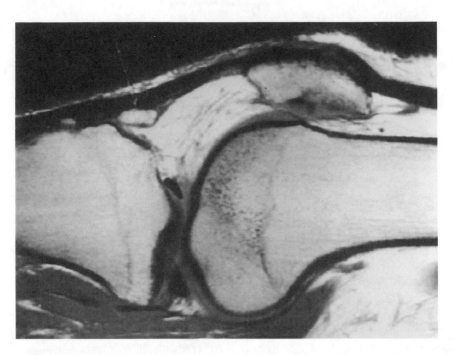

Figure 7–1 Osgood-Schlatter's Condition. An occasional ossicle is noted in the tendon near the tibial tuberosity, which is consistent with the concept of traction apophysitis. Courtesy of Douglas Hertford, MD, and Corinthian Diagnostic Radiology, New York, New York.

lack of inflammation. He has reported that a regimen of strengthening exercises within pain tolerance works best for him, and he occasionally immobilizes the leg for up to 4 weeks.

BIPARTITE PATELLA

Bipartite patella is a condition whereby radiographically the patella appears to consist of two parts. It was first described by Gruber[12] in 1883 and was further described as a potentially painful condition by Green[13] and Weaver[14] in the 1970s. Investigators believe that the etiology of bipartite patella is rooted in the embryological development of the patella. The patella develops as a cartilage mass in the ninth week of embryonic life, and it ossifies from a single ossification center between the age of 3 and 6 years (see Chapter 2). There can be secondary ossification centers, especially laterally. Failure of fusion of such an accessory ossification center to the main body of the patella is currently believed to be the

cause of the bipartite patella. Green noted a nine-to-one ratio of males to females.[13]

Saupe[15] in 1943 described three types of bipartite patella. In type I, the fragment is inferior and may not be a bipartite patella at all but rather a variation on the Sinding-Larsen-Johansson syndrome (see Chapter 8), as no secondary ossification center exists inferiorly.[3] In type II, the "bipartite" fragment consists of the entire lateral margin of the patella. In type III, the superolateral corner is involved. Most bipartite patellae fall into the type III category (Figure 7–2).

Ishikawa et al[16] have noted that axial views of the patella taken with the patient squatting can demonstrate separation of the fragment in certain cases.

Some investigators have advocated excision of the fragment.[13,16] Ogata[17] noted that type II fragments require internal fixation whereas type III fragments can heal if the tendinous attachment of the vastus lateralis to the fragment is lengthened. Rohlderer[18] noted spontaneous

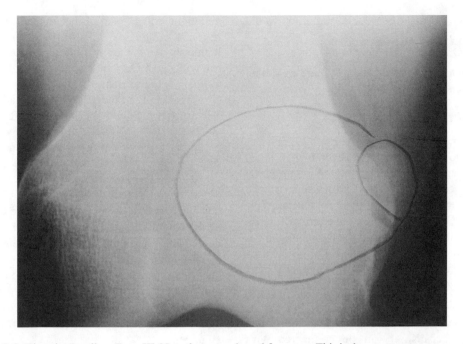

Figure 7–2 Bipartite Patella—Type III. Note the superolateral fragment. This is the most common type of bipartite patella.

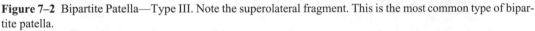

fusion of a bipartite patella after a release of the lateral retinaculum. Mori[19] performed a lateral release and excised a strip of retinaculum. The rationale for the lateral release or the lengthening of the vastus lateralis tendon is based on the premise that the superolateral secondary ossification center has not healed to the main body of the patella because of excessive pull of the vastus lateralis. If that pull is eliminated or sufficiently diminished, perhaps the small fragment can unite with the larger one. This appears to be true in a number of cases. The "pull of the vastus lateralis" may simply be a tight lateral retinaculum. I suspect that, if it was specifically sought upon examination, abnormal patellar tilt would be found in a number of these cases.

THE DORSAL DEFECT

The dorsal defect presents radiographically as a hole in the bone. The differential diagnosis includes a Brodie's abscess and a neoplastic con-

dition. The dorsal defect is located at the superolateral portion of the patella, and the histology consists of fibrous tissue. The combination of these two factors makes the dorsal defect less likely to be a tumor and more likely to represent a failure of ossification—a condition more related to the bipartite patella.

Patients need not be symptomatic, and spontaneous resolution of dorsal defects has been documented[20-22] (another strike against the neoplastic hypothesis). At the other extreme, some lesions involve the articular surface,[20,22,23] and others recur.[24]

In symptomatic patients, a technetium bone scan is usually positive,[3,20,25,26] but not always.[24] When nonoperative treatment fails, treatment consists of curettage and grafting.

PATELLAR DUPLICATION

The following three forms of duplication have been reported.[27-30]

1. One patella lies proximal to the other.

2. One patella lies dorsal (anterior) to the other.

3. One patella lies next to the other.

As pointed out by Fulkerson,[27] there may be a phylogenetic component.

PATELLAR TENDINITIS

True patellar tendinitis (jumper's knee) is not related to malalignment. However, in my experience, there are times when pain at the tip of the patella can be a referred pain secondary to malalignment that can only improve with a regimen that takes into account the entire picture including this malalignment. Such malalignment can include patella alta or simple tilt. See Chapter 8 for further discussion of true jumper's knee.

PATELLAR TENDON RUPTURE

Patellar tendon rupture is mentioned in this chapter because it can be connected with malalignment. By definition, a patellar tendon ruptures only if the tensile (pulling) stresses within the tendon are greater than the stresses it can withstand. Only two general conditions lead to this: (1) the presence of excessive stresses or (2) a weakening of the tendon. What leads to excessive stress? Playing basketball puts considerable stress on the patellar tendon, but very few basketball players rupture their tendon. Excessive weight for size could certainly place excessive stress. The second condition—weakening of the tendon—occurs if the tendon is diseased; this is the case in patellar tendinitis (see Chapter 8). Patella alta is also a cause of weakening of the tendon. The high patella places the extensor mechanism at a mechanical disadvantage. The quadriceps has to work harder (ie, contract with more force), with resultant increased tensile stresses within the patellar tendon. Kelly et al[31] have reported such a correlation in a review of 10 patients.

REFERENCES

1. Osgood RB. Lesions of the tibial tubercle occurring during adolescence. *Boston Med J.* 1903;148:114.

2. Schlatter C. Verletzungen des schnabelformigen fortsatzes der oberen tibiaepiphyse. *Beitr Klin Chir.* 1903;38:874.

3. Stefko JM, Fu F. Patellar problems in the young patient. In: Scuderi GR, ed. *The Patella.* New York: Springer-Verlag. 1995:169–200.

4. Mital MA, Matza RA, Cohen J. The so-called unresolved Osgood-Schlatter's lesion. *J Bone Joint Surg.* 1980;62A:732.

5. Hughston J, Walsh WM, Puddu G. *Patellar Subluxation and Dislocation.* Philadelphia: WB Saunders; 1984: 8. Saunders Monographs in Clinical Orthopaedics. Vol 5.

6. Jakob RP, Gumppenberg S, Engelhardt P. Does Osgood-Schlatter disease influence the position of the patella? *J Bone Joint Surg.* 1981;63B:579.

7. Krause L, Williams JPR, Catterall A. Natural history of Osgood-Schlatter disease. *J Pediatr Orthop.* 1990; 10:65.

8. Konsens RM, Seitz WH. Bilateral fractures through "giant" patellar tendon ossicles: a late sequela of Osgood-Schlatter disease. *Orthop Rev.* 1988;17:797–800.

9. Batten J, Menelaus MB. Fragmentation of the proximal pole of the patella. *J Bone Joint Surg.* 1985;67B:249–251.

10. Buckwalter JA. Pharmacological treatment of soft-tissue injuries: current concepts. *J Bone Joint Surg.* 1995;77A:1902–1914.

11. Micheli LJ. Patellofemoral disorders in children. In: Fox JM, Del Pizzo W, eds. *The Patellofemoral Joint.* New York: McGraw-Hill; 1993:105–121.

12. Gruber W. In bildungsanomalie mit bildungshemmung begrundete bipartition beider patellae eines jungen subjektes. *Wirchows Arch Pathol Anag.* 1883;94:358.

13. Green WT. Painful bipartite patella: a report of three cases. *Clin Orthop.* 1975;110:197.

14. Weaver JK. Bipartite patella as a cause of disability in the athlete. *Am J Sports Med.* 1977;5:137.

15. Saupe H. Primaire knochenmark seilerung die kneischeibe. *Dtsch Z Chir.* 1943;258:386.

16. Ishikawa H, Sakurai A, Hirata S, et al. Painful bipartite patella in young athletes. *Clin Orthop.* 1994;305:223–228.

17. Ogata K. Painful bipartite patella. *J Bone Joint Surg.* 1994;76A:573–578.

18. Rohlderer K. L'arthrose de la surface articulaire de la rotule. *Rev Chir Orthop.* 1964;50:361–368.

19. Mori Y, Okumo H, Iketani H, et al. Efficacy of lateral retinacular release for painful bipartite patella. *Am J Sports Med.* 1995;23:13–18.

20. Denham RH. Dorsal defect of the patella. *J Bone Joint Surg.* 1984;66A:116.

21. Haswell DM, Berne AS, Graham CB. The dorsal defect of the patella. *Pediatr Radiol.* 1976;4:238.

22. Sueyoshi Y, Shimozaki E, Matsumoto T, et al. Two cases of dorsal defect of the patella with arthroscopically visible cartilage surface perforations. *Arthroscopy.* 1993;9:164.

23. Hunter LY, Hensinger RN. Dorsal defect of the patella with cartilaginous involvement: a case report. *Clin Orthop.* 1979;143:131.

24. Merchan ECR, Olarte A, Lopez-Barea F, et al. Recurrent dorsal defect of the patella: case report. *Contemp Orthop.* 1995;30:237–241.

25. Gamble JG. Symptomatic dorsal defect of the patella in a runner. *Am J Sports Med.* 1986;14:425.

26. Goergen TG, Resnick D, Greenway G, et al. Dorsal defect of the patella (DDP): a characteristic radiographic lesion. *Radiology.* 1979;130:333.

27. Fulkerson JP. *Disorders of the Patellofemoral Joint.* 3rd ed. Baltimore: Williams & Wilkins; 1997:130–131.

28. Vallois H. Etude anatomique de l'articulation du genou chez les primates. Montpellier, France; 1914. Thesis.

29. Vallois H. La valeur morphologique de la rotule chez les mammifères. *Bull Mem Soc Anthrop.* 1917.

30. Haenisch F. Verdoppelung der patella in sagitaller richtung. *Fortschr Roentgenst.* 1925;33:678.

31. Kelly DW, Carter VS, Jobe FW, Kerlan RK. Patellar and quadriceps tendon ruptures—jumper's knee. *Am J Sports Med.* 1984;12:375–380.

CHAPTER 8

Patellar Pain Not Related to Malalignment: Differential Diagnosis

Although patella malalignment is commonly missed (ie, mistaken for a torn meniscus, a plica, etc), the converse is also true: patients are labeled as having "chondromalacia" (or a modern equivalent) when, in fact they have a well-defined problem unrelated to patella malalignment. Unfortunately, all of the conditions discussed below can coexist with patellar malalignment, and sorting out the source(s) of pain can be difficult. By and large, most of these conditions can be diagnosed with a careful physical exam and/or plain radiographs. Although several of these diagnoses are fairly straightforward, they can be easily missed if the practitioner does not think to look for them.

NEUROMA

A patient who has sustained blunt trauma to the knee (eg, a dashboard knee, a fall onto the knee) is a candidate for developing one or more neuromas.[1] A neuroma is a traumatic, painful irritation of a subcutaneous nerve. Patients with any kind of prior surgery including an arthroscopy can also suffer from neuromas. Telltale signs include skin that is locally sensitive to simple palpation and gentle squeezing (see Chapter 4). There is often a Tinel sign.

The nerve most commonly involved with a neuroma is the infrapatellar branch of the saphenous nerve. Its course is variable as it comes around the front of the knee from the medial side. Mochida and Kikuchi[2] noted that when

practitioners perform an arthroscopy, there is only a 10-mm perfectly safe zone medial to the patellar tendon at the level of the distal pole of the patella. Intra-articular pathology sometimes dictates portals outside this zone.

The diagnosis can be confirmed by a subcutaneous injection of lidocaine. Treatment includes a corticosteroid injection or surgery.

ILIOTIBIAL TENDINITIS

The iliotibial band (ITB) or iliotibial tract is a complex structure (see Chapter 2) that spans the hip and the knee joint. As with the hamstrings and quadriceps, it is susceptible to tightness, which can be tested via the Ober test (see Chapter 4).

In activities involving repeated, unrelenting flexion and extension of the knee, the ITB can rub along the lateral epicondyle. The patient presents with pain about the knee that can include pain in the anterior portion of the knee.

On physical examination, there is localized tenderness over the ITB as it crosses the lateral femoral condyle.

Treatment consists of nonsteroidal anti-inflammatory medication[3]; stretching as needed; modalities (eg, ultrasound); injection; and, quite rarely, surgery. The ITB is an important structure both as a static and dynamic stabilizer of the knee, so during surgery one does not simply divide it. A transverse cut can be made through a portion of the ITB, a cruciate incision can be made through the ITB at the level of the lateral epicondyle, or a Z-plasty (a Z-shaped incision) can be carried out. The latter is more complex than it would appear at first glance, because the ITB is attached anteriorly to the patella and posteriorly to the femur. It is not a free-standing tendon or ligament. Incising the ITB at the level of the greater trochanter can be considered, especially if there are also symptoms about the hip.

PLICA SYNDROME

A widened, thickened, inflamed plica can cause pain about the anterior knee.[4,5] Of the many possible plicae about the knee (see Chapter 2), it is the medial patellar plica that is associated with plica syndrome. Classically plica syndrome presents with anteromedial knee pain and a snapping sensation as the inflamed, thickened plica snaps over the medial femoral condyle. To diagnose this condition, a palpable cord should be palpated medial to the patella as the knee flexes and extends. It is possible to mistake the plica syndrome for a torn meniscus or patella subluxation (popular diagnoses of the 1970s and early 1980s).[6–11] Conversely, it is possible to diagnose a plica syndrome when, in fact, the patient suffers from patellar subluxation. This is easy to do when the diagnosis of patella malalignment is not appreciated during the physical exam and a medial plica is noted at the time of arthroscopy.

The medial plica has a static, medializing effect on the patella, and the excision of a medial plica can have an effect on patellar tracking. There has been at least one report of new patellar subluxation following medial plica excision.[12]

PATELLAR TENDINITIS (JUMPER'S KNEE)

Patellar tendinitis causes pain at the anterior knee, and it is therefore frequently construed as "patellar pain." Investigators believe that this condition is secondary to overuse in athletes who frequently participate in sports involving jumping, cutting, or rapid acceleration/deceleration. Richards et al[13] have specifically studied

high-performance volleyball players and have correlated patellar tendinitis with deep-knee flexion angles and substantial tibial external torsional moments. Tall patients may be at increased risk.[14] Duri and Aichroth[14] noted that 5 of the 21 patients in their series had experienced Osgood-Schlatter's disease. The pathology is often at the osteotendinous junction, where visible changes are not always present. However, even in these cases, Ferretti and colleagues noted "pseudocystic cavities with myxomatous and hyaline metaplasia at the border between mineralized fibrocartilage and bone."[15(p58)] Puddu et al[16] have described three categories of tendinitis:

1. The peritenon is inflamed and infiltrated with plasma cells. The tendon belly itself is intact.
2. The peritenon is intact but the tendon itself is pathological: it is wider, thicker, more yellow than normal and is adherent to the paratenon. There can be cavities and calcified areas.
3. A combination of 1 and 2.

The presenting complaint is pain. In the milder stages, it is relieved by warm-up exercises prior to sports and rest following sports; however, in the more severe stages, it is present with most types of activity and even at rest. On exam, the patient has point tenderness over the inferior pole of the patella. This finding differentiates patellar tendinitis from the so-called Hoffa syndrome, where it is the fat pad that is inflamed and tender. The differentiation between the two conditions is not always clear, because the fat pad has been implicated in some of the more generalized symptoms associated with patellar tendinitis (eg, crepitus).[14,17]

On rare occasion, patellar tendinitis can be a reflection of underlying knee pathology.[18] The pathology can sometimes be seen on magnetic resonance imaging (MRI)[19] (Figure 8–1), computed tomography (CT), and ultrasound.[14,20,21] Ultrasound is recommended as the first line of testing (when available) because of its ease and relatively low cost.[21,22]

Nonoperative treatment can include rest and anti-inflammatory medications. Exercise regi-

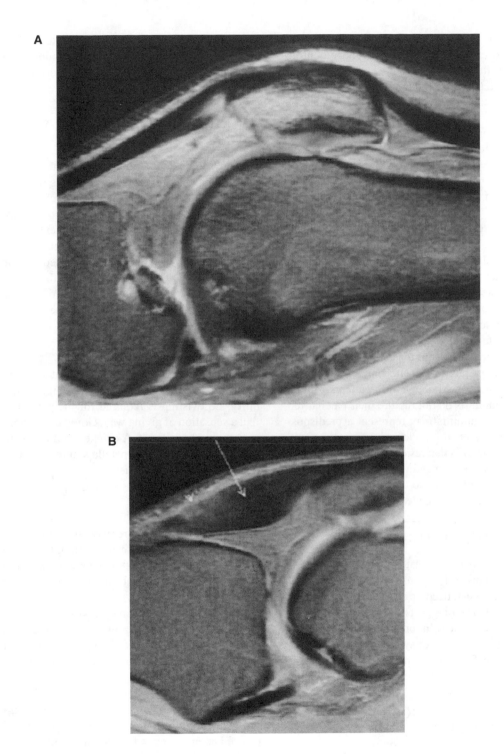

Figure 8–1 Patellar Tendinitis. (**A**) A signal change is noted within the proximal portion of the tendon. (**B**) Abnormal thickening of the patellar tendon. Courtesy of Douglas Hertford, MD, and Corinthian Diagnostic Radiology, New York, New York.

mens are controversial. Some have recommended exercises involving eccentric contractions of the quadriceps as a way to take tension off the tendon,[23] although overly vigorous, eccentric exercises (eg, jumping) can cause the condition in the first place.[22] Despite the risk of tendon rupture,[24,25] the administration of a steroid injection in select cases has been described.[14,26]

When nonoperative management fails, surgery can be successful. The tendon can be "combed" in the direction of its fibers as with the Achilles tendon ("peignage"), the tip of the patella can be curetted or drilled,[26] a portion of patellar tendon can be excised,[27] or the central third of the tendon can be excised proximally along with a piece of bone. Benazzo[26] reported a success rate of about 80% in a relatively large series of 46 cases. The more severe the degeneration, the less favorable the results.

The most worrisome aspect of patellar tendinitis is its possible connection with a patellar tendon rupture. Although most patients with patellar tendinitis do not rupture their patellar tendon, the tendinitis may represent a predisposition. Kelly et al[28] reviewed 10 patients with severe tendinitis that resulted in a patellar tendon rupture. Rosenberg and Whitaker[29] reported on a similar case. Systemic disease (obvious or latent) may create an added risk for rupture.[30,31]

FAT PAD SYNDROME

The fat pad is intimately associated with the patellar tendon, lying just behind and on either side of it. It can become enlarged, inflamed, and tender.[14,32] The diagnosis can be made by injecting an anesthetic solution directly into it and observing a resolution of symptoms. On rare occasions, the fat pad can become ossified, but it need not be ossified to be a source of pain.

SINDING-LARSEN-JOHANSSON SYNDROME

This condition is similar in presentation to patellar tendinitis and is seen in adolescents.[33,34] On lateral radiographs, calcification is noted within the proximal portion of the patellar tendon. This gives an elongated appearance to the distal pole of the patella.

ANTERIOR CRUCIATE LIGAMENT TEAR

Both patella subluxation and an anterior cruciate ligament tear can give symptoms of instability. In both cases, the instability can occur with planting of the foot and twisting of the upper body. The anterior cruciate ligament tear is likely to be noted on MRI scans, while the patella subluxation can easily be missed on the same study (see Chapter 5). Although the patella subluxation is more likely to be missed than the ligament tear, this is not uniformly true.

QUADRICEPS ATROPHY

Quadriceps atrophy gives the patient a feeling of instability, but this is usually a straight instability: no twisting is required for the patient to feel a sensation of giving way. Going down steps is particularly difficult. A chicken-and-egg situation can develop when patella subluxation and quadriceps atrophy coexist.

TUMORS

Patellar tumors are extremely rare, and the clinician can be forgiven for not putting this diagnosis at the top of any list. But patients with patellar tumors can indeed present with anterior knee pain.

The patient may feel pain and swelling, but these symptoms are common to knee conditions (see Chapter 4). The presenting sign can be a pathological fracture from 10% to 20% of the time.[35–37]

Tumors that have been reported include metastases, giant cell tumors that are usually aggressive[36,38] (Figure 8–2), chondroblastoma,[35,36] osteoblastoma, osteoid osteoma,[36] solitary osteochondroma, chondroma, ganglion,[36] simple bone cyst,[39] aneurysmal bone cyst (ABC),[36]

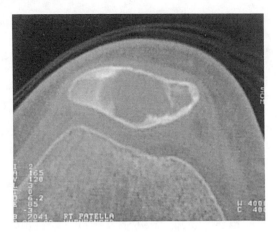

Figure 8–2 Giant Cell Tumor. *Source:* Reprinted with permission from PC Ferguson, AM Griffin, and RS Bell, Primary Patellar Tumors, *Clinical Orthopaedics and Related Research*, Vol 336, p 201, © 1997, Lippincott–Raven Publishers.

brown tumor, lymphoma, hemangioma,[40] hemangioendothelioma,[36] unicameral bone cyst, osteosarcoma (Figure 8–3), and plasmacytoma.[36] Treatment varies from curettage to amputation, depending on the nature and stage of the lesion.

Soft tissue tumors can also occur about the extensor mechanism (eg, hemangiomas).

RHEUMATOLOGICAL CONDITIONS

Inflammatory arthritis can initially present with anterior knee pain. In fact, inflammatory arthritis can initially present with radiographically and arthroscopically confirmed unicompartmental arthritis of the patellofemoral joint.

OSTEOCHONDRITIS DISSECANS

Sir James Paget discovered this condition, which he termed "quiet necrosis," in 1870.[41,42] Osteochondritis dissecans is a relatively uncommon condition; it is defined as partial or total separation of an intra-articular bone fragment with overlying articular cartilage in the absence

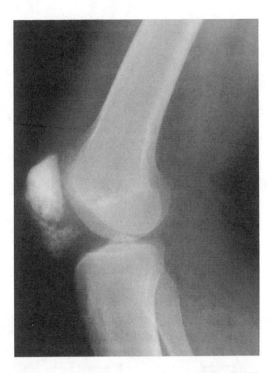

Figure 8–3 Osteosarcoma. *Source:* Reprinted with permission from PC Ferguson, AM Griffin, and RS Bell, Primary Patellar Tumors, *Clinical Orthopaedics and Related Research*, Vol 336, p 202, © 1997, Lippincott–Raven Publishers.

of acute trauma. It is associated with seemingly spontaneous bone necrosis. The knee is the most common site for this uncommon condition, but the patella itself is an infrequent site for it (Figure 8–4).

Etiology

König[43] believed that the necrosis associated with osteochondritis dissecans is secondary to trauma (perhaps repetitive) and that a subsequent inflammatory response leads to a separation of the fragment. In 1887 he coined the term *osteochondritis dissecans*. The tibial spine has been implicated as a source of "trauma," especially for the most common lesions (those of the lateral aspect of the medial femoral condyle). Fairbank introduced this theory in 1933, when

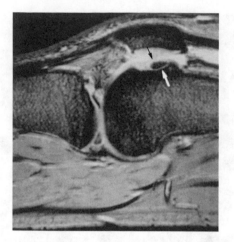

Figure 8–4 Osteochondritis Dissecans. The patello-femoral joint is a rare site for this condition, and the prognosis is more guarded than for lesions of the medial femoral condyle. *Source:* Reprinted with permission from JS Parisien, *Current Techniques in Arthroscopy*, 2nd ed, © 1996, Current Medicine/Churchill Livingstone.

he postulated that with internal rotation of the tibia a tibial spine could impinge on the medial condyle. Abnormal ossification, endocrine factors, and genetic factors have also been invoked.

Naturally, the "tibial spine–impingement" theory does not explain the occurrence of osteochondritis dissecans in other parts of the knee such as the patella. Hellstrom[44] in 1923 suggested that impaction of the medial aspect of the patella against the medial femoral condyle could be a cause of patellar osteochondritis dissecans.

Presentation

The history and exam for the diagnosis of osteochondritis dissecans are nonspecific. The onset of pain can be gradual or sudden. Pain, swelling, crepitus, effusion, and quadriceps atrophy are all present to a certain degree. Catching or locking can occur if the lesion is partially detached. If the fragment is completely detached, the symptoms are identical to those of any loose body.

In the advanced stages, the osteochondritis dissecans lesion is seen on plain X-rays, but in the earlier stages MRI can better detect lesions. MRI is also the best imaging modality when trying to assess the integrity of the fragment, a major factor in the decision about treatment.

Osteochondritis dissecans usually occurs in the distal half of the patella.[45–47] Schwarz[46] found fully two thirds of lesions in the distal half. This area corresponds to the portion of the patella that articulates with the trochlea in the first 45 degrees of flexion. Because most activities of daily living involve flexion in this range, the implications of this finding are not clear. Osteochondritis dissecans can also be present in the trochlea.[48]

Treatment and Prognosis

Principles of treatment for osteochondritis dissecans are the same as for other parts of the knee. When the lesion is found early and the patient is young (open growth plate), the patient can be treated nonoperatively and the prognosis is probably good—as it is in the rest of the knee. Micheli[49] has reported good results in two children treated with casting. If the fragment is partially detached, the bed can be curetted or drilled to stimulate a bleeding and healing response, and the fragment can then be fixed to the bony bed with a variety of fixation devices (wire, absorbable pins, Herbert screw[50]). Edwards and Bentley[51] reported good to excellent results in four cases treated with open drilling. This drilling can be done arthroscopically.[45,52] Desai et al[45] studied 13 athletes with this condition, 11 of whom were treated by excision of the fragment and drilling of the bed. Of these patients, 10 had good to excellent results at a follow-up ranging from 18 months to 19 years (average 4 years and 8 months). These authors found that prognosis could be correlated with the size of the lesion, with larger lesions not faring as well as smaller ones. The two patients who were not operated on because of the early stage of the disease ("no subchondral sclerosis on X-ray") did well. Not all results have been so sanguine. In Schwarz's review of 31 operative cases in 25 patients, 70% still had pain and 60% complained of some functional deficit.[46]

In short, osteochondritis dissecans of the patella is as mysterious here as it is in other parts of the knee. Treatment principles are the same as they are elsewhere. Closed, stable lesions in the younger child do best; detached, large fragments in the young adult fare worst.

LYME DISEASE

Lyme disease can produce an antigen-antibody response that leads to joint inflammation. It is very unusual for anterior knee pain to be the presenting symptom of this disease, but it remains a possibility. If the most difficult thing about Lyme disease is considering it in the differential diagnosis, the second most difficult thing is interpreting the results of a Lyme titer. There can be false-negative and false-positive results. Clinical judgment must be used with respect to obtaining an infectious diseases consultation.

REFLEX SYMPATHETIC DYSTROPHY AND RSD-LIKE CONDITIONS

Reflex sympathetic dystrophy (RSD) can exist regardless of whether surgery has been performed and should be considered when the patient appears to have more pain than is warranted. Typically, the pain is severe, burning, and unrelenting. The skin of the affected knee may be warmer or cooler than that of the other knee and may be hypersensitive to light touch or palpation. See Chapter 15 for a more complete discussion of these conditions.

INFECTION

Osteomyelitis of the patella is rare.[53] It can present as acute or subacute osteomyelitis. The acute form is generally obvious, as the patient presents with the classic signs and symptoms of infection. With subacute osteomyelitis, how-

ever, the patient simply has pain. Fever, redness, swelling, and abnormal serum laboratory values can all be absent. Radiographs feature a radiolucent lesion, which must be differentiated from a tumor. Even the culture can be negative, and the diagnosis is made on histological analysis.[53]

Even more rare is tuberculosis (TB) of the knee that involves only the patella (only nine cases have been reported in the English-language literature[54]). TB ("the Great Masquerader") can present not with typical boggy synovitis but as an osteolytic lesion. Patients living in or coming from areas where TB is pandemic and patients who are immunocompromised are most at risk.

REFERRED PAIN

Hip pathology can cause pain that is referred to the knee (usually the medial or anterior aspect). Although most commonly noted in the pediatric population, it can also occur in adults. When knee pain is actually referred pain, there is no tenderness anywhere about the knee or patella and there are no visible abnormalities. Ranging the hip often exacerbates the pain. A lumbar radiculopathy, which can vary in its presentation, can contribute to pain about the knee.

OVERUSE

Overuse pain is strictly the result of excessive or inappropriate activity without the slightest hint of malalignment. I have very rarely seen this. Malalignment is often the reason why one person develops overuse pain about the patella and another person does not. Treatment for this condition is relatively straightforward. The clinician should thoroughly question the patient about his or her exercise regimen to pinpoint the offending activity, and then the patient must modify that activity.

STRESS FRACTURE

Stress fracture is a very rare cause of patellar pain.[55] Stress fractures can be transverse or vertical, and they often heal well. However, on occasion, they can be stubborn and surgery may be necessary. They tend to be associated with athletic activity, but they have not yet been correlated with patella malalignment.

OTHER CAUSES OF PATELLAR PAIN

For discussion of the dorsal defect and bipartite patella, see Chapter 7. For discussion of psychosomatic pain, see Chapter 15.

REFERENCES

1. Pinar H, Özkan M, Akseki D, et al. Traumatic prepatellar neuroma: an unusual cause of anterior knee pain. *Knee Surg Sports Traumatol Arthrosc.* 1996;4:154–156.

2. Mochida H, Kikuchi S. Injury to infrapatellar branch of saphenous nerve in arthroscopic knee surgery. *Clin Orthop.* 1995;320:88–94.

3. Buckwalter JA. Pharmacological treatment of soft-tissue injuries: current concepts. *J Bone Joint Surg.* 1995;77A:1902–1914.

4. Dupont JY. Synovial plicae of the knee. *Knee.* 1994;1:5–19.

5. Patel D. Arthroscopy of the plicae—synovial folds and their significance. *Am J Sports Med.* 1978;6:217.

6. Broom MJ, Fulkerson JP. The plica syndrome: a new perspective. *Orthop Clin North Am.* 1986;17:279.

7. Hardaker WT, Whipple TL, Bassett FH. Diagnosis and treatment of the plica syndrome of the knee. *J Bone Joint Surg.* 1980;62A:211.

8. Munzinger U, Ruckstuhl J, Scherrer H, et al. Internal derangement of the knee due to pathologic synovial folds: the mediopatellar plica syndrome. *Clin Orthop.* 1981;155:59.

9. Nottage WM, Sprague NF, Auerbach BJ, et al. The medial patellar plica syndrome. *Am J Sports Med.* 1983;11:211.

10. Muse GL, Grana WA, Mollingsworth S. Arthroscopic treatment of medial shelf. *J Arthrosc Rel Res.* 1983; 102:67.

11. Pipkin G. Knee injuries: the role of suprapatellar plica and suprapatellar bursa in simulating internal derangements. *Clin Orthop.* 1971;74:161.

12. Limbird TJ. Patellar subluxation following plica resection. *Orthop Rev.* 1988;17:282.

13. Richards DP, Ajemian SV, Wiley P, et al. Knee joint dynamics predict patellar tendinitis in elite volleyball players. *Am J Sports Med.* 1996;24:676–683.

14. Duri ZAA, Aichroth PM. Patella tendonitis: clinical and literature review. *Knee Surg Sports Traumatol Arthrosc.* 1995;3:95–100.

15. Ferretti A, Ippolito E, Mariani P, et al. Jumper's knee. *Am J Sports Med.* 1983;11:58.

16. Puddu G, Cipolla M, Cerullo G. Tendinitis. In: Fox JM, Del Pizzo W, eds. *The Patellofemoral Joint.* New York: McGraw-Hill; 1993:177–192.

17. Duri ZAA, Aichroth PM, Dowd G. The fat pad: clinical observations. *Am J Knee Surg.* 1996;9:55–66.

18. Maddox PA, Garth WP. Tendinitis of the patellar ligament and quadriceps (jumper's knee) as an initial presentation of hyperparathyroidism. *J Bone Joint Surg.* 1986;68A:288.

19. Bodne D, Quinn SF, Murray WT, et al. Magnetic resonance images of chronic patellar tendonitis. *Skeletal Radiol.* 1988;17:24.

20. Davies SG, Baudoin CJ, King JB, et al. Ultrasound, computed tomography, and magnetic resonance imaging in patellar tendonitis. *Clin Radiol.* 1991;43:52.

21. Fritschy D, de Gautard R. Jumper's knee and ultrasonography. *Am J Sports Med.* 1988;16:637–640.

22. Stefko JM, Fu F. Patellar problems in the young patient. In: Scuderi GR, ed. *The Patella.* New York: Springer-Verlag; 1995.

23. Parker RD, Calabrese GJ. Anterior knee pain. In: Fu FH, Harner CD, Vince KG, eds. *Knee Surgery.* Baltimore: Williams & Wilkins; 1994:939.

24. Ismail AM, Balakrishmann R, Rajakamur MK. Rupture of the patellar ligament after steroid infiltration. *J Bone Joint Surg.* 1969;51B:503.

25. Kennedy JC, Willes RB. The effect of local steroid injections on tendons. *Am J Sports Med.* 1991;4:11.

26. Benazzo F, Stennardo G, Valli M. Achilles and patellar tendinopathies in athletes: pathogenesis and surgical treatment. *Bull Hosp Joint Dis.* 1996;54:236–240.

27. Karlsson J, Lundin O, Lossing IW, et al. Partial rupture of the patellar ligament: results after operative treatment. *Am J Sports Med.* 1991;19:403.

28. Kelly DW, Carter VS, Jobe FW, et al. Patellar and quadriceps tendon ruptures—jumper's knee. *Am J Sports Med.* 1984;12:375.

29. Rosenberg JM, Whitaker JH. Bilateral infra-patellar tendon rupture in a patient with jumper's knee. *Am J Sports Med.* 1991;19:94.

30. Kricun R, Kricun ME, Arangio GA, et al. Patellar tendon ruptures with underlying systemic diseases. *Am J Radiol.* 1980;135:803.

31. Martin JR, Wilson CL, Mathews WH. Bilateral rupture of the ligamenta patellae in a case of disseminated systemic lupus erythematosus. *Arthritis Rheum.* 1958; 1:548.

32. McConnell J. Fat pad irritation—a mistaken patellar tendinitis. *Sport Health.* 1991;9(4):7–9.

33. Larsen S. En little ukjendt sygdom i patella. *Norsk Mag Laegevid.* 1921;19:856–858.

34. Johansson S. En förut icke beskriven sjukdom i patella. *Hygiea.* 1922;84:161–166.

35. James RL, Shelton ML, Sachdev RK. Chondroblastoma of the patella with a pathologic fracture: a case report. *Orthop Rev.* 1987;16:834.

36. Mercuri M, Casadei R, Ferraro A, et al. Tumours of the patella. *Int Orthop.* 1991;15:115–120.

37. Kransdorf MJ, Moser RP, Vinh TN, et al. Primary tumors of the patella. *Skeletal Radiol.* 1989;18:365–371.

38. Linscheid RL, Dahlin D. Unusual lesions of the patella. *J Bone Joint Surg.* 1966;48A:1359–1366.

39. Saglik Y, Ucar DH, Yildiz HY, Dogan M. Unicameral bone cyst of the patella. *Int Orthop.* 1995;19:280–281.

40. Bansal VP, Singh R, Grewal DS, et al. Haemangioma of the patella. *J Bone Joint Surg.* 1974;56:139–141.

41. Paget J. On the production of some loose bodies in joints. *St Barth Hosp Rep.* 1870;6:1.

42. Obedian RS, Grelsamer RP. Osteochondritis dissecans of the distal femur and patella. *Clin Sports Med.* 1997;16:157.

43. König F. Über freie Korer in den Gelenken. *Dtsch Z Chir.* 1887;27:90–109.

44. Hellstrom J. Beitrag zur kenntnis ders osteochondritis dissecans in kniegelenk. *Acta Orthop Scand.* 1923;55: 190–221.

45. Desai SS, Patel MR, Michelli LJ, et al. Osteochondritis dissecans of the patella. *J Bone Joint Surg.* 1987; 69B:320–325.

46. Schwarz C, Blazina ME, Sisto DJ, et al. The results of operative treatment of osteochondritis dissecans of the patella. *Am J Sports Med.* 1988;16:522.

47. Stanitski CL. Osteochondritis dissecans of the knee. In: Stanitski CL, DeLee JC, Drez D, eds. *Pediatric and Adolescent Sports Medicine.* Philadelphia: WB Saunders Co; 1994:387–405.

48. Kurzweil PR, Zambetti GJ, Hamilton WG. Osteochondritis dissecans in the lateral patellofemoral groove. *Am J Sports Med.* 1988;16:308.

49. Micheli LJ. Patellofemoral disorders in children. In: Fox JM, Del Pizzo W, eds. *The Patellofemoral Joint.* New York: McGraw-Hill; 1993:105–122.

50. Marandola MS, Prietto CA. Arthroscopic Herbert screw fixation of patellar osteochondritis dissecans. *Arthroscopy.* 1993;9:214–216.

51. Edwards DH, Bentley G. Osteochondritis dissecans patellae. *J Bone Joint Surg.* 1977;59B:58–63.

52. Pfeiffer WH, Gross ML, Seeger LL. Osteochondritis dissecans of the patella: MRI evaluation and a case report. *Clin Orthop.* 1991;271:207–211.

53. Alexeeff M, Macnicol MF. Subacute patellar osteomyelitis. *Knee.* 1995;1:237–239.

54. Dhillon MS, Rajasekhar C, Nagi ON. Tuberculosis of the patella: report of a case and review of the literature. *Knee.* 1995;2:53–56.

55. Orava S, Taimela S, Kvist M, et al. Diagnosis and treatment of stress fracture of the patella in athletes. *Knee Surg Sports Traumatol Arthrosc.* 1996;4:206–211.

ADDITIONAL READINGS

Ferguson PC, Griffin AM, Bell RS. Primary patellar tumors. *Clin Orthop.* 1997;336:199–204.

Lundy DW, Aboulafia AJ, Otis JB, et al. Myxoid liposarcoma of the retropatellar fat pad. *Am J Orthop.* 1997;26:287–289.

Popp JE, Yu JS, Kaeding CC. Recalcitrant patellar tendinitis: magnetic resonance imaging, histologic evaluation, and surgical treatment. *Am J Sports Med.* 1997;25:218–222.

CHAPTER 9

Classification of Patellofemoral Disorders

Many classifications of patellofemoral disorders have been published. Some address the specific source of the pain, some address only the appearance of the chondral lesions, some factor in the radiographic appearance of the patellofemoral joint, some combine all of these elements. This chapter outlines some of the existing classifications and presents a proposed classification.

NOMENCLATURE AND CLASSIFICATION OF CHONDRAL LESIONS

What to call a traumatic or degenerative abnormality of articular cartilage is a source of controversy. *Chondromalacia* is not always technically correct and has too many negative connotations (see Chapter 1). *Chondritis* implies an inflammation, which is not present. *Chondropathy* is better suited to metabolic disorders. For the moment, the term *chondral lesion* seems most suitable.

A number of classifications of chondral lesions have been described, most of which feature four stages of cartilage degeneration. The fourth stage usually implies degeneration down to visible subchondral bone.

Outerbridge Classification

In 1961, Outerbridge[1] proposed the following stages of "chondromalacia patellae":

- *Stage I*: change of color from glistening white to dull and yellowish white; abnormal softening
- *Stage II*: fissuring and fragmentation, less than 1.25 cm
- *Stage III*: fissuring and fragmentation, greater than 1.25 cm
- *Stage IV*: erosion down to bone

Outerbridge found this pathology to be most common on the medial facet and attributed it to an abnormal ridge superomedial to the trochlea.

Ficat and Hungerford Classification

The Ficat and Hungerford[2] classification is based on "axial X-rays" (actually arthrography).

1. chondromalacia of the lateral facet
2. chondromalacia of the odd facet
3. central chondromalacia with symmetric extension medially and laterally
4. bipolar chondromalacia involving "the central portion of the two facets separated by a normal median ridge"
5. global chondromalacia or total chondromalacia involving the "totality of both facets"

Ficat and Hungerford characterized chondral lesions as *early* and *late*,[3] defined as follows:

- *Early*: "closed chondromalacia" with swelling and blistering; found most commonly on the lateral portion of the patella and attributed to excessive pressure

- *Late*: open lesion with fissures or ulcerations

Goodfellow Classification

Goodfellow et al[4] developed the following classification system:

- Grade I: Blister formation with basal degeneration; most commonly at distal part of ridge separating medial and lateral patella (Note: This ridge is not always present, see Chapter 2.)
- Grade II: Superficial degeneration most commonly along the odd facet thought to be secondary to decreased contact; starts with flaking and progresses to fibrillation and fissure formation
- Grade III: ulceration
- Grade IV: crater formation and subchondral eburnation

Insall Classification

Insall developed the following classification system[5,6]:

- I: softening and swelling (blister)
- II: deep fissuring down to subchondral bone
- III: fibrillation ("crab meat")
- IV: thinning, coarse granular appearance of cartilage, exposure of subchondral bone

Casscells Classification

In 1982, Casscells[7] proposed the following classification system for "chondromalacia":

- I: superficial erosion ≤ 1 cm
- II: involvement of deeper cartilage layers (1 to 2 cm)
- III: complete erosion of cartilage with exposure of subchondral bone (2 to 4 cm)
- IV: completely destroyed cartilage "wide area"

Bandi Classification

Bandi[6,8] proposed the following classification system for "chondromalacia" in 1982:

- I: softening, cartilage edema
- II: fragmentation and fissuring down to subchondral bone
- III: exposure of subchondral bone with sclerosing

Bentley Classification

Bentley[9] proposed the following classification system for "chondromalacia" in 1984:

- I: fibrillation or fissuring < 0.5 cm
- II: fibrillation or fissuring 0.5 to 1 cm
- III: fibrillation or fissuring 1 to 2 cm
- IV: fibrillation with or without exposed subchondral bone > 2 cm

Bauer and Jackson Classification

In 1988, Bauer and Jackson[10] developed the following classification system for femoral condyle lesions:

- Acute traumatic condyle lesions
  - I: linear crack
  - II: stellate fracture
  - III: flap
  - IV: crater
- Degenerative condyle lesion
  - V: fibrillated
  - VI: degradation

Noyes and Stabler Classification

Noyes and Stabler[11] developed the following system for grading articular cartilage lesions at arthroscopy:

- I: cartilage surface intact
- IA: softening < 1 cm
- IB: softening (deformation) ≤ 1.5 cm

- II: cracks, fissuring, fibrillation, fragmentation
- IIA: cracks, fissuring, fibrillation, fragmentation < ½ thickness
- IIB: cracks, fissuring, fibrillation, fragmentation > ½ thickness

- III: bone exposed
- IIIA: bone surface intact
- IIIB: bone surface excavation

(Note: Blunt trauma to the knee may not cause visible injury to the articular cartilage. Nevertheless, damage can be caused to the deeper layers.[12–14] At the time of publication, this damage is not visible on any form of imaging including magnetic resonance imaging. This deep layer damage can eventually be associated with more extensive damage to an extent that is not currently predictable.)

NOMENCLATURE AND CLASSIFICATION OF PATELLOFEMORAL DISORDERS

Patellofemoral disorders can be classified in a number of ways. The main differential diagnosis in my opinion is whether the pain is related to malalignment. There is a gray area to the extent that some conditions such as patellar tendinitis and Osgood-Schlatter's condition can only occasionally be linked to malalignment.

There are many parameters to consider in putting together a classification: the status of the patellofemoral articular surface, the three-dimensional positional position of the patella within the patellofemoral joint, abnormalities of the limb above and below the patella, and structural abnormalities about the patellofemoral joint itself.

Outerbridge Classification

Outerbridge[15] classified "chondromalacia patellae" in 1975 in the following manner:

A. Trauma (directly to the patella)
B. Dislocation (acute or recurrent; with or without a tear of the medial capsule, a medial patellar fracture, or an osteochondral "flake")
C. Malalignment syndrome with patellar subluxation
   1. factors increasing quadriceps bowstring effect
     a. female, wide pelvis
     b. valgus knees
     c. excessive laterally placed tibial tubercle

     d. congenitally flattened lateral femoral condyle
     e. patella alta
   2. lax medial capsular retinaculum
     a. tear following dislocation
     b. stretching secondary to
       i. tight lateral capsular retinaculum
       ii. chronic joint fluid
       iii. repetitive subluxation
   3. inefficient vastus medialis muscle
     a. congenitally high insertion
     b. atrophy of disuse
   4. congenitally tight lateral capsular retinaculum
   5. acute dislocation of athletes
D. Normal knee alignment with osteochondral ridge
E. Increased cartilage vulnerability
   1. congenital
   2. postarthrotomy rehabilitative period
   3. postcasting rehabilitative period
F. Occupation hazards
   1. military and athletic trainees
   2. jobs requiring excessive kneeling and squatting

Fulkerson-Schutzer Classification

Fulkerson and Schutzer[16,17] have devised a classification combining chondral changes and three-dimensional patellar positioning.

- Type I
  A. patellar subluxation with no articular lesion
  B. patellar subluxation with grade 1–2 chondromalacia
  C. patellar subluxation with grade 3–4 arthrosis
  D. patellar subluxation with a history of dislocation and minimal or no chondromalacia
  E. patellar subluxation with a history of dislocation, with grade 3–4 arthrosis
- Type II
  A. patellar tilt and subluxation with no articular lesion

B. patellar tilt and subluxation with grade 1–2 chondromalacia
C. patellar tilt and subluxation with grade 3–4 arthrosis
- Type III
  A. patellar tilt with no articular lesion
  B. patellar tilt with grade 1–2 chondromalacia
  C. patellar tilt with grade 3–4 arthrosis
- Type IV
  A. no malalignment and no articular lesion
  B. no malalignment and grade 1–2 chondromalacia
  C. no malalignment and grade 3–4 arthrosis

Merchant Classification (Abridged)

Merchant[18] developed the following classification for patellofemoral disorders:

I. Trauma (conditions caused by trauma in the otherwise normal knee)
   A. acute trauma
   B. repetitive trauma (overuse syndromes)
      1. patellar tendinitis (jumper's knee)
      2. quadriceps tendinitis
      3. peripatellar tendinitis (anterior knee pain of the adolescent secondary to hamstring tightness)
      4. preoperative patellar bursitis (housemaid's knee)
      5. apophysitis (Osgood-Schlatter, Sinding-Larsen-Johansson)
   C. late effects of trauma (eg, arthritis, patella infera, reflex sympathetic dystrophy)
II. Patellofemoral dysplasia
   A. lateral patellar compression
   B. chronic subluxation of the patella
   C. recurrent dislocation of the patella
      1. associated fractures (osteochondral, avulsion)
      2. secondary chondromalacia
      3. secondary arthritis
III. Idiopathic chondromalacia patellae

IV. Osteochondritis dissecans
V. Synovial plicae (symptomatic)

HISTOLOGY

One of the hallmarks of patellar malalignment is a change in the articular cartilage of the patella. This change is to a certain extent visible—and, thus, the name *chondromalacia*. Again it must be emphasized that pain from patellar malalignment can be present even if there are no visible changes in the articular cartilage. Furthermore, there can be significant histological changes in the absence of any grossly discernible changes in articular cartilage.[12] These changes can also be noted on electron microscopy.[19]

When edema is present, there is a decrease in cell density, a reduced and uneven level of fast green (SO) staining down to the deepest areas of cartilage, and a suggestion that proteoglycan synthesis is greatly decreased.[12] In advanced lesions, Mori et al have noted a large number of undifferentiated mesenchymal cells and fibroblast-like cells about the fissures. These features are absent in patients with osteoarthritis unrelated to patella malalignment.[12]

PROPOSED CLASSIFICATION OF PATELLOFEMORAL SYMPTOMATOLOGY

Rather than include all elements of the classification of patellofemoral symptomatology in one table, it is perhaps better to divide the classification into subgroups. This concept was first proposed by Merle d'Aubigné[20] in 1954 for describing hip function (his subgroups were pain, motion, and activities). Lewandrowski et al[6] also recently used this concept when they broke down articular cartilage lesions of the knee into six groups: appearance, depth, area, clinical stage (ie, acute/chronic), location, and severity.

I propose a classification divided into three subgroups: etiology (source of pain), radiology, and a description of the chondral lesions.

I. Patellofemoral classification by source of pain.

    A. patellofemoral pain and/or instability not related to the extensor mechanism
        1. neuroma
        2. plica
        3. iliotibial band tendinitis
        4. inflammatory arthritis
        5. primary synovial process (benign or malignant)
        6. referred pain
        7. cruciate ligament tear
        8. loose body
        9. meniscal tear
      10. quadriceps atrophy
      11. scar

    B. patellofemoral pain without malalignment
        1. trauma
           a. trauma 1 (contusion, fracture)
           b. trauma 2 (dislocation)
           c. trauma 3 (patellar tendon or quadriceps tendon rupture)
        2. apophysitis
           a. Osgood-Schlatter's condition
           b. Sinding-Larsen-Johansson condition
        3. overuse
           a. patellar tendinitis
           b. iliotibial band tendinitis
           c. quadriceps tendinitis
        4. chondral lesion not related to malalignment (eg, osteoarthritis)
        5. osteochondritis dissecans of the patella
        6. tumors (eg, hemangioma)
        7. reflex sympathetic dystrophy

    C. patellofemoral symptomatology with malalignment
        1. abnormal tilt (present, absent)
        2. visible subluxation (present, absent)
        3. lateral facet tenderness (present, absent)
        4. medial facet tenderness (present, absent)
        5. retinacular tenderness (present, absent)
        6. apprehension (Fairbanks) (present, absent)
        7. giving way (instability) (present, absent)
        8. quadriceps (Q) angle (normal, increased, decreased)
        9. laxity (normal, increased)
      10. limb alignment (normal, varus, valgus)
      11. squinting patella (present, absent)
      12. flat feet (present, absent)
      13. Osgood-Schlatter's condition (present, absent)

II. Patellofemoral classification by radiological aspect

    A. patellar tilt
        1. lateral (lateral side down)
        2. medial (lateral side up)

    B. patellar translation
        1. lateral
        2. medial
        3. lateral/medial (lateral at a certain degree of flexion, medial at another degree of flexion)
        4. superior (alta)
        5. inferior (baja, infera)

    C. dysplasia
        1. trochlear
           a. none
           b. present (minor, moderate, severe)
        2. patellar
           a. none
           b. Hunter's cap
           c. pebble
           d. bipartite patella

III. Patellofemoral classification by assessment of chondral lesions

    A. nature
        1. blistering
        2. fibrillation
        3. crabmeat
        4. erosion

B. visible depth (Pathology may be deeper than can be appreciated through usual inspection)
  1. superficial
  2. partial thickness
  3. down to bone
C. location/size
  1. superolateral sector
  2. superocentral sector
  3. superomedial sector
  4. centrolateral sector
  5. centrocentral sector
  6. centromedial sector
  7. inferolateral sector
  8. inferocentral sector
  9. inferomedial sector

REFERENCES

1. Outerbridge RE. The etiology of chondromalacia patellae. *J Bone Joint Surg.* 1961;43B:752.

2. Ficat RP, Philippe J, Hungerford DS. Chondromalacia patellae: a system of classification. *Clin Orthop.* 1979;144:55–62.

3. Ficat RP, Hungerford DS. *Disorders of the Patellofemoral Joint.* 2nd Ed. Baltimore: Williams & Wilkins: 1977:128.

4. Goodfellow J, Hungerford DS, Woods C. Patello-femoral joint mechanics and pathology, II: chondromalacia patella. *J Bone Joint Surg.* 1976;58B:287.

5. Insall JN, Falvo K, Wise D. Chondromalacia patellae—a prospective study. *J Bone Joint Surg.* 1976;58A:1.

6. Lewandrowski KU, Ekkernkamp A, David A, et al. Classification of articular cartilage lesions of the knee at arthroscopy. *Am J Knee Surg.* 1996;9:121–128.

7. Casscells SW. Chondromalacia of the patella. *J Pediatr Orthop.* 1982;2:560–564.

8. Bandi W. Chondromalacia of the patella: etiology and pathogenesis, clinical aspects, therapy and prognosis. *Z Unfallmed Berufskr.* 1982;75:155–160.

9. Bentley G, Dowd G. Current concepts of etiology and treatment of chondromalacia patellae. *Clin Orthop.* 1984;189:209–228.

10. Bauer MD, Jackson RW. Chondral lesions of the femoral condyles: a system of arthroscopic classification. *Arthroscopy.* 1988;4:97–102.

11. Noyes FR, Stabler CL. A system for grading articular cartilage lesions at arthroscopy. *Am J Sports Med.* 1989;17:505.

12. Mori Y, Kubo M, Okumo H, et al. Histological comparison of patellar cartilage degeneration between chondromalacia in youth and osteoarthritis in aging. *Knee Surg Sports Traumatol Arthrosc.* 1995;3:167–172.

13. Thompson RC, Vener MJ, Griffiths HJ, et al. Scanning electron-microscopic and magnetic resonance imaging studies of injuries to the patellofemoral joint after acute transarticular loading. *J Bone Joint Surg.* 1993;75A:704–713.

14. Armstrong CG, Mow VC, Wirth CR. Biomechanics of impact-induced microdamage to articular cartilage: a possible genesis for chondromalacia patella. In: Finerman G, ed. *American Academy of Orthopaedic Surgeons Symposium on Sports Medicine: The Knee.* St. Louis, MO: CV Mosby Co; 1985:70–84.

15. Outerbridge RE, Dunlop J. The problem of chondromalacia patellae. *Clin Orthop.* 1975;110:177–193.

16. Schutzer SF, Ramsby GR, Fulkerson JP. Computed tomographic classification of patellofemoral pain patients. *Orthop Clin North Am.* 1986;17:235–248.

17. Fulkerson JP. *Disorders of the Patellofemoral Joint.* 3rd ed. Baltimore: Williams & Wilkins; 1997.

18. Merchant AC. Classification of patellofemoral disorders. *Arthroscopy.* 1988;4:235–240.

19. Mori Y, Kubo M, Okumo H, et al. A scanning electron microscopy study of the degenerative cartilage in patellar chondropathy. *Arthroscopy.* 1993;9:247–264.

20. Merle d'Aubigné R, Postel M. Functional results of hip arthroplasty with acrylic prosthesis. *J Bone Joint Surg.* 1954;36A:451.

ADDITIONAL READINGS

Deutsch AL, Shellock FG, Mink JH. Imaging of the patellofemoral joint: emphasis on advanced techniques. In: Fox JM, Del Pizzo W, eds. *The Patellofemoral Joint.* New York: McGraw-Hill; 1993:75–104.

Outerbridge RE. Further studies on the etiology of chondromalacia patellae. *J Bone Joint Surg.* 1964;46B:179.

CHAPTER 10

Examination of the Patellofemoral Joint: The Physical Therapist's Perspective

THE PATIENT'S HISTORY

The initial part of the examination of the patient involves obtaining a detailed history, so a differential diagnosis can be proposed. The diagnosis is later confirmed or modified by the physical findings. When taking the patient's history, the clinician needs to elicit the area of pain; the type of activity precipitating the pain; the history of the onset of the pain; the behavior of the pain; and any other symptoms such as clicking, giving way, or swelling.[1,2] This information gives an indication of the structure involved and the likely diagnosis. Table 10–1 lists the possible areas of pain and the likely structures that may be implicated. For example, if the activity that precipitated the patient's pain involves eccentric loading, such as jumping in basketball or increased hill work during running, patellar tendinitis would be suspected. On the other hand, if the athlete reports pain following flip turns or vigorous kicking in the swimming pool, or on delivery of a fast ball in cricket, an irritated fat pad would be suspected.[3] In both these conditions, the complaint is of inferior patellar pain. Exhibit 10–1 outlines the signs and symptoms of fat pad irritation and patellar tendinitis to help clinicians with the differential diagnosis. The patient with an irritated fat pad is aggravated by straight leg raise exercises. It is therefore essential for the therapist to recognize the condition so that the appropriate management can be implemented to enhance, rather than impede, recovery. The clinical diagnosis of patellar tendinitis can be confirmed with diagnostic ultrasound or magnetic resonance imaging (MRI). These investigations may show evidence of acute inflammation with a thickened tendon and associated fluid, cyst formation within the tendon, or a partial tear within the substance of the tendon.[1] In conditions of extreme chronicity, degeneration of the tendon occurs with little inflammation. This is referred to as patellar tendonosis.

SYMPTOMS

The patient with patellofemoral pain usually complains of a diffuse ache in the anterior part of the knee, which is exacerbated by stair climbing. For many, the knee aches after sitting for prolonged periods with the knee flexed (the movie sign). Some patients may have crepitus; this condition is often a source of concern for them because they believe that the crepitus is indicative of arthritis. However, crepitus is usually due to tight deep lateral retinacular structures and can be improved with treatment. Abernathy et al[4] examined the knees of first-year medical students ($n = 123$) and found that asymptomatic patellofemoral crepitus was present in 62% of the students.

Some patients may experience "giving way" or a buckling sensation of the knee. This occurs during walking or stair climbing (ie, movements in a straight line) and is a reflex inhibition of the quadriceps muscle. It must be differentiated

Table 10–1 Areas of Pain and the Structures That May Be Implicated

Pain Area	Involved Structure
Lateral	Small nerve injury of the lateral retinaculum
Medial	Recurrent stretching of the medial retinaculum; occasionally, medial plica
Inferior	Irritation of the infrapatellar fat pad; patellar tendinitis
Retropatellar	Probable articular cartilage damage; stress borne on subchondral bone
Superior	Quadriceps tendon; hemangioma (this is rare but must be considered)

from the giving way experienced when turning, which usually is indicative of an anterior cruciate deficient knee. Locking is another symptom that must be differentiated from intra-articular pathology. Patellofemoral locking is usually only a catching sensation where the patient can actively unlock the knee (unlike loose body or meniscal locking, where the patient is either unable to unlock or can only passively unlock the knee).

Mild swelling due to synovial irritation may also occur with patellofemoral problems. Mild swelling causes an asymmetric wasting of the quadriceps muscle, whereby the vastus medialis obliquus (VMO) is inhibited before the vastus lateralis (VL) and rectus femoris (RF).[5–7] A patient with primary intra-articular pathology, such as a meniscal or ligamentous injury, may have great difficulty resolving the subsequent secondary patellofemoral problem, particularly if it is not identified.

When considering the possible differential diagnoses, the clinician must remember that the lumbar spine and the hip can refer symptoms to the knee. For example, the prepubescent male with a slipped femoral epiphysis may present with a limp and anterior knee pain and may initially be misdiagnosed as having patellofemoral pain.

Neural tissue may also be a source of symptoms around the patellofemoral joint. Lack of mobility of the fifth lumbar (L-5) and first sacral (S1) nerve roots and their derivatives can give rise to posterior or lateral thigh pain. Symptoms

from neural tissue can be fairly easily differentiated from patellofemoral symptoms, because the pain will be exacerbated in sitting—particularly when the leg is straight rather than in the classic movie sign position of a flexed knee. The slump sitting test, as described by Maitland,[8] will quickly verify the neural tissue as being a source of the symptoms. Similarly, a peripheral nerve may scar down or become entrapped following arthroscopic surgery. The most common example is the infrapatellar branch of the saphenous nerve. Symptoms are sharp pain inferomedially with or without slightly altered sensation laterally. The symptoms are reported on deep squatting and jumping and thus are frequently confused with patellar tendinitis symptoms because of the proximity to the tendon. Pain can be reproduced with the patient prone, flexing the knee and externally rotating the tibia to stretch the nerve. Reproduction of the patient's symptoms with certain testing procedures usually confirms the diagnosis.

CLINICAL EXAMINATION

The clinical examination establishes the diagnosis and determines the underlying causative factors of the patient's symptoms so the appropriate treatment can be implemented.

Examination of Patient in Standing Position

The patient is initially examined in the standing position to determine the alignment of the

Exhibit 10–1 Fat Pad Irritation or Patellar Tendinitis

Fad Pad Irritation Signs and Symptoms	*Patellar Tendinitis Signs and Symptoms*

• tenderness at inferior patella
• "puffy" knees
• pain exacerbated by:
  –prolonged standing
  –negotiating stairs
• hyperextended/locked back knees
• pain when going up stairs as weight-bearing leg extends, when acute
• pain reproduced on extension or on over-pressure
• tenderness at inferior pole
• posterior displacement of inferior pole
	• tenderness at inferior patella
	• knees not "puffy"
	• pain exacerbated by:
	  –jumping
	  –mid to full squat
	• straighter quadriceps (Q) angle (< 15 degrees for females, < 12 degrees for males)
	• pain when at 3/4 to full squat; pain on jumping
	• no pain on extension or on overpressure
	• tenderness at inferior pole
	• no displacement of inferior pole

lower extremity. Biomechanical faults are noted so that the clinician has a reasonable indication of how the patient will move. The clinician assesses the femoral position, which is easier to see when the patient has the feet together. A position of internal rotation of the femur is a common finding in patients with patellofemoral pain. (The term *internal femoral rotation* is preferred to *femoral anteversion*, because *rotation* implies not only the bony position, but also the soft tissue adaptation that occurs as a result of the femoral anteversion. The soft tissue changes are quite amenable to change by conservative management. In addition, these patients usually present without hip X-rays, and a true diagnosis of femoral anteversion should not be given without radiographic confirmation.)

The internal femoral rotation often causes a squinting of the patellae (Figure 10–1), but if the lateral structures of the patellofemoral joint are tight, the patella may appear straight. The clinician assesses for the presence of an enlarged fat pad, which indicates that the patient is standing in hyperextension or a "locked-back" position of the knees (ie, the knees are resting at end-range of extension). The muscle bulk of the VMO is observed and compared with the other side. The VL and iliotibial band (ITB) are palpated to de-

termine the resting tension. Tightness in the ITB will lead to lateral tracking of the patella, particularly at 20 degrees of knee flexion, where it is maximally taut.[9] Presence of varus/valgus or torsion of the tibia is noted, because tibial malalignment will affect the pull of the soft tissues on the patella, giving rise to patellofemoral problems.

The clinician assesses the foot position, because the presence of pronated feet has been associated with patellofemoral symptoms (see Chapter 13). An abnormal valgus vector force is created by the excessive pronation that results in an increase in the dynamic quadriceps (Q) angle. The Q angle represents the line of pull of the rectus femoris muscle. It is the angle that is formed when a line from the anterior superior iliac spine to the midpole of the patella is bisected with a line from the tibial tubercle to the midpole of the patella (see Chapter 13). The outer limit for the Q angle is 15 degrees for females and 12 degrees for males. This measurement is only a static measurement. What is of more interest is the dynamic Q angle—what happens to the patella relative to the femur when the person moves. To determine whether the patient has an increase in compensatory pronation in standing, the talus is palpated on the medial and lateral sides to check

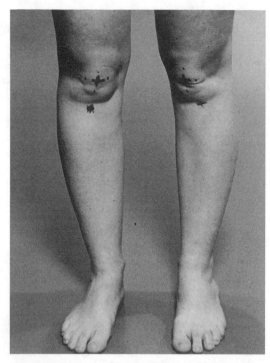

Figure 10–1 Internal Femoral Rotation. This patient demonstrates internal femoral rotation and the consequent squinting patellae appearance.

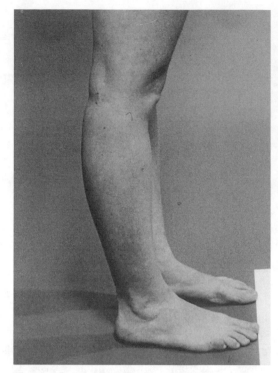

Figure 10–2 Locked-Back Knee Viewed from the Side.

for symmetry of position. In relaxed standing, the subtalar joint should be in midposition. The shape of medial and lateral longitudinal arches is noted. If, for example, the medial longitudinal arch is flattened, then the patient exhibits prolonged pronation during walking. The great toe and first metatarsal are examined for callus formation as well as position. If the patient has callus on the medial aspect of the first metatarsal or the great toe, or has a hallux valgus, then the clinician should expect the patient to have an unstable push-off in gait. When examined prone, this patient will have a forefoot deformity.

From the side, the clinician can check pelvic position to determine whether there is an anterior tilt, posterior tilt, or a swaybacked posture. Position of hyperextension or "locked-back" knees can be verified looking from the side (Figure 10–2). From behind, the level of the posterior superior iliac spine is checked, gluteal bulk

is assessed, and the position of the calcaneus is observed. If the clinician finds that the calcaneus is in a relatively neutral or inverted position and the talus is more prominent on the medial side, then the clinician could anticipate that the patient may have a stiff subtalar joint. Thus, from a person's static alignment, the clinician can have a reasonable idea of the dynamic picture and can anticipate how the patient will move. Any deviations from the anticipated movement give a great deal of information about the muscle control of the activity.

Dynamic Examination

The aim of the dynamic examination is not only to evaluate the effect of muscle action on the static mechanics, but also to reproduce the patient's symptoms so the clinician has an objective reassessment activity to evaluate the effectiveness of the treatment. The least stressful activity of walking is examined first. For example, at heel strike, individuals with patellofemoral pain who stand in hyperextension do not exhibit the necessary shock absorption at the knee. Consequently, the femur internally rotates and the quadriceps does not function well in inner range due to lack of practice. If the patient's symptoms arc not provoked in walking, then the clinician evaluates more stressful activities such as stair climbing. If symptoms are still not provoked, then squat and one-leg squat may be examined and used as a reassessment activity. When assessing an athlete with patellofemoral symptoms, it can be difficult for the clinician to reproduce the symptoms during the examination, so the control ("wobbliness factor") of the one-leg squat is of great interest. Improvement of control of the one-leg squat during treatment generally indicates that the athlete's patellofemoral symptoms will be improved for the athletic activity, so muscle control is an important reassessment sign.

Examination of Patient in Supine Position

With the patient in the supine position, the clinician assesses the soft tissue structures and begins to confirm the diagnosis. Gentle, careful palpation should be performed on the soft tissue structures around the patella. The joint lines are palpated to exclude obvious intra-articular pathology. Palpation of the retinacular tissues reveals whether any part of the retinaculum is under chronic recurrent stress and is the source of the patient's symptoms. Pain in the infrapatellar region indicates that the infrapatellar fat pad may be the source of the symptoms, particularly if the patient has no history of eccentric loading of the quadriceps muscle. To verify whether the infrapatellar fat pad is the culprit, the clinician should shorten the fat pad by lifting it toward the patella. If, on further palpation, the pain is gone, then the clinician can be relatively certain that the patient has a fat pad irritation. If the pain remains, then the patient has patellar tendinitis. The diagnosis of fat pad irritation can be con-

firmed by performing a passive extension maneuver on the knee, which often reproduces the patient's infrapatellar pain. Passive flexion of the knee compromises the patellofemoral joint and provides compression to the menisci, which may be symptomatic if damaged. Passive movements of the knee allow the clinician to ascertain any guarding movements.

With the patient in the supine position, the clinician tests the length of the hamstrings, iliopsoas, rectus femoris, tensor fasciae latae (TFL), gastrocnemius, and soleus muscles. Tightness of any of these muscles has an adverse effect on patellofemoral joint mechanics and must be addressed in treatment. Soft tissue tightness is particularly prevalent during the adolescent growth spurt in which the long bones are growing faster than the surrounding soft tissues.[10] This leads not only to problems of lack of flexibility, but also to muscle control problems where the short muscles cannot maneuver the long levers of the limbs.

Tightness of the hamstrings or gastrocnemius causes a lateral tracking of the patella by increasing the dynamic Q angle.[11] When an individual with tight hamstrings runs, there is an increase in knee flexion at heel strike. Because the knee cannot straighten, an increased dorsiflexion is required to position the body over the planted foot. If the range of full dorsiflexion has already occurred at the talocrural joint, further range is achieved by pronating the foot, particularly at the subtalar joint. This causes an increase in the valgus vector force and hence an increase in the dynamic Q angle.[11]

If the ITB is tight, the patella will be drawn laterally when it is supposed to be centering in the trochlea, because the ITB is maximally tight at 20 degrees of knee flexion. Tightness of the ITB causes a lateral tracking and tilting of the patella and often a weakness of the medial retinaculum.[12]

The iliopsoas, rectus femoris, and TFL may be tested using the Thomas test. The patient stands with the ischia touching the end of the treatment table. One leg is pulled up to the chest to flatten the lumbar lordosis; then the patient lies down on the table, keeping the flexed leg close to the chest. The other leg should be resting so that the hip is in a neutral position (ie, on the table, at the same width as the pelvis), and the knee should be flexed to 90 degrees. If the hip is in neutral position but the knee cannot be flexed, the rectus femoris is tight. If the hip is flexed, but lying in the plane of the body, the iliopsoas is tight. But if the hip remains flexed and abducted, the TFL is tight. Lack of flexibility of the TFL can be further confirmed in sidelying by Ober's test. The Thomas test should be performed on both legs to allow comparison between legs. Hamstring flexibility may be examined by a passive straight leg raise, once the lumbar spine is flattened on the table and the pelvis is stable. Normal length hamstrings should allow 80 to 85 degrees of hip flexion when the knee is extended and the lumbar spine is flattened.

An essential part of evaluating the patient in the supine position is assessing the orientation of the patella relative to the femur. The clinician's goal is to maximize the surface area of contact so that, for the same amount of force, there is less pressure being distributed through the overloaded part of the joint. In order to maximize the area of contact of the patella with the femur, the patella should be in the optimal position before it enters the trochlea. The clinician needs to consider the patellar position not with respect to the normal, but with respect to the optimal, because articular cartilage is nourished and maintained by evenly distributed, intermittent compression.

An optimal patellar position is one where the patella is parallel to the femur in the frontal and the sagittal planes, and the patella is midway between the two condyles when the knee is flexed to 20 degrees. The position of the patella is determined by examining four discrete components in a static and dynamic manner: glide, lateral tilt, anteroposterior tilt, and rotation. Determination of the glide component involves measuring the distance from the midpole of the patella to the medial and lateral femoral epicondyles. The patella should be sitting equidistant (± 5 mm) from each epicondyle when the

knee is flexed to 20 degrees (Figure 10–3). A 5 mm lateral displacement of the patella causes a 50% decrease in VMO tension.[13] The patella may sit equidistant to the condyles, but moves laterally, out of the line of the femur when the quadriceps contracts, indicating a dynamic problem. The dynamic glide examines the effect of the quadriceps contraction on patellar position as well as the timing of the activity of the different heads of quadriceps. The VMO should be activated at the same time or slightly earlier than the VL. In patients with patellofemoral pain, the VMO activity can be delayed.

If the passive lateral structures are too tight, the patella will tilt so that the medial border of the patella is higher than the lateral border and the posterior edge of the lateral border is difficult to palpate. This is a lateral tilt; if severe, this condition can lead to excessive lateral pressure syndrome. When the patella is moved in a medial direction, it should initially remain parallel to the femur. If the medial border rides anteriorly, the patella has a dynamic tilt problem that

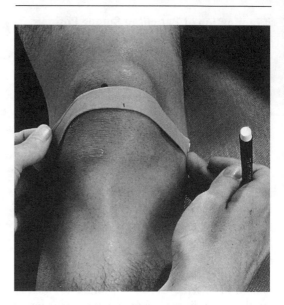

Figure 10–3 Assessment of Glide Position. The therapist can measure the distance from the middle of the patella to the medial femoral epicondyle and the lateral femoral condyle. The two distances should be equal.

indicates that the deep lateral retinacular fibers are too tight, affecting the seating of the patella in the trochlea.

When the patella is in an optimal position, it is parallel to the femur in the sagittal plane. A most common finding is a posterior displacement of the inferior pole of the patella. This results in fat pad irritation and often manifests itself as inferior patella pain, which is exacerbated by extension maneuvers of the knee (Figure 10–4). A dynamic posterior tilt problem can be determined during an active contraction of the quadriceps muscle as the inferior pole is pulled posteriorly, particularly in patients who hyperextend.

To complete the ideal position, the long axis of the patella should be parallel to the long axis of the femur. If a line is drawn between the medial and lateral poles of the patella, it should be perpendicular to the long axis of the femur. If the inferior pole is sitting lateral to the long axis of the femur, the patient has an externally rotated patella (Figure 10–5). If the inferior pole is sitting medial to the long axis of the femur, then the patient has an internally rotated patella. The

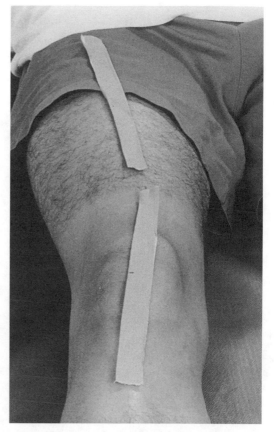

Figure 10–5 Assessment of Rotation. The long axis of the patella and the long axis of the femur should be parallel. Here the patient has an external rotation of the patella, as the inferior pole is lateral to the superior pole, relative to the line of the femur.

presence of a rotation indicates that a particular part of the retinaculum is tight. Tightness in the retinacular tissue compromises the tissue and can be a source of symptoms.

Examination of Patient in Sidelying Position

When the patient is lying on the side, the retinacular tissue can be specifically tested for elasticity. With the knee flexed to 20 degrees, the patella is moved in a medial direction. The clinician should be able to expose the lateral femoral condyle (Figure 10–6). The superficial

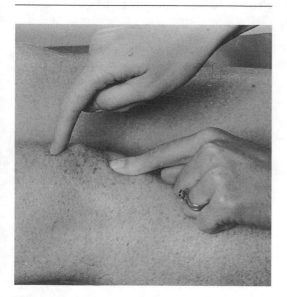

Figure 10–4 Assessment of Anteroposterior Tilt. This is determined by palpating the inferior pole of the patella and the superior pole. The soft tissue depth around each pole should be similar.

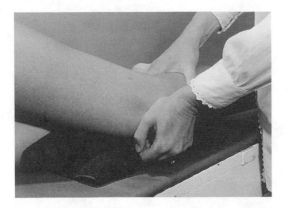

Figure 10–6 Testing the Superficial Lateral Retinacular Structures. With the patient in the sidelying position, the patella is displaced medially.

retinacular fibers are implicated if the lateral femoral condyle is not readily exposed. To test the deep fibers, the clinician places his/her hand on the middle of the patella, takes up the slack of the glide, and applies an anteroposterior pressure on the medial border of the patella. The lateral femoral condyle should move freely away from the femur, and on palpation the tension in the retinacular fibers should be similar. This test can also be used as a treatment technique.

ITB tightness may be confirmed by Ober's test. The patient lies on his/her side, with the leg that is being tested uppermost. The lower leg is flexed to stabilize the pelvis. The knee of the upper leg is flexed to 90 degrees, while the hip is abducted and slightly extended. If the ITB is of normal length, the thigh should drop to the table. However, if the band is shortened, the thigh remains abducted when the leg is released.

Examination of Patient in Prone Position

When the patient is prone, the clinician may examine the foot to determine whether the patient has a primary foot deformity that is contributing to the patellofemoral symptoms. Such a deformity should be addressed with orthotics or specific muscle training. When the patient is in the prone position, the clinician can evaluate the flexibility of the anterior hip structures by examining the patient in a figure-of-four position. This position is created when the hip being tested is abducted and externally rotated while the knee of that leg is flexed. The foot of that leg is placed underneath the other leg (which is straight) at the level of the tibial tubercle. The result is that the legs look like the figure 4. This position tests the available extension and external rotation at the hip, which is often limited because of chronic adaptive shortening of the anterior structures as a result of the underlying femoral anteversion. The distance of the anterior superior iliac spine from the table is measured, so the clinician has an objective measure of change. A modification of the test position can also be used as a treatment technique.

The quadriceps may be tested for tightness in the prone position. It will confirm the findings of the Thomas test for rectus femoris tightness. A lumbar spine palpation can be performed at this stage of the examination if the clinician believes that the knee symptoms have been referred from a primary pathology in the lumbar spine. A summary of the examination process is listed in Exhibit 10–2. Once the patellofemoral joint has been thoroughly examined and the primary problems have been identified, the patient is ready for treatment.

Exhibit 10–2 Examination Checklist

ASSESSMENT IN STANDING POSITION

Examine for biomechanical abnormalities. Observe alignment from:

1. front
   - normal standing
     –position of the feet with respect to the legs
     –Q angle
     –tibial valgum/varum
     –tibial torsion
     –talar dome position
     –navicular position
     –Morton's toe
     –hallux valgus
   - feet together
     –squinting patellae
     –vastus medialis obliquus bulk
     –vastus lateralis tension
2. side
   - pelvic position—tilt
   - hyperextension of the knees
3. behind
   - posterior superior iliac spine position
   - gluteal bulk
   - calf bulk
   - calcaneal position

DYNAMIC EVALUATION

Evaluate the effect of the bony alignment and soft tissue on the following dynamic activities:

1. walking, if no pain
2. steps, if no pain
3. squat, if no pain
4. one-leg squat

ASSESSMENT IN SUPINE POSITION

Determine the causative factors of the symptoms and formulate a diagnosis.

1. palpation of the tibiofemoral joint line and soft tissue structures of the patellofemoral joint
2. tibiofemoral tests
3. meniscal tests
4. ligament tests
5. Thomas test—psoas, rectus femoris, tensor fasciae latae
6. tests for hamstrings, gastrocnemius
7. slump test for dural length, particularly indicated if the patient complains of lateral knee pain when sitting with the legs out straight
8. hip tests (if applicable)
9. orientation of the patella
   A. glide, dynamic glide
   B. lateral tilt
   C. anteroposterior tilt
   D. rotation

ASSESSMENT IN SIDELYING POSITION

Tests for tightness of the lateral structures include the following:

1. medial glide—tests superficial lateral structures
2. medial tilt—tests deep lateral structures
3. Ober's test for iliotibial band tightness

ASSESSMENT IN THE PRONE POSITION

1. lumbar spine palpation if applicable (ie, dural test positive)
2. foot assessment
3. hip rotation
4. femoral nerve mobility

REFERENCES

1. Brukner P, Khan K. *Clinical Sports Medicine*. New York: McGraw-Hill; 1993.

2. Fulkerson J, Hungerford D. *Disorders of the Patellofemoral Joint*. 2nd ed. Baltimore: Williams & Wilkins; 1990.

3. McConnell J. Fat pad irritation—a mistaken patellar tendinitis. *Sport Health*. 1991;9(4):7–9.

4. Abernathy PJ, Townsend P, Rose R, Radin E. Is chondromalacia a separate clinical entity? *J Bone Joint Surg*. 1978;60B:205–210.

5. Stokes M, Young A. Investigations of quadriceps inhibition: implications for clinical practice. *Physiotherapy*. 1984;70:425–428.

6. Spencer J, Hayes K, Alexander I. Knee joint effusion and quadriceps reflex inhibition in man. *Arch Phys Med*. 1984;65:171–177.

7. de Andrade J, Grant C, Dixon A. Joint distension and reflex muscle inhibition in the knee. *J Bone Joint Surg*. 1965;47A:313.

8. Maitland GD. *Vertebral Manipulation*. London: Butterworths; 1986.

9. Fulkerson JP. Awareness of the retinaculum in evaluating patellofemoral pain. *Am J Sports Med*. 1982; 10:147–149.

10. Subotnik S. The foot and sports medicine. *J Orthop Sports Phys Ther*. 1980;2:53–54.

11. Root M, Orien W, Weed J. *Clinical Biomechanics*. Vol. 2. Los Angeles: Clinical Biomechanics Corp; 1977.

12. Tiberio D. The effect of excessive subtalar joint pronation on patellofemoral mechanics: a theoretical model. *J Orthop Sports Phys Ther*. 1987;9:160–165.

13. Ahmed A, Shi S, Hyder A, Chan K. The effect of quadriceps tension characteristics on the patellar tracking pattern. Transactions of the 34th Orthopaedic Research Society; Atlanta: 1988; 280.

CHAPTER 11

Conservative Management of Patellofemoral Problems

Patellofemoral conditions are usually managed successfully with conservative treatment. However, without patient compliance, progress is slow or nonexistent, as there are no "quick-fix solutions" to patellofemoral problems. Patient education is therefore one of the key factors in the management of patellofemoral pain. The patient must have a clear understanding of why the symptoms have occurred and what needs to be done to improve the symptoms. If the clinician significantly reduces the patient's symptoms during the initial visit, the patient is generally receptive to the clinician's suggestions and follows through with them—at least for a short period of time.

The aims of the conservative approach are twofold: (1) to optimize the patellar position within the trochlea so that the patient's symptoms are significantly decreased, and (2) to improve the lower limb mechanics so that the condition is less likely to recur. An optimal patellar position is achieved by stretching the tight lateral structures (the lateral retinaculum and the iliotibial band) and changing the activation pattern of the vastus medialis obliquus (VMO). The VMO centralizes the patella in the trochlea during the first 30 degrees of knee flexion. Centralization of the patella in the trochlea can be facilitated if the hip, knee, and foot are aligned in the frontal plane. This alignment should decrease the dynamic quadriceps (Q) angle and minimize excessive lateral displacement of the patella. If the clinician does not improve the patient's hip, foot, and pelvic function, and the alignment of the lower extremity remains poor, the VMO may have to function at a greater percentage of its maximum oxygen consumption ($VO_{2\ max}$) to overcome the valgus vector force created by the increased dynamic Q angle. With the VMO working at a greater percentage of its $VO_{2\ max}$, it may become more readily fatigued, so it may be difficult for a patient to remain symptom free after prolonged activities. Therefore, patellofemoral management not only must focus on improving patellar movement and control, but also must address the problems of poor pelvic and foot mechanics to enhance a long-term symptom-free period for the patient. However, the first priority in treatment should be to gain a significant reduction in the patient's symptoms.

SYMPTOM REDUCTION

Symptom reduction should be immediate and long lasting. Symptom reduction occurring for the duration of the treatment and until the patient walks into the parking lot does not inspire the patient with the confidence that the clinician has the condition under control. A strategy for minimizing the symptoms must be given to the patient, because lingering pain can be extremely tiring and depressing. One way of decreasing the patient's symptoms is to optimize the entry of the patella into the trochlea. This can be achieved by taping the patella to correct the abnormal tracking, as well as by stretching the tight retinacular structures. The therapist can massage and friction the lateral retinacular tissue to improve the mobility of the area. This procedure is usually performed when the patient is in the sidelying position, with the therapist tilting the medial border of the patella posteriorly before commencing the soft tissue work (Figure 11–1). If part of the lateral retinaculum is particularly tight and difficult to loosen, the stretching process can be helped by injecting 5 mL of local anesthetic into the tightest portions of the lateral retinaculum. Immediately following the injection, the soft tissue should be firmly massaged. To maintain the stretch of the lateral structures, the patient may be shown how to self-stretch the retinacular tissue to further decrease the lateral patellar tilt (Figure 11–2).

The proximal part of the iliotibial band (ITB)—the tensor fasciae latae (TFL)—may also be stretched. The TFL is often difficult to stretch well. Many types of stretches for the TFL/ITB have been described in the literature, which have varying degrees of success. The cli-

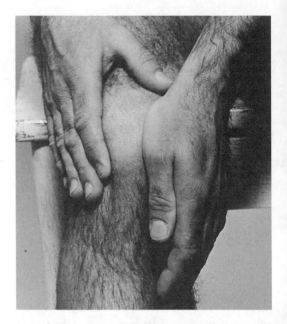

Figure 11–2 Self-Mobilization of the Deep Lateral Retinacular Tissues. While sitting, the patient tips the medial border of the patella to lift the border away from the femur. The patient uses the thenar eminence part of the hand to do this, and the other hand massages the lateral structures (moisturizer or oil must be used to lubricate the skin area). The knee is generally flexed about 60 degrees.

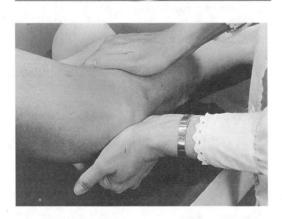

Figure 11–1 Massage of Lateral Retinacular Tissue. With the patient sidelying with the knee flexed to 30 degrees, the therapist first glides the patella medially then tilts the medial border of the patella posteriorly to stretch the deep lateral retinacular structures. The therapist faces the patient and places the elbow of the mobilizing arm into the side of the body so the mobilizing requires minimal effort on the part of the therapist. The therapist's other hand may be used to massage the tight deep structures.

nician may need to show a patient several different TFL stretches before determining the most suitable stretch for that patient.

To provide a more permanent elongation of the adaptively shortened retinacular tissue, a sustained low load is required to cause creep in the viscoelastic collagen material (ie, the soft tissue elongates over time). A number of investigators have documented that the length of soft tissues can be increased with sustained stretching.[1-4] The magnitude of the increase in displacement depends on the duration of the applied stretch; if the stretch is applied for long periods displacement increases.[3,4] It is hypothesized that the tape may enable creep to occur in the lateral structures, but only if it can be maintained for a prolonged period of time without becoming loose. A rigid, nonstretch tape made

Exhibit 11–1 Skin Problems Associated with Taping

Friction Rub

- friction on medial aspect of knee due to patella trying to move laterally and the tape pulling medially
- occurs within 1 week; becomes less of a problem as the skin toughens
- common (80% of patients experience friction rub to some extent)

Allergic Reaction

- raised, itchy rash all over the knee where the tape has been
- occurs within 1 day if there has been previous exposure; occurs after 10 days if patient not previously exposed
- rare (5% of patients experience a reaction; usually a history of skin allergy; sometimes individuals with fair skin and red hair or individuals with an Asian background have problems)

Source: Reprinted with permission from J McConnell, Problems of Patella and Other Soft Tissue Injuries, in *Athletic Injuries and Rehabilitation*, Zachazewski, McGee, and Quillen, eds, © 1996, WB Saunders.

Exhibit 11–2 Solutions for Skin Problems Associated with Taping

Friction Rub

- When taping, lift the skin on the medial aspect of the knee.
- Remove tape carefully. Peel back slowly and use the other hand to decrease the pull on the skin.
- Use a tape remover.
- Rub hand cream into medial aspect of knee once the tape is removed.
- If the skin breaks down, leave the tape off or cover with nonstick gauze and tape over that.

Allergic Reaction

- Leave tape off. Apply ice to relieve the itch.
- If severe, put cortisone cream over inflamed area.
- If possible, identify at-risk individuals. For these patients, use hypoallergenic tape alone.
- Tape for short periods of time only.

Source: Reprinted with permission from J McConnell, Problems of Patella and Other Soft Tissue Injuries, in *Athletic Injuries and Rehabilitation*, Zachazewski, McGee, and Quillen, eds, © 1996, WB Saunders.

of rayon fabric is required. This type of tape is unlike most other strapping tapes, because it is more difficult to remove from the roll due to its enhanced adhesive properties. In addition, it is more difficult to tear because the rayon fabric has some pliancy in all directions, enabling it to withstand higher stresses. As a consequence, the tape can cause the skin to break down from friction or from an allergic reaction. The skin can be protected by adequate skin preparation before applying the tape and by use of hypoallergenic tape under the rigid strapping tape. Exhibits 11–1 and 11–2 summarize skin problems associated with taping and the solutions to these problems. True allergic reaction is rare, affecting only about 5% of the patients who require patellofemoral taping. When this occurs, the entire tape area is raised and itchy. The most likely

skin problem is the friction rub, where the skin breaks down on the medial side of the knee. The skin is the intermediary between the laterally tilted patella and the medially directed firm tape. However, with adequate skin preparation, the tape can be worn for a prolonged period of time. Taping and training of the VMO to actively change the patellar position should have a significant effect on patellofemoral mechanics.

Taping the patella in patellofemoral pain syndrome sufferers has been found to do the following:

- reduce pain[5,6]
- increase the quadriceps muscle torque[7,8]
- increase eccentric quadriceps femoris muscle strength[6]

- increase tolerance to knee joint loading[5]
- provide a mechanical advantage to the quadriceps muscle[8]

The order of correction and the tension of the tape is tailored for each individual, based on the assessment of the patellar position. The worst patellar component is always corrected first, and the effect of each piece of tape on the patient's symptoms should be evaluated by reassessing the painful activity. The tape should always improve the patient's symptoms immediately. To achieve this goal, it is often necessary to correct more than one patellar component.

If the inferior pole of the patella is displaced in a posterior direction, it must be corrected first, because taping over the inferior pole of the patella will aggravate the fat pad and exacerbate the patient's pain. The tape must be placed on the superior third of the patella, either at the lateral border or in the middle of the patella so glide and/or lateral tilt are corrected at the same time as the posterior tilt. The tape should tip the inferior pole of the patella out of the fat pad (Figure 11–3).

A 5-mm lateral displacement is a significant glide problem that can be improved by placing a piece of nonstretch tape from the lateral patellar border and firmly pulling it to just past the medial femoral condyle (Figure 11–4). At the same time, the soft tissue on the medial aspect of the knee is lifted toward the patella to create a tuck or fold in the skin superomedially. This provides a more effective correction of the glide component and also minimizes the friction rub (friction between the tape and the skin), which is relatively common in patients with extremely tight lateral structures.

Patients with tight deep lateral retinacular tissue present with a laterally tilted patella and often complain of lateral knee pain. Taping from the middle of the patella to the medial femoral condyle provides some stretching to these tight structures, by lifting the lateral border of the patella anteriorly so that it is more parallel with the femur in the frontal plane (Figure 11–5). The stretching effect from the tape should be supplemented by mobilization of the deep lateral retinacular tissues as shown in Figure 11–1.

If there is an asymmetrical restriction in the mobility of the lateral retinacular structures, the patella will rotate externally if the distal fibers are tight and internally if the proximal fibers are tight. External rotation is more common; to correct this problem, the clinician pulls the tape with one hand from the inferior pole upward and

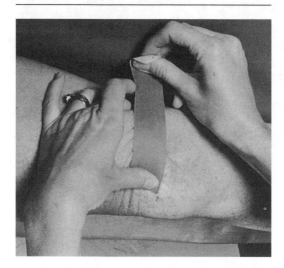

Figure 11–3 Patellar Taping. Correction of an anteroposterior tilt component of the patella involves placing tape on the superior aspect of the patella to tip the patella out of the fat pad.

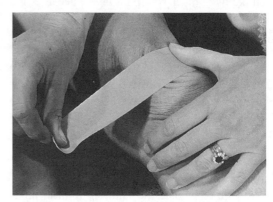

Figure 11–4 Correction of a Glide Component. Place tape on the lateral border of the patella, lift the skin on the medial side toward the patella, and pull the tape medially just short of the hamstrings tendons.

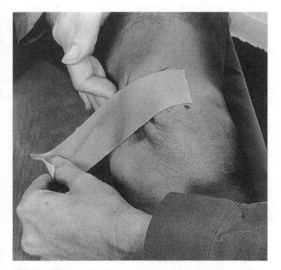

Figure 11–5 Correction of a Tilt Component. Place tape in the middle of the patella, lift the skin on the medial side toward the patella, and pull the tape medially just short of the hamstrings tendons. This tilts the lateral border of the patella away from the femur.

medially toward the opposite shoulder while the other hand rotates the superior pole laterally. Care must be taken so that the inferior pole is not displaced into the fat pad (Figures 11–6 and 11–7). Internal rotation, on the other hand, is

corrected by taping from the superior pole downward and medially.

After each piece of tape is applied, the symptom-producing activity is reassessed. The clinician's goal is at least a 50% decrease in symptoms. If this has not been achieved, further correction may be necessary with ongoing evaluation of patellar position (correction of one component may change the other components). If the clinician is unable to change the patient's symptoms at all with tape, then one of the following must be considered:

- The patient requires other tape to further unload the soft tissues.
- The tape was poorly applied.
- The assessment of patellar position was inadequate.
- The patient has other knee pathology that is inappropriate for taping.

UNLOADING

The principle of unloading is based on the premise that inflamed soft tissue does not respond well to stretching. For example, in a patient with a sprained medial collateral ligament,

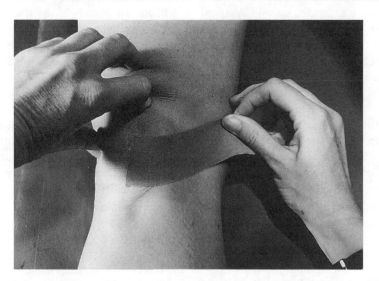

Figure 11–6 Correction of an External Rotation Component. Place tape on the inferior pole of the patella, rotate the superior pole of the patella outward, and use the tape to rotate the inferior pole inward.

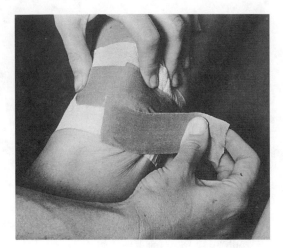

Figure 11–7 Another Correction of External Rotation. It is difficult to correct external rotation first because there is usually a lot of soft tissue slack that is taken up by correcting the other components. Rotation correction is usually one of the last components to be corrected.

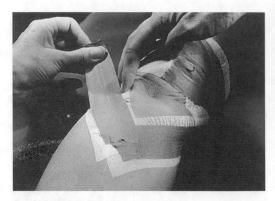

Figure 11–8 Unloading the Fat Pad. Start the tape at the tibial tubercle and lift the soft tissue toward the patella while firmly pulling the tape to the medial and lateral joint lines.

applying a valgus stress to the knee will aggravate the condition, whereas a varus stress will decrease the symptoms. The same principle applies for patients with an inflamed fat pad, an irritated ITB, or a pes anserinus bursitis. The inflamed tissue needs to be shortened or unloaded. To unload the fat pad, the tape starts at the tibial tubercle and comes out in a wide V to the medial and lateral joint lines. As the tape is being pulled toward the joint line, the skin is lifted toward the patella, thus shortening the fat pad. To unload the ITB for the treatment of iliotibial friction syndrome, a V tape is applied above and below the lateral joint line to the middle of the femur and tibia, respectively. The soft tissue is lifted toward the patella (Figure 11–8).

As well as being used to unload painful soft tissue structures, tape can be used to facilitate or inhibit a muscle contraction. This can be done by applying the tape in the direction of the muscle fibers (*facilitation*) or applying the tape across the muscle belly (*inhibition*). To unload a painful structure, the tape should shorten the inflamed or damaged soft tissue. When it is necessary to facilitate a muscle contraction, the tape

needs to shorten the muscle tissue and should be placed in the direction of the muscle fibers. To minimize excessive muscle activity, tape is placed firmly across the muscle belly.

The patient should never train with or through pain or effusion, as it has been shown quite conclusively that effusion has an inhibitory effect on muscle activity.[9–11] If the patient experiences a return of the pain, then the tape should be readjusted. If the activity is still painful, the patient must cease the activity immediately. The tape will loosen quickly if the lateral structures are extremely tight or the patient's job or sport requires extreme amounts of knee flexion. The tape should be applied each day and removed with care in the evening. This practice allows the skin time to recover.

The tape is kept on all day, every day, until the patient has learned how to activate the VMO at the right time. The tape is like training wheels on a bicycle and can be discontinued once the patient masters the skill of keeping the patella centered in the trochlea during all weight-bearing activities.

MUSCLE TRAINING

Successful management of patellofemoral conditions involves altering the activation pattern of the medial and lateral quadriceps muscles and the hip musculature (gluteals and TFL). The position of the patella in the trochlea, particularly in the first 30 degrees of knee flexion, is determined by the interaction of the VMO and vastus lateralis (VL).[12] It has been hypothesized that the VMO, which has a smaller cross-section than the VL, must receive a feed-forward enhancement of its excitation level to track the patella optimally.[13–14] Most studies on individuals with patellofemoral pain have supported this hypothesis by demonstrating that the electromyographic (EMG) activity and reflex onset time of the VMO relative to the VL is different than the ratio of activity and onset time found in asymptomatic individuals.[15–18] However, there is some controversy in the literature regarding the onset and activation pattern of the VMO and the VL in symptomatic and asymptomatic individuals.[17–19] Some of this disagreement is due to the different methodologies employed to collect and analyze the data.[17–22] Little consensus exists in the literature regarding the most appropriate computer algorithm for determining the onset of EMG activity. Methods for determining onset may vary in terms of EMG processing (low-band pass filtering at 10, 50, and 500 Hz), threshold value (1, 2, and 3 standard deviations beyond the mean of baseline activity), and the number of samples for which the mean must exceed the defined threshold (20, 50, and 100).

Gilleard and colleagues[23] recently reported that during stair ascent and descent, taping the patella of symptomatic individuals so that the symptoms were diminished by 50% altered the onset of the VMO and VL muscles such that the VMO was activated earlier and the VL was delayed. Fourteen symptomatic subjects completed a stair ascent and descent task with the affected patella untaped and taped to reduce pain symptoms by at least 50%. During step-up, VMO onset occurred significantly earlier ($F_{1,13} = 18.657$) in the movement when taped (75.71 degrees, SD 0.89) compared to the untaped condition (71.43 degrees, SD 1.19) and significantly earlier than VL onset (75.11 versus 72.54 degrees) ($F_{1,13} = 10.907$). During step-down, VMO onset occurred significantly earlier ($F_{1,13} =$

5.751) when taped (29.64 degrees, SD 1.28) compared to untaped (31.90 degrees, SD 1.30). VL onset was significantly delayed ($F_{1,13} = 15.144$) from 30.93 degrees (SD 1.98) when untaped to 36.77 degrees (SD 1.65) when taped. When taped, the VMO activated significantly earlier than the VL (29.64 versus 36.77 degrees) ($F_{1,13} = 13.043$) during step-down.

Rehabilitation must be aimed at optimizing the timing and function of the various heads of quadriceps. Improvement in the timing of the contraction of the VMO may be difficult if the VL is particularly overactive. Unless the VL can be inhibited in some way, it will be reinforced with all load-bearing activities and the VMO may not necessarily be activated; this will further increase the imbalance. It is possible to decrease the activity in the VL by using very firm tape across the muscle belly (Figure 11–9). Taping, along with the appropriate exercise program, should more effectively facilitate the VMO.

Clinicians need to be familiar with the different types of training and their effects before prescribing an exercise regimen. When prescribing exercises, clinicians should consider the issues of training and context specificity, rather than focusing on the muscle strength alone. The goal is to enhance the coordination and skill of the movement not just to improve the strength of the muscles. Strength can be defined in three ways:

1. *isometric strength*—the maximum force that can be exerted against an immovable object
2. *isotonic (concentric) strength*—the maximum weight that can be lifted
3. *isokinetic strength*—the maximum torque that can be generated against a resistance, moving at a constant velocity

However, coordinated movement requires not maximum but optimal activity so that the appropriate muscles are selected (spatial pattern) and stimulated at the right time (temporal pattern).[24] The spatial and temporal requirements in training make rehabilitation more challenging and rewarding for the clinician and patient alike.

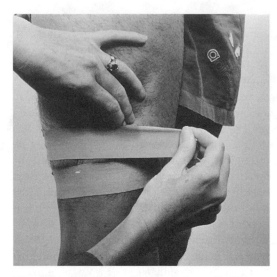

Figure 11–9 Inhibiting the Vastus Lateralis. This requires firm tape on the belly of the muscle from mid-thigh anterior lateral to mid-thigh posterior. The muscle is squashed into submission. Generally two or three pieces of tape along the thigh are required.

SPECIFICITY OF TRAINING

No longer is it sufficient simply to prescribe a series of straight-leg-raise procedures in the hope that this may decrease the patient's symptoms. Straight-leg-raise activities have no effect in preferentially activating the VMO over any of the other quadriceps muscles, regardless of the hip rotation bias.[25–26] This should not come as a surprise, because the VMO has no role in extending the knee but keeps the patella aligned in the trochlea by providing a medial force on the patella. It is this action that needs to be improved and retained in treatment—and, thus, the need for specificity in training. When considering specificity of training, the clinician must be aware that training effects are specific to the limb position; joint angle; as well as type, force, and velocity of contraction. This means that if a muscle is trained in one postural position, there will be increases in strength in that position and not in other positions. So, training the VMO with the patient supine—as in the straight-leg-raise maneuver—does not mean that the VMO

will have improved function going up and down stairs.

One of the first studies on specificity of training reported that after an 8-week isometric training program to the elbow flexors in the standing position, the participants demonstrated a significant increase in isometric elbow flexor torque in standing; however, when tested in the supine position, the study participants demonstrated relatively little increase in the isometric elbow flexor torque.[27] Isokinetic training has been found to be velocity specific; that is, if a muscle is trained at one velocity it becomes stronger at that velocity (and less so at other velocities). Rutherford and Jones reported that after 12 weeks of concentric and eccentric training, subjects recorded a mean increase of 180% in isokinetic strength, but a mean increase of only 11% in isometric strength.[28]

Training causes changes within the nervous system that allows an individual to better coordinate the activation of muscle groups. It is the clinician's responsibility to facilitate the changes within the patient's nervous system. The goal is for these changes to become automatic with practice, indicating a change in the motor program. The motor program, a predetermined set of neural commands, is controlled by the situational context where the movement is performed.[29,30]

ENVIRONMENT

The *situational context* means that a task must be considered in terms of the environment, whether the environment is moving (open skill) or stationary (closed skill).[30] An identical task has different requirements if performed in a different environment. For example, the task of standing reading a book is different if it is performed at the bus stop (closed skill) or on the bus (open skill). If one stands on the bus reading a book the same way that one stands reading at the bus stop, one will end up going through the windshield every time the bus brakes and accelerates in the traffic. The closed skill is concerned with the spatial control of the activity, whereas

the open skill has temporal requirements because the movement is externally paced and the
timing is determined by the external environment.[30] The challenge in rehabilitation is to ensure that the rehabilitation, particularly in late
stage, is designed with the appropriate environment in mind. For example, the late-stage rehabilitation of a runner with a patellofemoral problem will be quite different than that of a tennis or
basketball player who has to anticipate and be
prepared for rapid changes of direction.

However, the emphasis in the early stages of
rehabilitation should be on the timing and intensity of the VMO contraction relative to the VL.
To overcome the tendency for lateral tracking of
the patella and to ensure that the patella seats
well in the trochlea, the VMO needs to activate
slightly earlier than the VL. Biofeedback devices, particularly dual-channel devices, are
extremely useful to expedite this process
because they give patients immediate feedback
and reinforcement when the correct pattern is
achieved.[31,32] EMG biofeedback training to the
VMO has been shown to have a significant effect on the seating of the patella in the trochlea.[33]

TRAINING THE VASTUS MEDIALIS OBLIQUUS

Training the VMO needs to be very specific
and precise to be effective. The VMO, which
does not extend the knee, is not activated by the
traditional straight-leg-raise maneuvers.[25] As the
VMO arises from the tendon of the adductor
magnus[34] and is supplied in most cases by a
separate branch of the femoral nerve,[35] the therapist can emphasize adduction of the thigh to facilitate a VMO contraction. Activation of adductor magnus significantly improves the VMO
contraction in weight bearing.[36] The adductors
are rarely required to perform forcible adduction, but are essentially synergists in the complex patterns of gait activity.[37] However, in non–
weight-bearing activities, a maximal contraction
of the adductor magnus is required before facili-
tating VMO activity.[36] Certainly adduction during straight-leg-raise exercises has no effect on

VMO activation.[26] The clinician must be aware
that many patients may initially internally rotate
rather than adduct the thighs, as internal rotation
is an easier maneuver for a patient to perform
and, if the hip is flexed, the adductors promote
an internal rotation movement.

Internal rotation of the hip increases the valgus vector force at the knee and can cause an increase in patellofemoral pain. Some patients
with marked internal femoral rotation may require a stretching of the anterior hip structures to
increase their available external rotation and to
help gluteal muscles work in inner range. This is
done in the prone position with the patient's hip
externally rotated, the foot of the externally rotated leg is underneath the extended leg. The patient is instructed to push along the length of the
thigh to try to flatten the pelvis against the treatment table (Figure 11–10). If this can be
achieved, the patient is instructed to keep the
pelvis on the table while lifting the knee of the
externally rotated leg off the table. This differentiates hip movement from lumbar spine movement and works the gluteus medius muscle in inner range. If the posterior portion of the gluteus
medius muscle is working well, there is less activity in the TFL; this results in a decreased pull
on the patella by the lateral retinacular fibers
and, therefore, an enhancement of VMO activity.[38] A patient who demonstrates extremely
poor balance and a gross inability to activate the
gluteus medius requires a more permanent facilitation of the gluteals. This can be done by
taping to shorten the gluteals (Figure 11–11).
The tape stays on for about a week and usually
needs to be replaced two or three times while the
muscle is getting the idea that it actually has to
do something. During this time, the patient
needs to be fairly diligent about training the
muscle so the new program can be effective.

Because training is specific to limb position, it
is essential that the gluteus medius is mainly
trained in weight bearing. This can be done extremely effectively by asking the patient to stand
side-on to a wall. The leg closest to the wall is
flexed at the knee so the foot is off the ground,
and the hip is in a neutral position. The patient

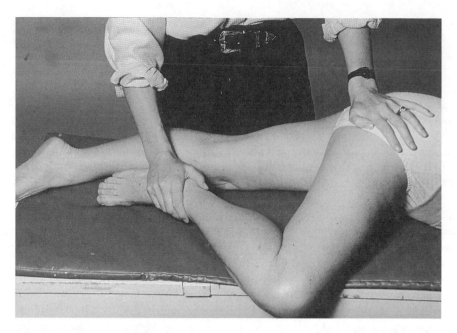

Figure 11–10 Anterior Hip Joint Structure Stretch. While the patient is prone, he or she flexes and abducts the hip so the malleolus can rest at the tibial tubercle. The patient is instructed to push along the length of the thigh to try to flatten the anterior superior iliac spine onto the table.

should have all the weight on the standing leg, which is flexed slightly. The patient externally rotates the standing leg without moving the foot or the pelvis and at the same time pushes the other leg into the wall. If the patient is doing this exercise correctly, he or she will feel a burning in the gluteus medius, especially if the contraction is sustained for at least 20 seconds (Figure 11–12). Common errors include flexing too far forward with the hips so the tension is felt in the ITB, flexing the knee too much so the quadriceps bears the brunt of the exercise, or rotating the hips so tension is felt in the back. Once the patient has felt the burning in the gluteal region, then he or she is ready for further weight-bearing training.

The therapist need not be concerned about commencing early weight-bearing activities, because with the appropriate positioning of the patella using tape, the patient should be pain-free. After all, the patient will be weight bearing when arriving for and leaving from treatment. Train-

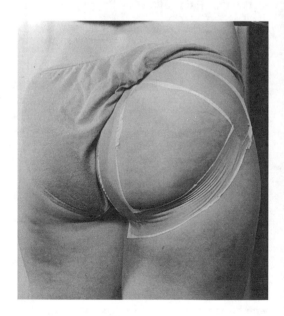

Figure 11–11 Stimulation of the Gluteals. The gluteals can be facilitated by taping the buttock so that the muscles fibers are shortened.

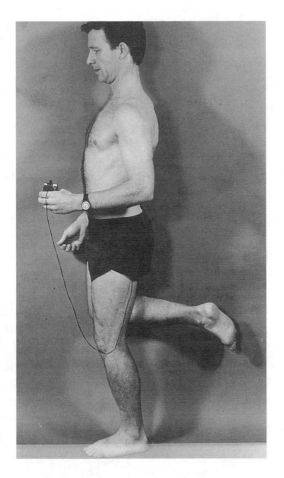

Figure 11–12 Gluteus Medius Training (Weight Bearing). The patient stands with one knee touching the wall. The lateral border of the foot of the standing leg is parallel to the wall, and the knee and the hip are in line with the foot. The knee of the standing leg is slightly flexed. The patient rotates the knee of the standing leg externally without moving the foot or the hip. A burning sensation should be felt in the gluteus medius posterior fiber region. A biofeedback device may be positioned on the gluteus medius.

ing in functional positions should accelerate recovery, as the best training is usually the carefully monitored practice of the activity itself.[1] Provided that the patient is relatively pain free in this position, a useful starting exercise is small-range knee flexion and extension movements (the first 30 degrees) in walk-stance position,

with the VMO constantly active. This position simulates the motion of the knee during the stance phase of walking and is also the position where VMO recruitment is poor and the seating of the patella in the trochlea is critical. If the patient is not pain free in the walk-stance position, small-range flexion and extension movements with the weight, either equally on both feet or partially through the symptomatic limb, should be commenced. The patient's pain may return during the course of treatment, indicating that the tape has loosened and needs readjusting. For a patient who is having difficulty contracting the VMO, muscle stimulation may be used to facilitate the contraction.

PROGRESSION OF TREATMENT

Training may be progressed from the walk-standing position to standing on one leg, where the pelvis is kept level and the lower abdominals and the glutei are worked together while the other leg is swinging back and forward, simulating the activity of the stance phase of gait. However, this does not necessarily improve the patient's ability to negotiate stairs. The patient should practice slowly stepping on and off a step, from a small height initially, in front of a mirror, so that changes in limb alignment can be observed and deviations can be corrected (Figures 11–13 and 11–14). The pelvis must remain parallel with the floor; the hip, knee, and foot should be aligned. Some patients may only be able to do one repetition before the leg deviates. This is sufficient for them to start with, as inappropriate practice can be detrimental to learning. The patient should increase the number of repetitions as the skill level improves because the VMO is a stabilizing muscle, so endurance training is the ultimate goal.[39] It is preferable for the therapist to emphasize quality, not quantity. Initially, small numbers of exercises should be performed frequently throughout the day. The aim is to achieve a carryover from functional exercises to functional activities. If a patient has been in pain for some time, there may be some habitual changes to the motor program, particularly with regard to steps. It may be necessary to teach the patient to flex the hips more when stepping off a step. This will result in a shortening of the lever arm of the quadriceps, so the knee can flex in a pain-free range during stepping. Increasing the amount of trunk flexion is suggested[40] to move the center of body mass anteriorly, placing it closer to the knee joint center and farther from the hip joint center. This decreases demand on knee extensors.

For further progression, the patient can move to a larger step, initially decreasing the number of contractions and slowly increasing them again. As the control improves, the patient can alter the speed of the stepping activity and may vary the place on descent where he or she stops going down. Weights may be introduced in the hands or in a backpack on the back. Again, the number of repetitions and the speed of the move-

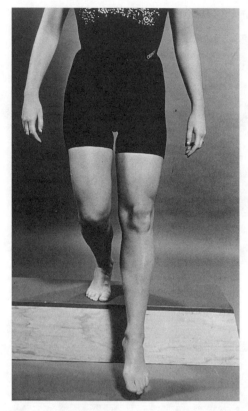

Figure 11–14 Stepping Off a Step with Adequate Pelvic Control. The hip should be parallel to the floor.

ment should be decreased initially and built back up again. Training should be applicable to the patient's activities/sport (eg, a jumping athlete should have jumping incorporated in the program). Figure-eight running, bounding, jumping off boxes, jumping and turning, and other pleometric routines are particularly appropriate for the high-performance athlete. However, the patient's VMO needs to be monitored at all times for timing and level of contraction relative to the VL. The number of repetitions performed by the patient at a training session depends upon the onset of muscle fatigue. The goal is to increase the number of repetitions that the patient can do before the onset of fatigue. Patients should be taught to recognize muscle fatigue or quivering so that they do not train through fatigue and risk exacerbating their symptoms.

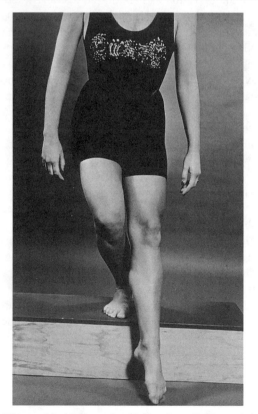

Figure 11–13 Stepping Off a Step Without Adequate Pelvic Control.

FOOT PROBLEMS

For some patients, muscle training of the hip and knee is not sufficient to control the symptoms, and management of abnormal foot posture is required. This may involve changing the way the ground sees the foot (ie, with orthotic prescription) or changing the way the foot sees the ground (ie, by mobilizing stiff joints and training specific muscles to control mobile joints).

Excessive or prolonged pronation causes an increase in the valgus vector force and hence an increase in the dynamic Q angle. The increase in pronation may be due to an intrinsic foot problem or to an external problem, such as tight hamstrings or gastrocnemius muscles. Tight hamstrings cause an increase in compensatory pronation by not allowing the knee to straighten when the foot hits the ground, especially during running; an increased amount of dorsiflexion is required to position the body over the planted foot. If the full range of dorsiflexion has already occurred at the talocrural joint, further range is achieved by pronating the foot, particularly at the subtalar joint. The full range of dorsiflexion at the talocrural joint is also affected when the gastrocnemius muscle is tight. Because 10 degrees of dorsiflexion is required during normal walking, further range can be achieved by pronating at the subtalar joint. In such cases, the excessive pronation may be corrected by stretching the tight muscles.

Intrinsic foot problems may be improved by muscle training. Patients who exhibit prolonged pronation during midstance in gait may be shown how to train the supinators of their feet. This should improve the stability of the foot for push-off and decrease the increased valgus vector force created at the knee by the abnormal foot pronation. The position of training is midstance. The patient is instructed to lift the arch while keeping the great toe on the ground, and then pushing the first metatarsal and great toe into the ground. The rationale behind this exercise is that if the base of the first metatarsal is lifted using the tibialis posterior muscle, the line of action of the peroneus longus is improved. The peroneus longus can then efficiently act on the first metatarsal and improve the stability of the first ray in preparation for push-off.[41] Tape may be used to facilitate the muscle activity and stabilize the unstable midfoot. The tape should dorsiflex and abduct the navicular to resupinate the midfoot (Figure 11–15). If the patient also has a stiff subtalar joint and is lacking the initial pronation required on heel strike, the clinician can mobilize the calcaneus (Figure 11–16). At the conclusion of treatment, tape may be applied to provide a constant low load on the calcaneus to increase the eversion at the joint (Figure 11–17). Tape may also be used to improve the stability of push-off by changing the line of action of the first metatarsophalangeal joint. This involves putting the first ray in a neutral position (Figure 11–18) but may also involve correcting a hallux valgus deformity, with the tape providing a gentle pull on the great toe to correct the malposition (Figure 11–19).

If the patient is unable to keep the first metatarsophalangeal joint on the ground when training the tibialis posterior muscle, then the foot deformity is too large to correct with training alone. Orthotics will be necessary to control the excessive pronation. See Chapter 13 for a more detailed explanation of orthotic prescription and fabrication.

WEANING FROM TAPE

The patient needs to wear the tape until the muscles have been endurance trained. This may take a considerable time for some individuals. The following is a suggested test sequence to determine if the patient is ready to be without the tape for daily activities:

1. 5 sets of 10 steps performed slowly and controlled with a 10-second rest between each set
2. 1-minute quarter squat against the wall
3. 1-minute half squat against the wall
4. an additional 5 sets of 10 continuous steps

The VMO and VL are monitored at all times. Deterioration in VMO activity relative to VL in-

A   B

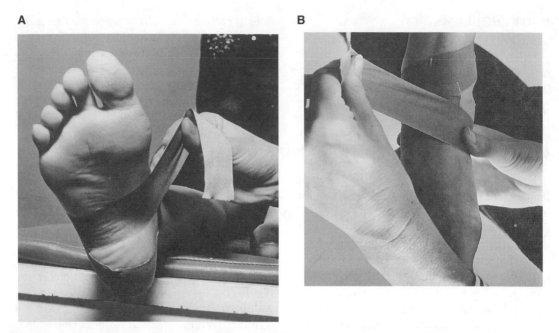

Figure 11–15 Correction of a Pronated Foot. (**A**) Begin taping on the top of the foot, coming laterally to the posterior surface, then progress medially on the sole of the foot to the navicular. (**B**) Correction of a midfoot collapse can be achieved by lifting the navicular up and back.

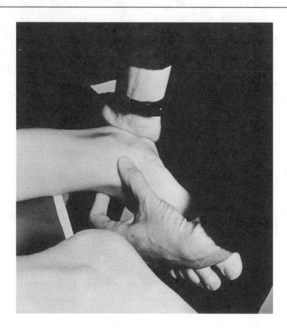

Figure 11–16 Mobilization of a Stiff Subtalar Joint. The patient is in the sidelying position, and the foot is held in dorsiflexion to simulate walk-standing. The clinician stabilizes the tibia with a seat belt or his or her leg and stabilizes the talus with the nonmobilizing hand. The calcaneus is everted during the mobilizing technique. This is an end-of-range procedure.

A

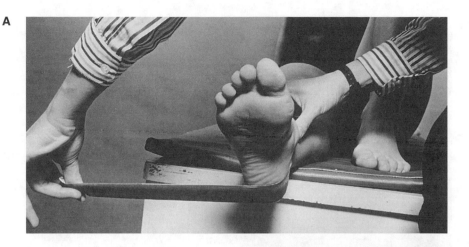

B

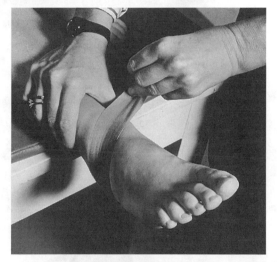

Figure 11–17 Taping To Increase the Range of Eversion Movement at the Calcaneus. (**A**) Tape is placed on the medial aspect of the calcaneus. The calcaneus is everted strongly. (**B**) Tape is anchored across the talocrural joint but should not interfere with movement at that joint.

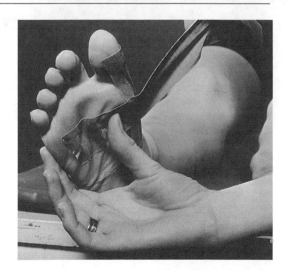

Figure 11–18 Taping To Improve the Stability of Push-Off. The first metatarsal head is dorsiflexed and interally rotated to aid push-off.

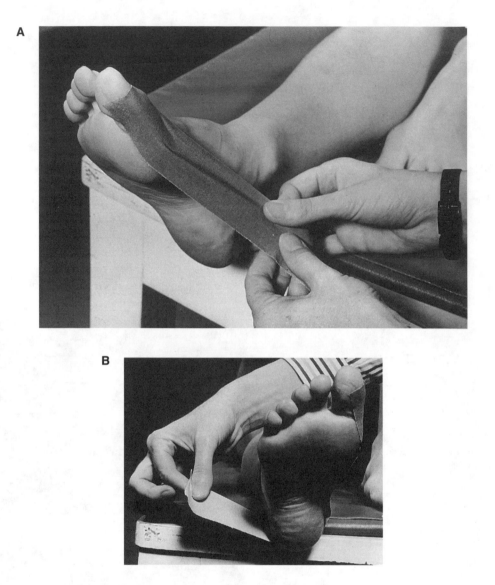

Figure 11–19 Correction of a Hallux Valgus Deformity. (**A**) Place tape distal to the interphalangeal joint of the great toe and (**B**) pull tape around to the fifth metatarsal. The amount of tension on the tape depends upon the amount of correction required and the amount of discomfort experienced when the toe is repositioned. It is often better to achieve a gradual change in position rather than attempt a full correction in one session.

dicates that the tape is not ready to come off. If the tape is ready to come off, then the patient should wear the tape on alternate days for 1 week. If the knee has survived that week with no recurrence of symptoms, the patient may take the tape off for daily activities. However, the pa-

tient should keep the tape on for sports. In some instances, the patient should apply fresh tape after sports, as the muscle is fatigued and the old tape has become loose. At this time, the patellofemoral joint is extremely vulnerable and symptoms may return. If the patient has been pain free for a month and is not taped for daily activities, the tape may be removed for sports, provided that the patient is able to complete the test described above without tape and without pain.

CONCLUSION

The need for surgery has almost been eliminated due to the improved understanding of the etiology of patellofemoral pain, the use of tape to reduce the symptoms, and the specific training of the VMO and the gluteals to change lower limb alignment. However, patient instruction and muscle training must be specific; otherwise, the patient's recovery is protracted and not sustained. If the patient fails a thorough conservative management program, appropriate surgery, followed by precise rehabilitation, is indicated to expedite recovery.

REFERENCES

1. Herbert R. Human strength adaptations: implications for therapy. In: Crosbie J, McConnell J, eds. *Key Issues in Musculoskeletal Physiotherapy.* Oxford, England: Butterworth-Heinemann; 1993.

2. Hooley C, McCrum N, Cohen R. The visco-elastic deformation of the tendon. *J Biomech.* 1980;13:521.

3. Taylor D, Dalton J, Seaber A. Visco-elastic properties of muscle-tendon units: the biomechanical effect of stretching. *Am J Sports Med.* 1990;18:300.

4. McKay-Lyons M. Low-load, prolonged stretch in treatment of elbow flexion contractures secondary to head trauma: a case report. *Phys Ther.* 1989;69:292.

5. Powers CM, Landel R, Sosnick T, Mengel K, et al. The effects of patellar taping on knee motion and stride characteristics in subjects with patellofemoral pain. In: *Proceedings of the 12th International Congress of the World Confederation for Physical Therapy.* Washington, DC; 1995:PL-RR-0913.

6. Sackos DT, Bilowith KL, Hurlburt M, Haskvitz EM. The effects of the McConnell taping technique on strength and pain in subject with symptoms of patellofemoral pain syndrome. In: *Proceedings of the 12th International Congress of the World Confederation for Physical Therapy.* Washington, DC; 1995:PO-RR-0238.

7. Conway A, Malone T, Conway P. Patellar alignment/ tracking alteration: effect on force output and perceived pain. *Isokinetics Exercise Sci.* 1992;2:9–17.

8. McConnell J. Promoting effective segmental alignment. In: Crosbie J, McConnell J, eds. *Key Issues in Musculoskeletal Physiotherapy.* Oxford, England: Butterworth-Heinemann; 1993.

9. de Andrade J, Grant C, Dixon A. Joint distension and reflex muscle inhibition in the knee. *J Bone Joint Surg.* 1965;47A:313.

10. Spencer J, Hayes K, Alexander I. Knee joint effusion and quadriceps reflex inhibition in man. *Arch Phys Med.* 1984;65;171–177.

11. Stokes M, Young A. Investigations of quadriceps inhibition: implications for clinical practice. *Physiotherapy.* 1984;70:425–428.

12. Fulkerson J, Hungerford D. *Disorders of the Patellofemoral Joint.* 2nd ed. Baltimore: Williams & Wilkins; 1990.

13. Wickiewicz T, Roy R, Powell P, Edgerton V. Muscle architecture of the human lower limb. *Clin Orthop Rel Res.* 1983;179:275–283.

14. Grabiner M, Koh T, Draganich L. Neuromechanics of the patellofemoral joint. *Med Sci Sports Exerc.* 1994;26:10–21.

15. Mariani P, Caruso I. An electromyographic investigation of subluxation of the patella. *J Bone Joint Surg.* 1979;61:169–171.

16. Perez PL, Gossman MR, Lechner D, Stephenson SX, et al. Electromyographic temporal characteristics of the vastus medialis oblique and the vastus lateralis in women with and without patellofemoral pain. In: *Proceedings of the 12th International Congress of the World Confederation for Physical Therapy.* Washington, DC; 1995:PO-RR-0239-T.

17. Voight M, Weider D. Comparative reflex response times of the vastus medialis and the vastus lateralis in normal subjects and subjects with extensor mechanism dysfunction. *Am J Sports Med.* 1991;10:131–137.

18. Witvrouw E, Sneyers C, Lysens R, T' Jonck L, et al. Comparative reflex response times of vastus medialis obliquus and vastus lateralis in normal subjects and subjects with patellofemoral pain syndrome. *J Orthop Sports Phys Ther.* 1996; 24:160–165.

19. Karst G, Willett G. Onset timing of electromyographic activity in the vastus medialis oblique and vastus lateralis muscles in subjects with and without patellofemoral pain syndrome. *Phys Ther.* 1995;75: 813–822.

20. Di Fabio RP. Reliability of computerized surface electromyography for determining the onset of muscle activity. *Phys Ther.* 1987;67:43–48.

21. Enoka R, Fuglevand A. Neuromuscular basis of the maximum voluntary force capacity of muscle. In: Grabiner M, ed. *Current Issues in Biomechanics*. Champaign, IL: Human Kinetics; 1993:215–236.

22. Hodges P, Bui B. A comparison of computer based onset determination methods. *J Electroencephalogr Clin Neurophysiol*. 1996;101:511–519.

23. Gilleard W, McConnell J, Parsons D. The effect of patellar taping on the onset of vastus medialis obliquus and vastus lateralis in patellofemoral pain syndrome. *Phys Ther*. (In press.)

24. Brooks V. Motor control. *Phys Ther*. 1983;63:664–673.

25. Soderberg G, Cook T. An electromyographic analysis of quadriceps femoris muscle setting and straight leg raising. *Phys Ther*. 1983;63:1434–1438.

26. Karst G, Jewett P. Electromyographic analysis of exercises proposed for differential activation of medial and lateral quadriceps femoris components. *Phys Ther*. 1993;73:286–295.

27. Rasch PJ, Moorehouse LE. Effect of static and dynamic exercises on muscular strength and hypertrophy. *J Appl Physiol*. 1957;11:29.

28. Rutherford O, Jones D. The role of learning and coordination in strength training. *Eur J Appl Physiol*. 1986; 55:100.

29. Singer R. *Motor Learning and Human Performance: An Application to Motor Skills and Movement Behaviors*. New York: Macmillan; 1980.

30. Gentile A. Skill acquisition: action, movement and neuromotor processes. In: Carr J et al, eds, *Foundations for Physical Therapy in Rehabilitation*. Gaithersburg, MD: Aspen Publishers; 1987:93–154.

31. Wild J, Franklin T, Woods GW. Patellar pain and quadriceps rehabilitation: an EMG study. *Am J Sports Med*. 1982;10:12.

32. Le Veau B, Rogers C. Selective training of the vastus medialis muscle using EMG biofeedback. *Physiotherapy*. 1980;60:1410–1415.

33. Ingersoll C, Knight K. Patellar location changes following EMG biofeedback or progressive resistive exercises. *Med Sci Sports Exerc*. 1991;23:1122–1127.

34. Bose K, Kanagasuntherum R, Osman M. Vastus medialis oblique: an anatomical and physiologic study. *Orthopedics*. 1980;3:880–883.

35. Lieb F, Perry J. Quadriceps function. *J Bone Joint Surg*. 1968;50A:1535–1548.

36. Hodges P, Richardson C. An investigation into the effectiveness of hip adduction in the optimization of the vastus medialis oblique contraction. *Scand J Rehab Med*. 1993;25:57–62.

37. Williams P, Warwick R. *Gray's Anatomy*. London: Churchill Livingstone; 1980.

38. Sahrmann S. The movement system balance theory: relationship to musculoskeletal pain syndromes. 1991. Unpublished research.

39. Richardson CA, Bullock MI. Changes in muscle activity during fast alternating flexion and extension movements of the knee. *Scand J Rehab Med*. 1986;18:51–58.

40. Durand A, Richards C, Malouin F, Bravo G. Motor recovery after arthroscopic partial meniscectomy. *J Bone Joint Surg*. 1993;75A:202–213.

41. Root M, Orien W, Weed J. *Clinical Biomechanics*. Vol. 2. Los Angeles: Clinical Biomechanics Corp; 1977.

CHAPTER 12

Surface Electromyography and Patellofemoral Dysfunction

OVERVIEW

Surface electromyography (SEMG) is the recording of muscle action potentials with skin surface electrodes. Intervention with SEMG has emerged as a popular topic in educational programs, and several controversies exist in the literature. This chapter reviews uses of SEMG for pain syndromes associated with faulty patellar alignment and tracking, here termed *patellofemoral pain syndrome* (PFPS). The concept of SEMG is introduced first, followed by review of uses of SEMG to discriminate patients from control subjects and investigate presumed motor control imbalances between the vastus medialis (VM) and vastus lateralis (VL). Exercises purported to have selective training effects on the VM are reviewed, and attempts to facilitate motor learning and rehabilitation with SEMG feedback are discussed. Case histories and a practical application guide are included to integrate clinical concepts.

SEMG BACKGROUND*

Motor activity is subserved by commands that are generated in the central nervous system and transmitted along alpha motor neurons to the periphery. Following chemical transmission across the neuromuscular junction, action potentials are produced along the sarcolemma, and electrical excitation becomes coupled to sarcomere shortening via complex chemical and micromechanical processes. Fundamentally, electrodes placed in the vicinity of excitable membranes will detect action potential events. SEMG electrodes detect the algebraic sum of voltages associated with muscle action potentials within their detection zone.[1] The SEMG signal represents the relative level of recruitment of an ensemble of motor units that underlay the electrodes.

Basics of the SEMG system have been described for clinicians in numerous sources.[1–6] Electrodes are usually in the shape of 0.5 to 1.0 cm discs coated with silver-silver chloride. Some SEMG configurations require a paste or gel to be placed as a conductive medium between the electrode detection surfaces and the skin, whereas others can be used "dry." Each recording channel is composed of two active electrodes and a reference electrode. Active electrodes tend to be spaced with their centers 1.0 to 3.0 cm apart. The difference in electrical charge between each active electrode and the reference makes for inputs to a differential amplifier with high input impedance (Figure 12–1). One of the amplifier input signals is inverted. This process has the effect of canceling elements of the signal that are common to both inputs (typically unwanted noise and artifacts) and passing muscle

This chapter is adapted from GS Kasman, JR Cram, and SL Wolf, *Clinical Applications in Surface Electromyography: Chronic Musculoskeletal Pain*, pp 363–401, © 1998, Aspen Publishers, Inc.

*This section is adapted from GS Kasman, *Surface EMG in Physical Medicine*, © 1990, Movement Systems.

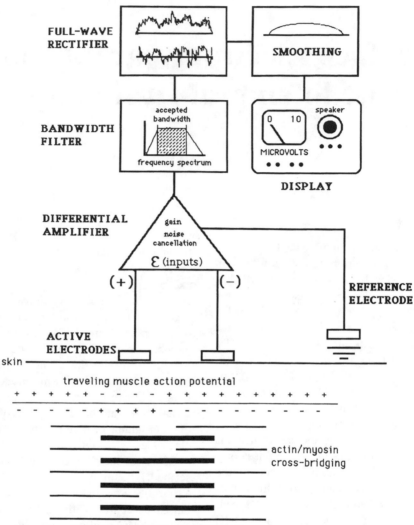
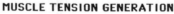

Figure 12–1 Schematic of a Basic Surface Electromyographic Recording System. Muscle action potentials travel along the sarcolemma, leading ultimately to actin/myosin cross-bridging and tension generation. Electrodes placed on the skin detect a voltage sum that results from the muscle action potentials of many motor units. Theoretically, electrical noise in the environment generates the same signal components at both of the active inputs of a differential amplifier. The differential amplifier sums inputs, one of which is made negative and the other positive, so that commonalities are canceled (conceptually, the sum of +1 and –1 is 0). Muscle action potentials cause a slightly different signal to be input at each of the positive and negative inputs, and a representative muscle signal is separated from noise. The amplifier boosts the small muscle voltage signal, providing gain with fidelity, to form an output capable of driving an electrical display of some sort. A bandwidth filter next passes frequencies that are associated with muscle activity and rejects frequencies associated with noise and artifacts. Typically, a full-wave rectifier "flips up" the bottom half of the alternating plus-minus waveform to ease inspection. The signal may also be smoothed to make it less "jumpy" for patient feedback. Contemporary SEMG systems that interface with a personal computer may skip the latter two steps. Finally, the representative muscle signal can be displayed with a variety of visual graphics and auditory arrays. *Source:* Reprinted with permission from GS Kasman, *Surface EMG in Physical Medicine,* © 1990, Movement Systems.

voltage components for amplification. The signal is next subjected to frequency bandpass filtering to enhance the signal-to-noise ratio. Surface voltages resulting from muscle action potentials can be decomposed into a specific frequency spectrum. Filters are used to pass frequencies related to muscle activity and to reject frequencies that are associated with noise. The SEMG signal may sometimes be processed further to ease interpretation of a visual or auditory display. Processing often includes full-wave rectification so that the plus-minus variations of the waveform are converted into a unidirectional signal. Several methods exist to smooth the peaks and valleys of the rectified waveform to ease inspection as well as to quantify the amplitude of the processed muscle signal.

Amplitude analyses are conducted to evaluate the magnitude and timing of muscle activity. Inferences are drawn regarding a muscle's role in effecting a particular posture or movement and how that role is altered by pathologic processes. The SEMG activity of a homologous muscle pair or that of an agonist, compared with its antagonists or synergists, is examined to assess muscle balance. Imbalance occurs when the relative stiffness of muscles that participate in concert to execute a specific movement is inappropriately coordinated.[7] Muscle imbalance is presumably a function both of faulty central nervous system motor control and of peripheral factors such as inefficient length-tension relationships and passive myofascial compliance. SEMG studies may therefore provide insight into the active component of muscle imbalance and can be linked by clinicians to the results of physical examination. Untoward motor programming may be influenced by nociception, perception, affect, beliefs, metabolic and nutritional issues, segmental and suprasegmental motor reflexes, sympathetically mediated reflexes, and a host of factors related to articular function and periarticular connective tissues. Analysis with SEMG can help clinicians to identify relationships between muscle impairments and other physical and psychologic impairments. Classification of impairments with observed functional limitations and disabilities can then

be used to drive treatment planning in a thoughtful way.[8] The effects of specific treatment procedures on muscle dysfunction also can be objectively verified, quantified, and documented with SEMG. Examination of SEMG amplitudes has been described for intervention with a wide variety of musculoskeletal disorders.[3,7]

Clinically less common than amplitude analyses, investigation of the frequency composition of SEMG signals is performed to study muscular fatigue. The frequency spectrum of the SEMG signal shifts in a reliable way with fatigue.[1] That is, the frequency spectrum becomes compressed toward slower values due to neuromuscular and metabolic changes associated with high-intensity isometric contractions. The shift begins as the contractions are sustained beyond a short time, preceding the actual loss of force, and continues as force declines. This means of fatigue monitoring may have certain advantages over other measures[9] and discriminates spinal pain patients from control subjects with impressive accuracy.[10–12]

A common use for the SEMG display, in addition to clinical and kinesiological evaluations, is to provide patients with feedback for motor learning.[7] Muscle cues produced by the SEMG device are far richer than those derived from a subject's intrinsic sensory apparatus. Initially, a patient may have little idea how to change the activity of a muscle that is not under intuitive voluntary control. The patient may not possess a suitable motor programming scheme to achieve the goal (for example, increased activation of one muscle relative to another) and may have difficulty distinguishing correct performance from error. Cues on the SEMG display are obvious and serve as a reference of correctness. Thus, the patient is able to evaluate various motor strategies for those that meet the goal. Successful strategies are repeated, and ineffective strategies are discarded. The patient identifies a progressively smaller subset of effective motor behaviors over time. SEMG feedback is used cognitively to label subtle intrinsic sensations as indicative of changes in muscle activity. Through the repeated association of artificial, extrinsic cues from the SEMG machine with natural kinesthetic sensations, an intrinsic reference of correctness is formed. The learner forms mature sensory identification and motor programming schema, and can then achieve the goal independently.

SEMG techniques offer distinct conveniences compared with other means of muscle monitoring. The methods are noninvasive and painless. Hence, use of SEMG tends to be readily accepted by patients and is generally quite safe. Although lead wires are used to connect the electrodes with the main instrument body (telemetry systems can be substituted if necessary), patients routinely are free to assume any position that is desired, including those for functional tasks. Recordings are feasible where dynamometers would be impractical, for example with in vivo discrimination of VM and VL functions. The SEMG display resolves changes in the magnitude and timing of muscle activity with far greater sensitivity than a clinician's or patient's eyes and hands. An entire range of activity levels can be captured for inspection, from voltages associated with activation of one or a few motor units to maximal effort recruitment. Within certain limits, the activity of particular muscles or muscle groups can be isolated. Setup becomes facile once the practitioner is experienced.

Technological advances have enabled commercial SEMG units to be miniaturized for ambulatory recordings of one to four channels of muscle activity. Patients can perform functional activities for a protracted time and the resultant SEMG data downloaded for analysis. Portable units are easily incorporated into therapeutic exercise programs in the clinic gym or prescribed for home programs. Commercial systems that incorporate a desktop computer are capable of simultaneous recordings from eight or more channels; sophisticated statistical processing of amplitude, timing, and frequency variables; and a plethora of options for patient feedback. Software engineers continue to develop more powerful products while exploiting graphical user interfaces so that operation becomes simpler. Manufacturers and vendors are able to deliver SEMG products to consumers with a cost value

that outstrips the pricing of earlier models. Like any other clinical agent, SEMG has limitations. Discussion of these qualifying factors is deferred to later in this chapter, after a context is set for SEMG approaches with PFPS.

SEMG AND THE PATELLOFEMORAL JOINT

Kinesiologic electromyographic studies of knee musculature have been conducted since the 1940s.[1] Muscles of the knee that are accessible for SEMG recordings include the rectus femoris, VM and VL components of the quadriceps, hamstrings—consisting of the lateral biceps femoris and medial semimembranosus/semitendinosus group—and gastrocnemius. The tensor fasciae latae can be selected for recording on the basis of its action at the knee through the iliotibial band and the relationship of the iliotibial band to the lateral retinaculum of the knee.[13] The sartorius, gracilis, adductor longus, adductor magnus, adductor brevis, and gluteal muscles contribute less directly to knee function. They are less often related to knee pathology evaluated with SEMG, although they bring about balanced muscle function throughout the lower extremity kinetic chain.

Elaborate synergistic and antagonistic relationships exist among all these muscles. For example, the VM and VL function synergistically to produce knee extension in the sagittal plane, but act antagonistically on the patella in the frontal plane. With the exception of the vastus muscles, each muscle's action crosses either the hip or ankle in addition to the knee. The ankle, knee, and hip form a closed kinetic chain when the foot is weight bearing on the ground; movement at one joint produces or constrains motion at the other joints. Ground reaction forces generated during stance are transmitted throughout the kinetic chain and met by the coordinated action of the uniarticular and biarticular musculature. When the lower extremity is engaged in the swing phase of gait, muscles acting on the knee must again contract in a manner that coordinates with hip and ankle control. Thus, motor programs must be implemented that regulate flex-ion-extension of the knee in a way that reconciles control of all joints of the lower-extremity kinetic chain.

Exhaustive discussion of the roles of lower-extremity musculature in control of the patellofemoral joint is beyond the scope of this chapter. The remainder of the chapter focuses on the quadriceps as the primary driver of the extensor mechanism and its dynamic influences on patellar alignment. This emphasis mirrors that of the existing clinical literature with SEMG. However, it is recognized that some clinicians perceive muscular imbalances involving the tensor fasciae latae and hamstrings as contributing to PFPS. In these cases, inappropriate dominance of the tensor fasciae latae or hamstrings (each relative to the quadriceps or its components) may result in untoward dissipation of the patellofemoral joint reaction force. Suspicions for these problems may be raised by observations of hamstring or tensor fasciae latae hypertrophy (often in conjunction with relatively diminished gluteal bulk), evidence of decreased extensibility with passive length tests for these muscles, and findings of hypomobility on accessory gliding of the patella. The interested reader is referred elsewhere for broad discussion of SEMG intervention with syndromes involving the tensor fasciae latae and hamstrings.[7]

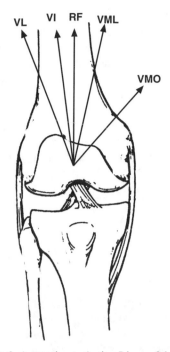

Figure 12–2 Approximate Action Lines of the Components of the Quadriceps. Vastus lateralis (VL), vastus intermedius (VI), rectus femoris (RF), vastus medialis longus (VML), and vastus medialis obliquus (VMO). *Source:* Reprinted from GS Kasman, JR Cram, and SL Wolf, *Clinical Applications in Surface Electromyography: Chronic Musculoskeletal Pain*, p 367, © 1998, Aspen Publishers, Inc.

Role of the VM and VL

The quadriceps femoris muscle acts in a concentric fashion to extend the knee and in an eccentric manner to decelerate knee flexion. The four components of the quadriceps—the VM, VL, vastus intermedius, and rectus femoris—act together to produce a knee extension moment. Each component generates tension with a particular magnitude and direction (Figure 12–2). The resultant force vector tends to displace the patella laterally as knee extension forces are created,[14,15] and this effect is in part attributable to the line of pull of the VL.[15] Lateral displacement of the patella is resisted by congruency of the lateral aspect of the patella with the lateral femoral condyle,[14] medial retinaculum,[16] medial patellofemoral and patellotibial ligaments,[16–18] and distal portion of the VM.[14,15,19,20]

Contrary to early descriptions, surface and intramuscular EMG studies have demonstrated that the VM is active throughout knee extension range of motion.[1,21,22] Along with the rest of the quadriceps, the VM is most active at terminal range during active knee extension in sitting and at the nadir of a closed-chain squat, with more activity displayed during the concentric than in the eccentric phase.[1,23] In contrast to the phasic action of the rectus femoris, and to a lesser extent to that of the VL, the VM is tonically active during rapid flexion-extension movements of the knee.[24]

On the basis of anatomic, physiologic, and mechanical criteria,[15,19,25] as well as of innervation and perhaps morphologic characteristics,[26] the VM can be functionally classified into two distinct portions. The proximal component, or vastus medialis longus, acts with a fiber orientation of 15 to 18 degrees medially from the longitudinal femoral axis, mechanically contributes to knee extension, and may share a common spinal and peripheral innervation with that of the vastus intermedius. The distal portion, or vastus medialis obliquus (VMO), is so named for its oblique fiber orientation of 40 to 60 degrees.[14,15] Fibers of the VMO originate from the adductor magnus tendon, medial intermuscular septum, and adductor longus tendon.[19,26] These fibers insert onto the patella and medial retinaculum, and superficially onto the rectus femoris tendon. The spinal and peripheral innervations of the VMO are distinct from that of the vastus medialis longus.[26] It is likely that the VMO does not contribute directly to knee extension torque, and its activity is not required to effect the "screw home" mechanism of the knee at terminal extension.[15] Rather, the VMO provides dynamic medial stabilization of the patella and is believed to be of primary importance in resisting lateral patellar displacement.[15,17,20] Some studies have targeted the VMO, whereas others have investigated the VM generally or have not specified the precise portion of the muscle tested. Through the remainder of this chapter, the designation VM will be used when reviewing literature unless the investigators reported specifically that they included the VMO.

The fibers of the VL attach to the patella at an angle between 12 and 15 degrees; unlike the rectus femoris, vastus intermedius, or vastus medialis longus, VL fibers are capable of direct lateral displacement of the patella.[15] Thus, these four muscles act synergistically to extend the knee, and the unique role of the VMO is to function as an antagonist to the lateral force of the VL. By balancing patellar tracking, the VMO increases the mechanical efficiency of the VL as a knee extensor[15] and reduces lateral patellar loading.[20] The capacities of VL and VMO to produce frontal plane forces are determined by their respective insertion locations on the patella, angles of fiber insertion, cross-sectional dimensions, morphologic characteristics, and properties relating to active neuromuscular recruitment. In addition to the anatomic differences discussed above, the cross-sectional area of the VL exceeds that of the VM, and a moderately greater proportion of type II fibers is found in the VL than in the VM.[27] It is obvious that a complex interplay of dynamic and passive factors contributes to balanced patellar tracking.

The quadriceps components, specifically including the VM, are reflexively inhibited by pain and joint effusion,[28,29] the effects being greater at terminal extension.[30] Spencer and colleagues[31] showed that the VM is inhibited after a saline injection of 20 to 30 mL into the knee joint space, whereas an injection of 50 to 60 mL is required to reach the threshold for reflex inhibition for the VL and rectus femoris. Some clinicians have suggested that the VMO atrophies first and is last to be rehabilitated.[32] Others[15] have argued that the prominence of the VMO is more apparent because of its thinner fascial covering and fiber obliquity, and that VMO atrophy simply reflects generalized quadriceps muscle weakness.

SEMG Discrimination of VMO:VL Function

SEMG is an attractive tool for clinicians in identifying VMO insufficiency. Because clinicians lack a practical way of isolating the force contributions of VMO and VL, and also lack a simple, reliable means of assessing patellofemoral kinematics, SEMG adds a unique dimension of information to the evaluation process. Recording with SEMG allows for relatively quick, low-cost assessment and collection of objective data regarding muscle function. If PFPS is truly a multifactorial problem, and if quadriceps insufficiency can be confidently ruled in or out for particular patients by analysis with SEMG, treatment might be directed to meet the specific needs of each patient. Insufficiency of the quadriceps or its components could be a contributory factor for some patients and not others. Patients who have PFPS with VMO insufficiency might need to work on VMO strengthening or improved motor control timing. Other patients might show depressed VMO as well as VL activity and participate in a program for general quadriceps conditioning. Alternatively, patients might demonstrate normal quadriceps function but presumably faulty lower-extremity kinetic chain mechanics and passive tightness. In an era of cost containment, SEMG assessment can help to assign the greatest resource value to each patient.

Results of early work with both surface and intramuscular electrodes established that VM and VL EMG activity tends to be relatively balanced in timing and magnitude during knee extension in healthy subjects.[1,21,30,33,34] Findings of other studies specifically targeting the VMO and VL were similar, with synchrony and symmetry of one muscle's recruitment relative to the other during routine quadriceps contraction.[22,35–48] Taken together, these investigations argue for similar VMO and VL EMG patterns as the norm. The investigators used a variety of recording techniques and quantification methods. Isometric, concentric, and eccentric quadriceps contractions were tested throughout joint range of motion, and many different open- and closed-kinetic-chain conditions were included.

Another methodologic approach has been to generate a mathematical ratio of VMO and VL EMG activity. This method has intuitive appeal as a basis for standardized patient and exercise comparisons, and it has been adopted by a number of investigators. Integrated or root-mean-square SEMG amplitude scores have been used most commonly to produce VMO:VL ratios.

Several groups have published results for healthy subjects. Souza and Gross[49] reported normalized VMO:VL SEMG amplitude ratios during 25% of maximal-volitional-effort isometric knee extension in sitting, stair ascent, and stair descent. SEMG ratios for VMO:VL function were approximately 1.0 ± 0.2, 1.1 ± 0.4, and 1.2 ± 0.2, respectively, or about 1.1 ± 0.3 overall across the three conditions. Cuddeford and associates[50] studied stationary bike, single-leg quarter squat, step-up, isometric quadriceps setting, straight leg raising, and short-arc knee extension exercises by using normalized VMO:VL activity ratios. SEMG ratios ranged from approximately 0.7 ± 0.5 (straight leg raising) to 1.2 ± 0.4 (bike) and averaged about 1.1 ± 0.4 across closed-chain exercises and 0.8 ± 0.4 across open-chain exercises. Karst and Jewett[25] used normalized data to calculate VMO:VL ratios ranging from approximately 0.8 ± 0.2 to 1.0 ± 0.1 during maximal-effort quadriceps setting and several submaximal variations of quadriceps setting plus straight leg raising. Kasman and colleagues[51] generated normalized VMO:VL activity ratios from subjects positioned in recumbent sitting as a function of isometric contraction intensity. VMO:VL ratios increased significantly as contraction intensity decreased, with ratio values ranging from approximately 0.8 ± 0.2 to 1.2 ± 0.5. Zakaria and associates[52] investigated maximal-effort quadriceps setting with ankle dorsiflexion in supine and maximal-effort hip adduction in supine, finding normalized VMO:VL activity ratios of about 1.0 and 0.9, respectively. Average SEMG activity ratios for VMO and VL derived from nonnormalized data have been reported at a similar level,[52–57] somewhat higher,[58,59] or somewhat lower,[49] although the range tends to be greater than that reported with normalized data. Normalized amplitude comparisons generated from fine-wire EMG recordings during a large number of knee extension exercises produced VMO:VL ratios ranging from 1.0 to 1.3.[60] Thus, results of study with both surface and intramuscular electrodes have proved to be broadly consistent for healthy subjects across diverse conditions, especially when normalization procedures have been included.

Dysfunctional Versus Healthy Knees

Many experimenters have attempted to discriminate between patients with PFPS and healthy subjects by using SEMG. Studies have differed in criteria for subject inclusion, contraction type, whether or not PFPS subjects had pain during the experimental tests, as well as complex variables related to SEMG measurement technique and data management; these studies have been reviewed in greater detail elsewhere.[7,61,62] The majority of reports revealed differences in SEMG activity between patient and control groups,[38,40,48,49,58,63–70] but some[71,72] failed to show any differences. Of experiments in which VM or VMO and VL activity was specifically compared with that of the VL, selective effects of PFPS were demonstrated on some occasions[38,49,58,65–67] but not others.[40,64,71,72] Nonselective effects tended to include a general depression of both VM or VMO and VL activity in knees with PFPS compared with control knees. Results of one additional study[73] that did not include a healthy control group documented responsiveness of VMO:VL ratios to a rehabilitation training program that was associated with patient improvement. Another group of investigators[74] reported that a 4-week exercise program was accompanied by a general increase in both VM and VL activity in symptomatic knees but not asymptomatic knees of the same subjects during a step-up/step-down task.

Within this body of work, SEMG activity was evaluated during seated isometric contractions,[38,40,48,49,58,64] standing isometric contractions,[70] step-up and step-down maneuvers,[49,74] seated isokinetic knee extension,[65,69] and treadmill running.[72] Seated patellar tendon reflex latencies were also investigated.[66,67,71] It may be that VMO and VL activity patterns are differentially affected by subtle but significant effects of joint angle, contraction intensity, open versus closed kinetic chains, and contraction type (isometric, concentric, or eccentric).[49,51,54,59] For example, SEMG deficits in patients with PFPS may be more pronounced during eccentric compared with concentric work,[65] or during closed chain contractions compared with open chain contractions.[70] In some of the studies, SEMG activity from the symptomatic knee was compared with that in the asymptomatic knee within the same patient.[40,49,63,65,69,74] In other cases, data recorded from healthy subjects were used for comparison against those of the affected knees of patients.[38,48,49,58,64,66–72] Two groups found that SEMG VMO:VL activity of each knee of unilaterally symptomatic patients was similar to each other but different from that in knees of healthy subjects.[49,67] Hence, sole use of the contralateral side for comparison in unilaterally symptomatic patients with PFPS may be inadequate.

PFPS may affect a heterogeneous patient population. Many different factors are believed to contribute to the disorder. For example, greater quadriceps (Q) angles are often found with this syndrome.[75] A larger Q angle is associated with a more lateral angle of the resultant quadriceps muscle force acting on the patella.[76] Increased Q angles in PFPS patients are associated with smaller VMO:VL activity ratios determined by SEMG. Because the Q angle affects VMO:VL activity ratios and because Q angles may vary with gender,[77] it may be important to match experimental groups on these variables. Gender effects have been suggested in experimental SEMG recordings of quadriceps components.[36] Further, age is a predictor of PFPS rehabilitation outcome and it may be important to match or stratify patients on this parameter.[78] It also seems unlikely that patients with recurrent subluxations would test the same as patients with hypomobility problems. Many of the investigators accepted PFPS subjects with a variety of clinical diagnoses or provided nonspecific clinical descriptions of their samples. Perhaps some subpopulations with this syndrome show altered VMO and VL activity and others do not. Finally, normalization of SEMG amplitude scores is an accepted practice to reduce data variance.[79,80] As alluded to above, such procedures may be useful in studying VMO and VL activity. Yet several of the investigators did not normalize their data for comparisons across recording sites and between subjects, and the normalization procedures used by others are potentially confounding.[49,72] Souza and Gross[49] provide a compelling argument that if the relative activities of VMO and VL are aberrant in the same way for the normalizing reference contraction as they are for the test activity, true differences between patients with PFPS and healthy subjects would be obscured.

The VMO:VL ratiometric approach may not be straightforward for a few more reasons. It can be speculated that the SEMG activity ratio has different biomechanical implications in different cases. Perhaps PFPS subjects with hypermobility should be trained to a greater VMO:VL ratio value to compensate with dynamic muscle con-

trol for deficient structural elements. That is, some patients with PFPS potentially require a greater VMO:VL ratio than that required by healthy subjects to achieve the same patellofemoral tracking efficiency (Figure 12–3).

The activity of each muscle is typically expressed as a percentage of maximal voluntary isometric contraction (%MVIC) for normalization before ratio calculation. A 5% MVIC VMO:5% MVIC VL ratio may not have the

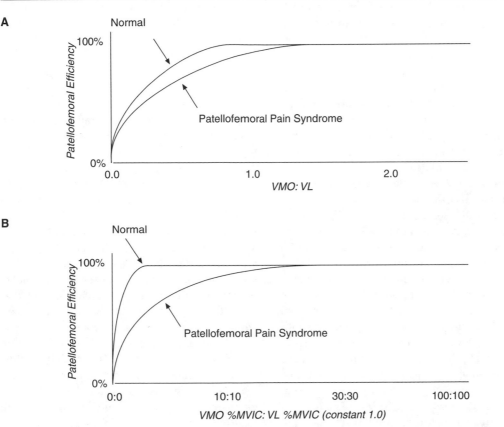

Figure 12–3 Speculative Effects of Vastus Medialis Obliquus (VMO) and Vastus Lateralis (VL) on Mechanical Efficiency of the Patellofemoral Joint. (**A**) Potential changes in the relationship between normalized VMO:VL SEMG ratios and patellofemoral efficiency in normal and dysfunctional conditions. (**B**) Absolute SEMG activity levels of VMO and VL—each expressed as a percentage of maximum voluntary isometric contraction (%MVIC)—vary. The VMO:VL ratio, however, remains constant at 1.0. Patients with patellofemoral dysfunction are represented as less efficient than healthy subjects at an equivalent %MVIC intensity, until a certain intensity is reached. Patients might gain efficiency by either increasing the VMO:VL ratio (**A**) or raising both VMO and VL activity levels to a greater intensity (**B**). *Source:* Reprinted from GS Kasman, JR Cram, and SL Wolf, *Clinical Applications in Surface Electromyography: Chronic Musculoskeletal Pain*, p 376, © 1998, Aspen Publishers, Inc.

same effect on dissipation of the patellofemoral joint reaction force as a 50% MVIC VMO:50% MVIC VL ratio, even though both ratios are computed as 1.0 (Figure 12–3). These models would account for many of the experimental findings discussed above. Patients with PFPS would be characterized as showing depressed activity of the VMO in relation to the VL, or nonspecific depression of quadriceps recruitment, depending on the patient and task type. In a patient with active pain and effusion, the VMO might be more inhibited, and a lower VMO:VL ratio would result. Decreases in both VMO and VL activity would be seen with maximal-effort contraction in the presence of quadriceps atrophy. This would occur because of neurophysiologic factors and loss of cross-sectional volume. However, greater nonspecific SEMG activity could be produced at submaximal loads to compensate for inefficient excitation-contraction coupling. Thus, a depressed VMO:VL ratio would indicate muscle imbalance, but a ratio approximating 1.0 would not in and of itself rule out muscle insufficiency.

Anecdotally, some patients with PFPS appear to produce extraordinarily high VMO:VL activity. Perhaps these individuals recruit the VMO to a greater degree in compensation for a faulty length-tension relationship. That is, if the patella were subjected to excessive lateral tracking in the trochlear groove of the femur, the fibers of the VMO could be lengthened beyond their optimally efficient range for actin-myosin cross-bridging. This loss of function could be opposed by increasing the excitability of motor units and produce a normal or higher than normal VMO:VL ratio seen with SEMG. The level of chronicity and relative contribution of static and dynamic factors toward patellar malalignment probably contributes to the degree to which this phenomenon becomes manifest. Simple amplitude comparisons may eventually be proved to be less sensitive and specific than other SEMG measures, at least if used without a valid and reliable classification system for patients.

Multiple investigators have commented on patellofemoral dysfunction from the perspective of faulty timing and neuromuscular control.[24,66,81] Their view is one of motor control imbalance through a functional range-of-motion arc rather than simple strength or SEMG peak amplitude differences. Indeed, peak SEMG activity from the VMO and VL is limited to about 5% of maximum while a patient arises from a partial squat,[42] making it unlikely that weakness is the pivotal factor in producing patellofemoral dysfunction during this motion. To the extent that the VMO and VL are antagonistic to each other for medial-lateral dynamic control of the patella and ultimately synergistic to the other quadriceps components for efficient biomechanical function of the knee, their recruitment levels must be appropriately timed to each other and to the other quadriceps components for any given functional task. Studies that limit testing to peak SEMG amplitude comparisons during isometric contractions may be insensitive to timing issues.

Karst and Willet[71] did not detect any onset timing differences of VMO and VL in PFPS patients and healthy subjects after tendon tap, nor after initiation of concentric knee extension in sitting or a concentric step-up task. However, Voight and Wieder[66] and Witvrouw and associates[67] identified altered VMO and VL reflex latency patterns in response to patellar tendon tap in patients with PFPS. Decrements in VMO/VL onset timing related to PFPS during voluntary contraction also have been reported.[82] Morrish and Woledge[48] found a time lag in the rise in SEMG activity for both VMO and VL, relative to force production, during isometric knee extension in sitting, as well as a reduction in knee extensor torque in patients compared with healthy controls. None of these studies attempted to track motor function throughout a functional range-of-motion arc. Souza and Gross[49] did find differences between PFPS patients and healthy control subjects in peak VMO:VL activity extracted during functional concentric and eccentric stepping tasks. MacIntyre and Robertson,[72] using an SEMG ensemble averaging technique throughout the gait cycle, could not demonstrate any changes in VM and VL function between PFPS patients and controls during treadmill running.

Perhaps the most thorough EMG study that addresses timing and function was reported by Powers and colleagues.[41] Intramuscular fine-wire electrodes were used to record EMG activity from the VMO, vastus medialis longus, VL, and vastus intermedius during free-speed-level walking, fast-level walking, stair ascent, stair descent, ramp ascent, and ramp descent. No differences in activity onset or cessation were detected among the muscles for either PFPS patients or healthy control subjects. In addition, there were no selective differences in VMO and VL mean intensities, each respectively normalized to seated maximal-effort contractions. However, the vastus muscles of patients with PFPS demonstrated generally decreased mean intensities, compared with findings in healthy subjects, during the level walking and ramp tasks. There was also a general delay in onset of vastus muscle activity in the PFPS group during fast-level walking and ramp descent, as well as a later cessation during stair descent. Thus, selective VMO:VL effects in PFPS patients were not supported, although nonspecific trends among the vastus muscles were observed.

An expert panel commentary that followed this report discussed a number of methodologic issues and implications.[83] One point of consensus among panel members was that patients with PFPS probably represent a heterogeneous population. Because of practical considerations, Powers and associates[41] did not attempt to discriminate among different types of patients with this syndrome. The same point has been raised regarding earlier investigations, and the development of a valid and reliable classification system is needed to resolve conflicting study results.

Another plausible explanation for selective VMO:VL effects is that the fatigue resistance of the VMO might be lower than that of the VL in PFPS patients. Runners with PFPS do not differ from healthy control subjects in isokinetic strength, but they do vary in isokinetic endurance parameters.[75] Large numbers of task repetitions have, for the most part, not been studied with SEMG and PFPS subjects. Fatigability can be assessed by analyzing the frequency spectrum of the SEMG signal. In brief, the frequency spectrum shifts toward lower values as fatigue is produced.[1] There are no selective differences in frequency analyses from VMO and VL recordings after repeated isometric contractions or terminal knee extension exercises in healthy subjects.[84] However, this issue has yet to be studied in PFPS patients, and none of the previously reviewed investigations attempted to monitor the effects of sustained or repeated contractions to a fatigue point.

The author has observed numerous PFPS cases wherein SEMG VMO:VL activity has seemed depressed in magnitude (Figure 12–4). Open-chain testing has been included, but emphasis has been primarily on the closed chain. Closed-chain tasks more appropriately reflect functional limitations in PFPS patients. Activities have included unilateral weight acceptance during gait, step-ups, step-downs, leg press exercises, partial squats, and lunge steps. At times, similar VMO and VL peak magnitudes have been observed, but the recruitment timing of the VMO has appeared altered relative to that of the VL through a functional range-of-motion arc. Sometimes such changes are observed only during closed-chain tasks, with relatively unremarkable activity during open-chain tasks (Figure 12–5). Other patients show changes in magnitude or timing relationships only during the eccentric phase of closed-chain maneuvers and particularly through range-of-motion arcs that correlate to subjective pain reports (Figure 12–6). Recommendations for SEMG assessment of PFPS patients are summarized in Appendix 12–A. Not all patients with this syndrome require SEMG evaluation.

Effects of Specific Exercises on VMO and VL Activity

Rehabilitative exercises have long been proposed for PFPS.[16,85] Assessed with SEMG recordings of symptomatic knees, conditioning

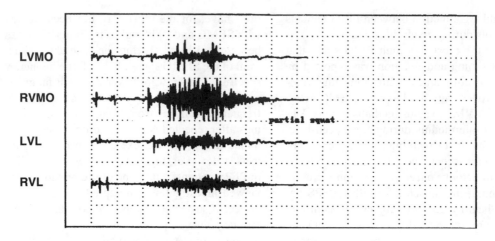

Figure 12–4 SEMG Activity of the Left (L) and Right (R) Vastus Medialis Obliquus (VMO) and Vastus Lateralis (VL) During a Bilateral Symmetric Partial Squat. Signals were recorded from a patient with chronic left patellofemoral pain syndrome. Lower extremity alignment and weight bearing were symmetric throughout the procedure. *Source:* Reprinted from GS Kasman, JR Cram, and SL Wolf, *Clinical Applications in Surface Electromyography: Chronic Musculoskeletal Pain*, p 378, © 1998, Aspen Publishers, Inc.

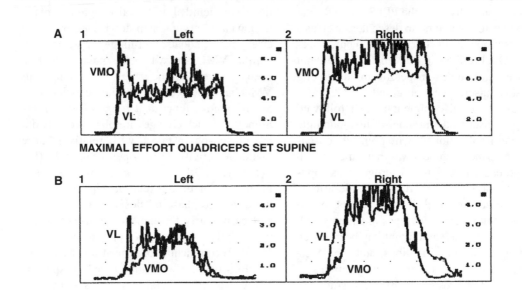

Figure 12–5 SEMG Activity of the Left (L) and Right (R) Vastus Medialis Obliquus (VMO) and Vastus Lateralis (VL), Recorded from a Patient with Chronic Bilateral Patellofemoral Pain Syndrome after Bilateral Lateral Release Surgery. (**A**) Activity for (**1**) left VMO and VL and (**2**) right VMO and VL during open-chain (supine) isometric quadriceps set at 0 degrees of knee flexion. (**B**) Activity for (**1**) left VMO and VL and (**2**) right VMO and VL during bilateral symmetric partial squat. Note the change in relative VMO and VL timing relationships from open- to closed-chain conditions. *Source:* Reprinted from GS Kasman, JR Cram, and SL Wolf, *Clinical Applications in Surface Electromyography: Chronic Musculoskeletal Pain*, p 378, © 1998, Aspen Publishers, Inc.

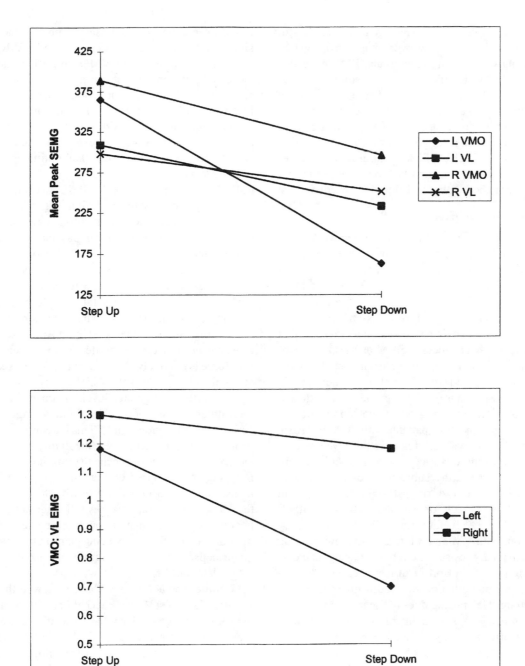

Figure 12–6 SEMG Activity of the Vastus Medialis Obliquus (VMO) and Vastus Lateralis (VL) During Step-Up (Concentric) and Step-Down (Eccentric) Maneuvers Recorded from a Patient with Chronic Left Patellofemoral Pain Syndrome. Note the change in relative VMO and VL activity patterns from concentric to eccentric conditions. *Source:* Reprinted from GS Kasman, JR Cram, and SL Wolf, *Clinical Applications in Surface Electromyography: Chronic Musculoskeletal Pain*, p 379, © 1998, Aspen Publishers, Inc.

exercises seem to produce general increases in VM and VL activity over time.[74] Investigators using surface and intramuscular EMG have also sought to identify particular positions or exercises that selectively enhance components of the quadriceps, and the VM or VMO in particular. The effects of a variety of open-kinematic-chain exercises are discussed below, followed by discussion of selected activities in a closed kinematic chain, and finally hip adduction procedures in both open- and closed-chain conditions.

Open-Chain Exercises

Early reports indicated that selective VM recruitment during knee extension could be facilitated by foot and ankle movements or tibial rotation in some persons, although no clear trend was identified across subjects and studies.[1,86–88] A subsequent body of work has emerged that has failed to identify any open-chain exercise that selectively enhances the VM or VMO in a consistent way. Results of systematic studies have not supported tibial rotation maneuvers in healthy subjects,[22,60,89,90] nor effects of ankle and foot position during quadriceps contraction in healthy subjects or patients with PFPS.[52,60] Also, there is no evidence for selective VMO recruitment during quadriceps setting at various joint angles in healthy subjects[22,60] or patients with PFPS,[39,60] nor during straight leg raising in healthy subjects or patients with knee pathology.[25,35,91–93] In fact, normalized peak activity from both VM and VL muscles is lower during maximally resisted straight leg raising than during maximal effort quadriceps setting.[92,93] Conscious combination of quadriceps setting with straight leg raising does not seem to make a difference.[25] A sustained training program with quadriceps setting produces general increases in SEMG activity, but it has no selective effects.[39] Conjoint lateral hip rotation with straight leg raising also does not increase VM, VMO:VL, or VMO:VML function, compared with standard straight leg raising.[1,25,43] Maximal hip lateral rotation is inferior to hip medial rotation positioning when terminal knee extension exercises are performed.[60] With healthy subjects, standard ter-minal knee extension exercises do not produce significant differences in fatigue-related SEMG frequency data between VMO and VL muscles,[84] do not improve patellar alignment as assessed by radiographic studies,[94] and do not selectively affect VMO or VL intramuscular EMG amplitudes.[35,60] Addition of hamstring coactivation to short-arc knee extension does not selectively change VMO or VL amplitudes in healthy subjects.[35]

Rehabilitative programs for PFPS that incorporate quadriceps setting, straight leg raising, and terminal knee extension exercises have been heavily promoted and seem to be associated with improvement for patients.[14,16,32,95–97] Despite this positive trend, there is no evidence that these exercises selectively enhance the function of the VMO relative to the VL. The rationale for use of quadriceps setting (in full extension), straight leg raising, and terminal knee extension exercises has been that the patellofemoral joint reaction force is relatively low, and that the exercises are well tolerated by patients.[43,85] Early studies also reported that greater levels of quadriceps recruitment are produced at the terminal range of active knee extension.[33,54,67,98] This latter effect is probably due to decreased mechanical efficiency of the extensor mechanism in the terminal range.[21] As stated earlier, there is no enhancement of VMO activity relative to that of the VL as the knee approaches full extension. It is generally agreed that although these exercise methods are useful in producing gains in general quadriceps strength, they are unlikely to affect VMO:VL balance.[25,39,60,84,89,94]

Grabiner and colleagues[61] have reviewed this apparent lack of selective EMG effect with common knee exercises. They have speculated that there might be some threshold level of VMO function required for satisfactory patellofemoral tracking. Atrophy might decrease the force-generating ability of all quadriceps components, including the VMO. According to this line of thinking, exercise results in general quadriceps recruitment and strength gain, which bring the VMO above its threshold level. Reports of non-selective alterations in VMO and VL EMG activity in knees of patients with PFPS versus knees of healthy subjects lend support to this view.[40,48,64]

Selective effects on SEMG amplitude VMO:VL ratios were, however, demonstrated by Sczepanski and associates[59] with isokinetic exercise in healthy subjects. These investigators noted a higher VMO:VL ratio with concentric contractions at 120 degrees per second, compared with eccentric contractions at 120 degrees per second or concentric contractions at 60 degrees per second. They also found a significantly greater VMO:VL ratio for the 60- to 85-degree arc of motion than the 35- to 60-degree arc, which in turn yielded a greater VMO:VL ratio than the 10- to 35-degree arc. The investigators concluded that arc of motion, as well as contraction type combined with angular velocity, are important parameters to consider.

Closed-Chain Exercises

The use of closed-chain rehabilitation has been strongly advocated and evaluated for PFPS.[85,99,100] McConnell[81,101,102] believes that it is appropriate to correct patellofemoral arthrokinematics with taping techniques and thus enable patients to tolerate functional closed-chain activities. She postulates that this method improves the length-tension relationship of the VMO. McConnell, along with Shelton and Thigpen,[85] emphasize that VMO retraining can be thought of in terms of motor skill acquisition, learning, and functional task performance. During certain closed-chain tasks, higher VM:VL or VMO:VL activity has been reported compared with traditional open-chain exercises.[49,50,53,103] This trend is consistent with the author's recommendations, favoring unilateral stance, step-up, squat, lunges, and leg press. The effect is not apparent, though, in two reports with the use of fine-wire intramuscular electrodes with both closed- and open-chain exercises.[35,60] As an aside, the SEMG activity of the VM is facilitated (and that of the medial gastrocnemius, semimembranosus, and rectus femoris is inhibited) when graded hip extension contractions are added to knee extension efforts in an open

chain.[104] Hip extension is naturally combined with knee extension in the closed chain, and perhaps there is a facilitory effect on the monoarticular extensors and the VM in particular.

Hip Adductor Exercises

Another area of uncertainty relates to the effect of adductor activity on VMO function. The potential role of hip adductor facilitation has received considerable, specific attention in the literature. Because fibers of the VMO take origin from the adductor tendons and disruption of these attachments has been identified in patients with recurrent patellar dislocations,[19,26] clinical use of hip adduction exercises has been proposed by several investigators.[19,36,42,81,89] Wheatley and Jahnke[88] recorded with surface electrodes and noted increased VM activity with adductor activation. Hanten and Schulties[89] used intramuscular electrodes to show that normalized VMO activity was significantly greater than VL activity during non–weight-bearing maximal-effort hip adduction. They tested adduction resistance applied to the distal aspect of the thigh, without a directed knee extension effort and without measuring knee extension torque. Grabiner and coworkers[105] also used intramuscular recordings and tested the effect of hip adduction on non–weight-bearing isometric knee extensor contractions at several intensities. Normalized VMO and VL activity levels were not changed by the addition of 50% maximum isometric hip adductor force to the knee extensor efforts. Andriacchi and associates[106] found that addition of graded abduction moments to a knee flexion moment produced changes in VM and VL intramuscular EMG activity at some knee joint angles. Although not directly compared, alterations in VM and VL activity in their report seem to follow parallel trends, without an apparent differential effect.

Using surface recordings, Karst and Jewett[25] did not find a facilitative influence of concomitant adductor contraction on VMO:VL or VMO:vastus medialis longus activity. These investigators supplied 5% body weight adduction resistance with a pulley apparatus affixed to the distal aspect of the leg. Adductor contraction was added to quadriceps setting plus straight leg raising with 5% body weight ankle cuff load. Adductor contraction did not have an effect when compared to quadriceps setting/straight leg raising alone or when compared to maximal effort quadriceps setting alone.

Zakaria and colleagues[52] used surface electrodes to investigate the effects of supine, maximal-effort hip adduction. A customized hip adduction bar was placed between the distal aspect of the thighs, and subjects were instructed to perform maximal-effort isometric hip adduction without a knee extension effort. There was no selective VMO facilitation with the hip adductor contractions compared with maximal-effort quadriceps set or quadriceps set plus ankle dorsiflexion.

Finally, Hodges and Richardson[53] studied VMO:VL SEMG activity in both weight-bearing and non–weight-bearing conditions with addition of 15%, 50%, and maximal hip adductor force to knee extension. Their weight-bearing position consisted of maintenance of 60 degrees of knee extension and 60 degrees of hip extension in a squat position. The non–weight-bearing position involved the same joint angles in supine without external load applied to the leg. There was no attempt to control for equivalent knee extensor loads. Average VMO:VL baseline activity was greater in the weight-bearing posture than in the non–weight-bearing position. Increased VMO:VL ratios were produced by addition of each of the adductor contractions in the weight-bearing position. However, only the maximal adductor contraction increased VMO:VL activity in the non–weight-bearing posture.

Collectively, this existing evidence runs contrary to the notion of adductor facilitation of VMO recruitment during open-chain knee extension, unless perhaps very-high-intensity contractions are used. Improved effects may be produced with closed-chain adductor exercise. None of the investigations included PFPS patients or a series of conditioning exercise sessions. Both might be important variables for study.

Implications for Exercise Prescription

The most effective method of exercise prescription for individual patients with VMO insufficiency may be to assess SEMG responses during trial of various movement tasks. SEMG evaluation of functionally relevant exercises in the closed chain should be emphasized. Assessed with SEMG, this is one practical aspect of exercise that supports higher VMO:VL activity with consistency.[49,50,53] Motor programming schema[107] for VMO and VL function will probably differ between purposeful closed-chain movements and open-chain exercises. Thus, exercise prescription can be viewed from the standpoint of neural adaptation and training in addition to peripheral conditioning effects.[108] This view is not meant to imply that open-chain exercises should be excluded but, rather, that exercise prescription should include functional considerations. If certain exercises act to facilitate the VMO selectively, they may be relatively patient-specific. Training recommendations are listed in Appendix 12–A. Additional perspective can also be found in a review of quadriceps exercise and PFPS by Callaghan and Oldham.[62]

SEMG Feedback Training

A number of investigators have promoted the use of SEMG feedback to retrain the VM or VMO.[73,81,85,86,94] SEMG feedback coupled with quadriceps exercise has produced outcomes superior to those with exercise alone or exercise combined with neuromuscular electrical stimulation (NMES) in patients with knee problems other than PFPS.[109–114]

McConnell[81,102] has suggested that VMO feedback training may be combined with patellofemoral taping. Taping has become popular with many physical therapists as part of a core approach to PFPS. Although taping techniques reduce symptomatic complaints, they do not seem to have an immediate effect on normalized VMO:VL activity assessed with fine-wire EMG electrodes.[60] Another study, using SEMG, failed to find any selective change between VM and VL activity across a 4-week conditioning period in patients treated with taping and exercise versus exercise alone.[74] However, this comparison could have been confounded by a lack of normalization across recording sites, subjects, and test days as well as by elements of the SEMG processing system. Other investigators reported increases in general quadriceps SEMG activity after taping the knees of patients with patellar hypermobility, but not after taping the knees of patients with PFPS and normal patellar mobility; each patient group differentiated on the basis of manual examination.[115] It may be that patellofemoral taping and SEMG feedback training can each be useful in rehabilitation, but perhaps through different mechanisms or in selective subpopulations. Several groups have proposed applying NMES to facilitate and strengthen the VMO,[97,116,117] and others have suggested combining SEMG feedback with NMES for knee rehabilitation programs.[7,110,118] Thus, quadriceps SEMG feedback is generally useful in rehabilitation, and options exist for innovative combination of SEMG training with other therapies.

Several investigators have systematically examined the effects of SEMG feedback training from VMO and VL with reference to PFPS. Wise and colleagues[73] trained patients diagnosed with PFPS to increase the activity of the VMO and maintain stable VL activity by using SEMG feedback. Patients used auditory and visual feedback during a progressive series of exercises. Phase I consisted of one to two orientation sessions of quadriceps setting and straight leg raising with the use of a 7.5:7.5 second work:rest cycle, as well as a supplementary home exercise program of 10 repetitions of each of these two exercises with the same timing two times per day. Phase II was implemented over two to six sessions and was similar to phase I, except that patients were instructed to increase VMO activity and maintain VL activity at baseline. Terminal knee extension exercises and resistive cuff weights were then added at the therapist's discretion. Once patients became pain free, they entered phase III, during which they practiced

VMO:VL training while bicycling, ambulating, and stair climbing. Total training lasted 4 to 6 weeks. Patients decreased their pain and returned to desired functional activities. Pretraining quadriceps setting VMO:VL ratios ranged from 0.38 to 0.79. Posttraining VMO:VL ratios ranged from 0.64 to 1.0. No attempt was made to normalize the SEMG data across recording sites, sessions, or subjects, and no formal statistical tests were reported. It is not clear whether data collection before and after training took place at equivalent contraction intensities. A control group was not included in the design.

LeVeau and Rogers[86] demonstrated that healthy subjects can be trained to increase the activity of the VM compared with that of the VL by using SEMG feedback. Subjects practiced for 30 minutes, 5 days per week for 3 weeks with seated isometric contractions. For each day of training, each subject's isometric one-repetition maximum load was determined, and 80% of that load was used as reference contraction for VM and VL SEMG activity levels. Each day's work consisted of five sets of six contractions, each set separated by a 30-second rest. Throughout the experiment, subjects received visual feedback when VM activity exceeded the VM training threshold, and auditory feedback when VL activity exceeded the VL threshold level. During the initial 2 weeks, subjects attempted to contract the VM to 25% or greater of that day's SEMG reference level while progressively reducing VL recruitment. Subjects had difficulty reducing VL activity without also decreasing VM activity. Hence, there was little change in relative balance over the training period. During the third training week, subjects succeeded in increasing VM recruitment while maintaining VL activity below threshold level, producing a significant training effect. The investigators therefore believed that uptraining the VM was a more successful strategy than downtraining the VL.

Also using healthy subjects, Ingersoll and Knight[94] showed that VMO feedback can result in improved patellofemoral alignment. They trained one group of subjects with the Daily Adjustable Progressive Resistive Exercise technique for four sets of 20-degree terminal knee extension exercises three times per week for 3 weeks. A second group of normal subjects worked three times per week for 3 weeks with an SEMG feedback program with the use of auditory and visual cues for VMO and VL feedback. Subjects receiving feedback increased SEMG activity of the VMO while minimizing that of the VL through a progressive series of exercises, including quadriceps setting, straight leg raising, terminal knee extension, stationary bicycle, ambulation, and stair climbing. A third group of normal subjects served as untrained control subjects. SEMG data were not reported, but subjects receiving feedback demonstrated significantly more medial radiographic patellofemoral congruence angle change between pretraining and posttraining periods as assessed with the quadriceps contracted, compared with the group training with terminal knee extension exercises alone. The radiographic patellar rotation angle during quadriceps contraction was changed between pretraining and posttraining periods in a more posterior direction for the feedback group compared with the control group. The investigators concluded that the SEMG feedback program produced changes in VMO:VL motor behavior, favoring improved medial patellar tracking and tilt, which were not obtained in the control group or the group receiving only terminal knee extension exercises. Unfortunately, it cannot be stated with certainty whether results in the group trained with SEMG were derived from the addition of feedback or from other training tasks.

Taken together, results of these reports seem to indicate that SEMG feedback can be used to change the relationship of the VMO to the VL, with potential consequences for patellofemoral function. Carefully controlled investigations with the use of SEMG feedback training with different types of PFPS patients are needed. If, as has been suggested, a key to managing VMO insufficiency is to view the problem as one of faulty motor control rather than as pure weakness, both amplitude and timing measures should be included in experimental designs. Analysis of SEMG frequency data and large numbers of task repetitions may also be useful during assessment. Functional outcomes measurement and comparison of SEMG training to other therapies, as well as combination treatments, would be helpful to determine optimal training programs.

Limitations of SEMG Methods

Thus far, the use of VMO and VL recordings to gauge dynamic medial and lateral control of the patella has been described. Throughout the chapter, limitations of SEMG techniques as a potential source of conflict in the literature have been alluded to. The discussion will now bring together and amplify some of those points. SEMG electrodes record the algebraic sum of muscle action potential voltages from their pickup zones.[1] This approach neglects passive patellar restraints. Therefore, the extent to which SEMG methods characterize resultant forces acting on the patella must be incomplete. To be meaningful, SEMG findings must be interpreted within the context of a complete history and relevant clinical tests.

SEMG recordings from specific portions of the quadriceps muscle may be vulnerable to signal cross-talk from nontargeted areas of the quadriceps and adjacent muscles. Cross-talk is influenced by muscle bulk dimensions, proximity to coactivated muscles, intervening tissue conductances between the skin and the target muscle as well as between coactivated muscles, electrode location, size and spacing, and other aspects of the recording and processing setup.[1,119,120] Recordings of VL activity may be contaminated by activity from the adjacent bulk of the vastus intermedius, rectus femoris, and hamstrings (less likely) during knee extension.[84] Because of the proximity of the adductor bulk and potential coactivation of the VMO and hip adductors, surface recordings of VMO activity may be subjected to signal contamination from the adductor muscles. This factor has gone uncontrolled in some studies during which the hip adductors might have been active in stabilizing weight-bearing limbs. No studies have been identified in which intramuscular recordings, which are far less susceptible to cross-talk, were compared directly with surface recordings specifically for the VMO and hip adductors. Investigators in two different studies anecdotally concluded that surface and intramuscular recordings from specific regions of the quadriceps produced similar results.[34,121] It is somewhat reassuring that in the larger body of existing literature, results obtained with intramuscular electrodes are consistent with results obtained with surface recordings under similar testing circumstances.

Although a linear or near-linear relationship between percentage of maximal SEMG activity and force output has been demonstrated under isometric nonfatiguing conditions for many muscles, the relationship may be influenced by sarcomere resting length, contraction velocity, proportionate amounts and geometric distributions of type I and II fibers, angle of insertion, fatigue, and neurophysiologic mechanisms.[3] How these factors specifically influence VMO versus VL activity detected by SEMG and their respective contributions to patellar stabilization is unknown. Investigators have advised caution in interpreting SEMG data with respect to VMO and VL functions, noting differences in muscle cross-sectional area, angle of fiber insertion, and morphologic characteristics.[61] The relationship between SEMG and force may be different for VMO and VL, and the relationship may be differentially affected by changes in contraction type, velocity, and intensity.

Because of the previously discussed issues and differences in electrical conductance, SEMG data should be normalized in some fashion before multisite or across-subject comparison. For example, different thicknesses of subcutaneous adipose tissue and skin impedances across subjects would differentially suppress the magnitude and frequency content of each subject's surface electrical signal.[1] Within subjects, the fascia overlying the VL is approximately twice as thick as that overlying the

VMO.[15] Other things being equal, this would tend to attenuate VL activity to a greater extent than VMO activity for surface recordings. SEMG amplitude scores of the VMO and VL during a test contraction arc most often expressed as a percentage of each muscle's respective score during maximal-effort quadriceps setting or seated knee extension. Conversion to a percentage of the maximum is intended to nullify the effects of unintended variations in electrode placement as well as between-site and between-subject differences in impedance and muscle geometry. SEMG scores during ambulatory activities can also be expressed as a percentage of the peak value obtained during the gait cycle, and this method has been used during a study of PFPS.[72] Any type of normalization procedure, however, has limitations for clinically relevant interpretation of SEMG values.[3,7,79,122,123] As was stated earlier, problems here can confound interpretation of SEMG studies of the VM and VMO in relation to the VL.[49,72]

In discussing SEMG studies of movement, it has been assumed that factors that enhance recruitment of the VMO relative to the VL lead to lasting changes in VMO:VL function if repeated in a training regimen. This may be a reasonable postulate,[25] but in much of the work to date no attempt has been made to monitor subjects over time. Caution must be used in extrapolating results of these experimental designs to patient training programs that target lasting gains in strength, motor skill, and functional activity performance.

Some clinical SEMG devices incorporate a frequency bandwidth filter with a low bandpass cutoff at 100 Hz. It is suggested that quadriceps SEMG activity be investigated with equipment that has a low cutoff of about 20 to 25 Hz and that devices with a low cutoff of 100 Hz not be used. The frequency spectrum of the SEMG signal typically includes a great deal of activity below 100 Hz. Thus, with a progressive left shift in power density plots during fatigue,[1] it is vitally important that bandwidth filters pass the appropriate range of frequencies during clinical work. Research findings have been reported on

VMO:VL activity detected by SEMG devices with a bandpass low cutoff of 100 Hz. The magnitude of effect, if any, is unknown.

SEMG assessment and feedback training for PFPS is best performed with units that have dual-channel capacity or greater. Although single-channel SEMG units are less expensive and easy to operate, there is no way to monitor directly the balance of VMO and VL activities. VM and VMO activity tends to parallel that of the other quadriceps components. Increased or decreased activity from a single VMO recording site does not imply that anything meaningful has happened in terms of VMO:VL balance, and selective gains in VMO function should not be assumed.[39,94]

Finally, it is recommended that clinicians who include SEMG feedback training to change the timing of muscle activity use sampling rates of at least 1000 Hz, line tracing visual displays, and minimal display smoothing. Systems with high temporal resolution and off-line software analysis are required to assess onset timing precisely. Karst and Willet[71] have emphasized that many handheld SEMG devices are wholly inadequate to detect subtle timing parameters. Thus, clinicians working in the temporal domain should expect to purchase more sophisticated equipment and (usually) be able to detect only gross changes through a range-of-motion arc.

CASE HISTORIES

Case History 1

A 43-year-old female urban taxi driver presented with right anterior knee pain of several months' duration. The patient began each day without pain but experienced progressive pain through the course of her work shift. Moving the foot from the accelerator to the brake pedal was definitely exacerbating, as was going up or down stairs or squat maneuvers in her home. She led a relatively sedentary lifestyle but had recently started a walk-jog exercise program. Knee pain was not reproduced during her walk-

jog sessions, although symptoms seemed to be reproduced earlier than usual during the following day if she was working. Asymmetrical shortness of the right rectus femoris and iliotibial band were noted on physical examination. Symptoms were reproduced with resisted knee extension under closed-chain conditions. Resisted knee extension in an open chain was well tolerated. A previously prescribed general stretching and quadriceps strengthening program had been ineffective at reducing symptoms. Pain was now causing time loss from work.

Peak SEMG activity recorded from the VMO was depressed on the symptomatic side compared with the asymptomatic side by more than 35% during bilateral squat as well as reciprocal lunge or step-up/step-down activities. VL activity was roughly symmetrical. Activity for each recording site was also normalized as a percentage of maximal-effort isometric SEMG value and then expressed as a VMO:VL ratio. The right VMO:VL ratio consistently ranged between 0.9 and 1.2 during submaximal contractions in non–weight-bearing activities—values similar to those for the asymptomatic side during performance of open- and closed-chain tasks. However, the right VMO:VL ratio fell to 0.7–0.8 during squat and stair activities. When pressing down with moderate force on a brake pedal after moving from an accelerator was simulated, the VMO:VL ratio initially was found to average about 0.6, and then increased slightly as the movement range was completed.

Treatment was provided with SEMG-triggered neuromuscular electrical stimulation over the VMO for 20 minutes. Trials were started in sitting and progressed quickly into weight-bearing and simulated driving movements. Next, electrical stimulation was withdrawn; SEMG retested with all activities showed a VMO:VL ratio greater than 0.9, accompanied by decreased symptoms. A home program was designed combining SEMG-triggered neuromuscular electrical stimulation, patellofemoral taping, and stretching, performed daily by the patient for 7 days. On retest 7 days later, the patient demonstrated independent carryover of VMO:VL SEMG ratios approaching 0.9 for all activities, symptoms were dramatically reduced, and the patient was able to drive a complete shift. SEMG-triggered neuromuscular electrical stimulation was discontinued, while taping and exercise were continued at home for another 4 weeks. SEMG feedback was also used during this period to help make changes in seat position and motor habit that decreased recruitment of the tensor fasciae latae and rectus femoris during simulated driving. In addition, manual techniques were applied for mobilization along fascial planes of the lateral thigh, lateral retinaculum of the knee, and iliotibial band insertion. The patient attended a total of five clinic visits over the active treatment period of $5\frac{1}{2}$ weeks. She was consistently symptom free and could perform all desired functional activities at the conclusion of the treatment period. The patient was discharged with instructions to continue therapeutic exercises and general conditioning as part of a health maintenance routine. She remained compliant with her maintenance home program, and no further complaints of knee pain were registered over a 2-year follow-up period.

Case History 2

A 39-year-old female was referred for additional physical therapy 8 months after reconstructive surgery for rupture of the right anterior cruciate ligament, and 2 months following knee flexion manipulation under anesthesia performed for capsular fibrosis. The patient had been treated with frequent physical therapy that included supervised exercise; a variety of thermal, electrical, and manual agents; and graded functional activity progression. Despite intensive and extensive effort, passive knee range of motion was restricted to 5 to 110 degrees, limited by perception of retropatellar and infrapatellar pain as well as general stiffness. Gait was profoundly dysfunctional with diminished right weight bearing, decreased right push-off and medial heel whip, decreased knee and ankle motion throughout, slow and dysrhythmic ca-

dence, asymmetric step length, and decreased arm swing. The patient admitted to being fearful of severely painful but transient "catching" sensations during ambulation. She remained at work as a school teacher but avoided aerobic and social dance, gym exercise, and outdoor activities with which she was previously active. Limb girth was decreased markedly over the right calf and thigh. Moderate effusion was present at the knee, with highly restricted patellar mobility. There appeared to be a condition of patella alta and shortness of the rectus femoris and single joint hip flexors. Knee extension peak torque was 55% lower on the right compared with the left, as measured on an isokinetic apparatus at 60 degrees per second.

Compared with the left side, SEMG activity of the right VMO was depressed by 79% and that of the VL by 40% during maximal-effort open-chain tasks. Nonnormalized VMO:VL activity during maximal-effort quadriceps set or isometric knee extension averaged about 0.4 on the right and 1.0 on the left. During bilateral squat, with equal weight bearing of the lower extremities ensured with a scale under each foot, nonnormalized VMO:VL activity peaked at 0.3 on the right and 0.7 on the left. Interestingly, when normalized to seated isometric maximal-effort contraction, VMO:VL activity during the squat was 0.8 on the right and 0.7 on the left. This later point illustrates the potential confusion caused by normalization to maximal-effort contraction, when maximal contractions are themselves likely to be deficient. The right VMO was activated to a higher percentage of maximum during the bilateral squat, presumably because of muscular and articular impairments. The normalized right VMO:VL value falls within expected limits but, when viewed in the larger context, can hardly be considered characteristic of healthy knee function. Thus, normalized comparisons to population standards may be supplemented by nonnormalized as well as percent asymmetry calculations.

Treatment was initiated with a program of SEMG feedback training to overcome what was believed to be profound inhibition of the quadriceps in general and VMO in particular. Therapeutic ultrasound was also applied over the peripatellar region, followed by manual mobilization. The patient received vigorous behavioral and cognitive support to ameliorate pain behaviors. Quota performance levels were established for each conditioning exercise and functional activity. Emphasis was placed initially on improving quadriceps recruitment and normalizing gait. As these issues improved, manual mobilization became more aggressive. SEMG feedback was also used to reduce guarding responses during passive flexion stretches. After about 6 weeks, the patient's exercise program closely resembled the program that had been attempted in her previous physical therapy course. Now, however, the patient was making documented progress at each treatment session. The patient believed that the difference resulted from identifying quadriceps inhibition, as well as her learned avoidance behaviors, and providing a nonthreatening feedback tool to reestablish conscious control. Regular therapy visits were tapered in frequency and discontinued after 16 weeks. At that time, the patient walked with an unremarkable gait, produced symmetrical quadriceps SEMG activity, demonstrated 0 to 135 degrees of passive motion, and participated in aerobic and artistic dance classes without difficulty.

Case History 3

A 33-year-old male presented with complaints of bilateral anterior knee pain produced during road or trail running, downhill hiking, uphill bicycling, in-line skating, rock climbing, and volleyball lunging. Symptoms had waxed and waned for years but now were at their worst and significantly limiting of athletic activity. Pain was produced some time after each activity was initiated and increased slowly with continued play. He was unable to specify any single traumatic event and was functioning at his typical level of sports activity when symptoms started to progress. The patient had undergone several courses of physical therapy over previous years. He had been prescribed a series of

conditioning exercises and received shoe orthotics for foot pronation. Control of pronation and medial hip rotation appeared much improved with his orthotics. He had also received instructions for exercises to promote general hip flexibility and especially hamstring flexibility. Movement of lumbar spinous processes was palpable at about 45 degrees of straight leg raise, with about 65 degrees of total straight-leg-raise mobility. No improvement in hamstring flexibility was produced, despite the fact that the patient had devoted considerable time and energy to his stretching exercises. The hamstrings appeared relatively hypertrophied and the gluteus maximus of relatively low bulk on the patient's lean frame. Considerable lateral patellar mobility was noted with passive gliding as well as mild patient apprehension. Shortening of the lateral retinaculum and iliotibial band did not seem contributory.

Maximal-effort seated knee extension in the clinic was not painful. SEMG activity from the VMO and VL appeared symmetric, right to left, and unremarkable overall during these maximal efforts. Deep lunges tended to exacerbate the patient's symptoms most readily and were important functional movement components for him. Thus, lunges were selected for patient-specific evaluation. SEMG activity from the VMO and VL during lunging was normalized to respective SEMG values generated with maximal-effort isometric contractions in 60 degrees of knee flexion in sitting. Normalized (as well as nonnormalized) VMO:VL activity during lunging without orthotics or shoes was calculated to be approximately 0.6 bilaterally, and slightly but consistently improved with shoes and orthotics. The patient next reproduced his hamstring stretching routine. Stretching exercises were accompanied by lateral hamstring SEMG activity averaging about 10% of maximum hamstring value.

Treatment was initiated to update the patient's orthotics, which had partially broken down. An exercise program was designed to facilitate general quadriceps strength, power, and endurance with both open- and closed-chain tasks. Careful instruction was provided in hamstring stretching technique. SEMG feedback was regarded as critical during this process. The patient incorporated contract/relax and abdominal breathing techniques to decrease active hamstring tone, and he used the SEMG signal as a cue for pacing and amplitude of stretch. He quickly learned to maintain a stable, quiescent SEMG baseline, yet felt he could move effectively to end range. The patient believed that SEMG feedback was pivotal in helping him to become aware of kinesthetic sensations associated with unconstructive hamstring contractions and to learn a new sensory scheme that characterized effective stretching. Quadriceps and hamstring exercises were combined with conditioning exercises for the gluteus maximus as well as a series of sports-specific training progressions for the trunk and lower extremities, all to be performed independently by the patient. He was also reinstructed in patellofemoral taping techniques. In previous therapy courses, tape application had given him a greater "sense of confidence" with his knee, but did not of itself seem to make a lasting difference in symptom provocation once the tape was discontinued.

The patient returned to the clinic for a total of eight visits over a 4-month period. Each time SEMG activity of the VMO, VL, lateral hamstrings, and gluteals was displayed. The patient oriented with open-chain isometric contractions and quickly made the transition to simulated sports maneuvers. His objectives were to identify body positions, equipment modifications, and cognitive strategies that would increase recruitment of the vasti and gluteus maximus relative to the hamstrings as well as the VMO relative to the VL. An elite athlete, the patient learned without much difficulty to facilitate the vasti and gluteus maximus relative to hamstrings. However, no specific changes in body position, equipment, or exercise could be found to immediately increase recruitment of the VMO relative to the VL. Nevertheless, over time he was able to use SEMG feedback and cognitive strategies to selectively uptrain the VMO. This became apparent by gradually improving VMO:VL activity patterns across sessions and,

during the final sessions, by observable increases within training periods.

Symptoms gradually abated over the treatment course. The patient noticed initially that he could perform a sport for a longer time before symptoms were reproduced. Ultimately, he participated in all routine activities without symptoms. Relatively mild symptoms were triggered with an unusually long or intense athletic event, but he felt he could easily manage such rare occurrences. At the time of discharge, peak SEMG values for the VMO and VL during maximal-effort contractions were increased relative to values recorded during the first visit. Submaximal activity had decreased for identical lunge and other sport tasks, and the lunge normalized VMO:VL ratio was approximately 0.8 bilaterally. Hamstring length had also improved, and he no longer utilized patellofemoral taping. The patient did continue with his shoe orthotics, functional activity modifications, and exercise regimen.

Notes on the Case Histories

Each of the above described patients was treated with multiple agents. The relative contribution of SEMG to the outcomes cannot be distinguished with certainty. Evaluation and feedback training with SEMG may possess unique benefits relative to other intervention strategies. Perhaps the most important points, though, are that practitioners routinely combine clinical techniques and the greatest strengths of SEMG may be found in integration with other approaches. When PFPS has become chronic, SEMG methods might then enable successful functional outcomes and patient satisfaction on a reasonable cost basis.

CONCLUSION

Knee extension is accompanied by a tendency to displace the patella laterally, which is dynamically opposed by the VMO. Imbalance of active and passive factors acting on the patella can lead to faulty compressive loading, cumulative trauma, and PFPS. Not all patients (and, in all likelihood, not the majority of patients) with PFPS have VMO insufficiency as a primary cause. The literature suggests substantial intersubject variability in terms of structural alignment and passive flexibility, quadriceps recruitment, and successful training regimens. Intramuscular and surface EMG have been used successfully in kinesiologic studies of the quadriceps as a unit and in studies of the actions of its component parts. The SEMG activity of the VMO has been qualified and quantified relative to that of the VL. Analysis of SEMG activity has been used to distinguish PFPS patients from healthy control subjects in terms of VMO:VL imbalance as well as general depression of vasti activity. However, there has been little consensus regarding guidelines for best practices, and additional study is required to discern techniques with optimal sensitivity and specificity.

Clinically, it seems logical to include SEMG examination of a patient during performance of functional activities that are known to exacerbate that patient's symptoms.

No open-chain exercise has been shown conclusively to facilitate the VMO in a selective manner. There have been favorable outcomes with knee extension and hip adduction maneuvers in the closed chain. Specific exercises may be evaluated with SEMG on a case-by-case basis to determine those with optimal effects for particular patients. SEMG feedback training has been used successfully to train the quadriceps in general and the VMO relative to the VL in particular. Training with SEMG feedback should be performed in patients with identifiable SEMG deficits, rather than applying a blanket PFPS protocol to all. Feedback training ought to be regarded as an adjunctive component of a comprehensive rehabilitation program.

REFERENCES

1. Basmajian JV, De Luca CJ. *Muscles Alive: Their Functions Revealed by Electromyography*. 5th ed. Baltimore: Williams & Wilkins; 1985.

2. Basmajian JV, ed. *Biofeedback: Principles and Practice for Clinicians*. 3rd ed. Baltimore: Williams & Wilkins; 1989.

3. Cram JR, Kasman GS. *Introduction to Surface Electromyography*. Gaithersburg, MD: Aspen Publishers; 1998.

4. Peek CJ. A primer of biofeedback instrumentation. In: Schwartz M, ed. *Biofeedback: A Practitioner's Guide*. New York: Guilford Press; 1987:45–95.

5. Soderberg GL, ed. *Selected Topics in Surface Electromyography for Use in the Occupational Setting: Expert Perspective*. Washington, DC: US Dept of Health and Human Services; 1992. NIOSH publication 91-100.

6. Turker KS. Electromyography: some methodological problems and issues. *Phys Ther*. 1993;73:698–710.

7. Kasman GS, Cram JR, Wolf SL. *Clinical Applications in Surface Electromyography: Chronic Musculoskeletal Pain*. Gaithersburg, MD: Aspen Publishers; 1998.

8. Jette AM. Physical disablement concepts for physical therapy research and practice. *Phys Ther*. 1994;74:380–386.

9. Ng JKF, Richardson CA, Jull GA. Electromyographic amplitude and frequency changes in the iliocostalis and multifidus muscles during a trunk holding test. *Phys Ther*. 1977;77:954–961.

10. Klein AB, Snyder-Mackler L, Roy SH, De Luca CJ. Comparison of spinal mobility and isometric trunk extensor forces with electromyographic spectral analysis in identifying low back pain. *Phys Ther*. 1991;71:445–454.

11. Roy SH, De Luca CJ, Emley M, Buijs RJC. Spectral electromyographic assessment of back muscles in patients with low back pain undergoing rehabilitation. *Spine*. 1995;20:38–48.

12. Gogia P, Sabbahi M. Median frequency of the myoelectric signal in cervical paraspinal muscles. *Arch Phys Med Rehabil*. 1990;71:408–414.

13. Puniello MS. Iliotibial band tightness and medial patellar glide in patients with patellofemoral dysfunction. *J Orthop Sports Phys Ther*. 1993;17:144–148.

14. Hughston JC, Walsh WM, Puddu G. *Patellar Subluxation and Dislocation*. Philadelphia: WB Saunders; 1984.

15. Lieb FJ, Perry J. Quadriceps function: an anatomical and mechanical study using amputated limbs. *J Bone Joint Surg*. 1968;50A:1535–1548.

16. Woodall W, Welsh J. A biomechanical basis for rehabilitation programs involving the patellofemoral joint. *J Orthop Sports Phys Ther*. 1990;11:535–542.

17. Hungerford DS. Patellar subluxation and excessive lateral pressure as a cause of fibrillation. In: Pickett JC, Radin EL, eds. *Chondromalacia of the Patella.* Baltimore: Williams & Wilkins; 1983:24–42.

18. Conlan T, Garth WP Jr, Lemons JE. Evaluation of the medial soft-tissue restraints of the extensor mechanism of the knee. *J Bone Joint Surg.* 1993;75A:682–693.

19. Bose K, Kanagasuntheram R, Osman MBII. Vastus medialis oblique: an anatomic and physiologic study. *Orthopedics.* 1980;3:880–883.

20. Goh JC, Lee PY, Bose K. A cadaver study of the function of the oblique part of vastus medialis. *J Bone Joint Surg.* 1995;77B:225–231.

21. Lieb FJ, Perry J. Quadriceps function: an electromyographic study under isometric conditions. *J Bone Joint Surg.* 1971;53A:749–758.

22. Signorile JF, Kacisk D, Perry A, Robertson B, et al. The effect of knee and foot position on the electromyographic activity of the superficial quadriceps. *J Orthop Sports Phys Ther.* 1995;22:2–9.

23. Komi PV, Kaneko M, Aura O. EMG activity of the leg extensor muscles with special reference to mechanical efficiency in concentric and eccentric exercise. *Int J Sports Med.* 1987;8S:22–29.

24. Richardson C, Bullock MI. Changes in muscle activity during fast, alternating flexion-extension movements of the knees. *Scand J Rehabil Med.* 1986;18:51–58.

25. Karst GM, Jewett PD. Electromyographic analysis of exercises proposed for differential activation of medial and lateral quadriceps femoris muscle components. *Phys Ther.* 1993;73:286–295.

26. Thiranagama R. Nerve supply of the human vastus medialis muscle. *J Anat.* 1990;170:193–198.

27. Johnson MA, Polgar J, Weightman D, Appleton D. Data on the distribution of fiber types in thirty-six human muscles: an autopsy study. *J Neurol Sci.* 1973;18:111–129.

28. de Andre J, Grant C, Dixon A. Joint distension and reflex inhibition in the knee. *J Bone Joint Surg.* 1965;47A:313–322.

29. Stokes M, Young A. Investigations of quadriceps inhibition: implications for clinical practice. *Physiotherapy.* 1984;70:425–428.

30. Stratford P. Electromyography of the quadriceps femoris muscles in subjects with normal knees and acutely effused knees. *Phys Ther.* 1981;62:279–283.

31. Spencer J, Hayes K, Alexander I. Knee joint effusion and quadriceps reflex inhibition in man. *Arch Phys Med Rehabil.* 1984;65:171–177.

32. Grana W, Kriegshauser L. Scientific basis of extensor mechanism disorders. *Clin Sports Med.* 1985;4:247–258.

33. Basmajian JV, Harden TP, Regenos EM. Integrated actions of the four heads of the quadriceps femoris: an electromyographic study. *Anat Rec.* 1972;172:15–20.

34. Pocock GS. Electromyographic study of the quadriceps during resistive exercise. *Phys Ther.* 1963;43:422–434.

35. Gryzlo SM, Patek RM, Pink M, Parry J. Electromyographic analysis of knee rehabilitation exercises. *J Orthop Sports Phys Ther.* 1994;20:36–43.

36. Brownstein BA, Lamb RL, Mangine RE. Quadriceps torque and integrated electromyography. *J Orthop Sports Phys Ther.* 1985;6:309–314.

37. Lange GW, Hintermeister RA, Schlegal T, Dillman CJ, et al. Electromyographic and kinematic analysis of graded treadmill walking and the implications for knee rehabilitation. *J Orthop Sports Phys Ther.* 1996;23:294–301.

38. Mariano P, Caruso I. An electromyographic investigation of subluxation of the patella. *J Bone Joint Surg.* 1979;61B:169–171.

39. Moller BN, Jurik AG, Tidemand-Dal C, Krebs B, et al. The quadriceps function in patellofemoral disorder: a radiographic and electromyographic study. *Arch Orthop Trauma Surg.* 1987;106:195–198.

40. Moller BN, Krebs B, Tidemand-Dal C, Aaris K. Isometric contractions in the patellofemoral pain syndrome. *Arch Orthop Trauma Surg.* 1986;105:24–27.

41. Powers CM, Landel R, Perry J. Timing and intensity of vastus muscle activity during functional activities in subjects with and without patellofemoral pain. *Phys Ther.* 1996;76:946–955.

42. Reynolds L, Levin TA, Mederios JM, Adler NS, et al. EMG activity of the vastus medialis oblique and the vastus lateralis in their role in patellar alignment. *Am J Phys Med.* 1983;62:61–70.

43. Wild J, Franklin T, Woods W. Patellar pain and quadriceps rehabilitation: an EMG study. *Am J Sports Med.* 1982;10:12–15.

44. Flynn TW, Soutas-Little RW. Mechanical power and muscle action during forward and backward running. *J Orthop Sports Phys Ther.* 1993;17:108–112.

45. Hsu A, Perry J, Gronley JK, Hislop HJ. Quadriceps force and myoelectric activity during flexed knee stance. *Clin Orthop.* 1993;288:254–262.

46. Miyagawa H, Furukawa R, Shimono T, et al. Electromyographic analysis of knee muscles during the lateral step-up exercise. *J Phys Ther Sci.* 1993;5:45–50.

47. Isear JA, Erickson JC, Worrell TW. EMG analysis of lower extremity muscle recruitment patterns during an unloaded squat. *Med Sci Sport Exer.* 1997;29:532–539.

48. Morrish GM, Woledge RC. A comparison of the activation of muscles moving the patella in normal subjects and in patients with chronic patellofemoral problems. *Scand J Rehab Med.* 1997;29:43–48.

49. Souza DR, Gross MT. Comparison of vastus medialis oblique: vastus lateralis muscle integrated electromyographic ratios between healthy subjects and patients with patellofemoral pain. *Phys Ther.* 1991;71:310–320.

50. Cuddeford T, Williams AK, Medeiros JM. Electromyographic activity of the vastus medialis oblique and vastus lateralis muscles during selected exercises. *J Orthop Sports Phys Ther.* 1996;4:10–15.

51. Kasman G, Cram J, Miller D. Electromyographic assessment of the distal vastus medialis and vastus lateralis as a function of contraction intensity. *J Orthop Sports Phys Ther.* 1994;19:72. Abstract.

52. Zakaria D, Harburn KL, Kramer JF. Preferential activation of the vastus medialis oblique, vastus lateralis, and hip adductor muscles during isometric exercises in females. *J Orthop Sports Phys Ther.* 1997;26:23–28.

53. Hodges P, Richardson C. The influence of isometric hip adduction on quadriceps femoris activity. *Scand J Rehabil Med.* 1993;25:57–62.

54. Simoneau GG, Wilk K. Electromyographic activity ratio between the vastus medialis and the vastus lateralis for four exercises. *Phys Ther.* 1993;73:S78.

55. Wilk KE, Simoneau G, McGraw J. The electromyographic activity of the quadriceps femoris vastus medialis/lateralis ratio during knee bend squats, knee extensions, and leg press exercises. *Phys Ther.* 1993;73:S80.

56. Schaub PA, Worrell TW. EMG activity of six muscles and VMO:VL ratio determination during a maximal squat exercise. *J Sport Rehabil.* 1995;4:195–202.

57. Rice MA, Bennett JG, Ruhling RO. Comparison of two exercises on VMO and VL EMG activity and force production. *Isokinetics.* 1995;5:61–67.

58. Boucher JP, King MA, Lefebvre R, Pepin A. Quadriceps femoris muscle activity in patellofemoral pain syndrome. *Am J Sports Med.* 1992;20:527–532.

59. Sczepanski TL, Gross MT, Duncan PW, Chandler JM. Effect of contraction type, angular velocity, and arc of motion on VMO:VL EMG ratio. *J Orthop Sports Phys Ther.* 1991;14:256–262.

60. Cerny K. Vastus medialis oblique/vastus lateralis muscle activity ratios for selected exercises in persons with and without patellofemoral pain syndrome. *Phys Ther.* 1995;75:672–683.

61. Grabiner MD, Koh TJ, Draganich LF. Neuromechanics of the patellofemoral joint. *Med Sci Sports Exerc.* 1994;26:10–21.

62. Callaghan MJ, Oldham JA. The role of quadriceps exercise in the treatment of patellofemoral pain syndrome. *Sports Med.* 1996;24:384–391.

63. Doxey GE, Eisenman P. The influence of patellofemoral pain on electromyographic activity during submaximal isometric contractions. *J Orthop Sports Phys Ther.* 1987;9:211–216.

64. Grabiner MD, Koh TJ, Andrish JT. Decreased excitation of vastus medialis oblique and vastus lateralis in patellofemoral pain. *Eur J Exp Musculoskel Res.* 1992;1:33–39.

65. Petschnig R, Baron R, Engel A, Chomiak J, et al. Objectivation of the effects of knee problems on vastus medialis and vastus lateralis with EMG and dynamometry. *Phys Med Rehab.* 1991;2;50–54.

66. Voight ML, Wieder DL. Comparative reflex response times of vastus medialis obliquus and vastus lateralis in normal subjects and subjects with extensor mechanism dysfunction: an electromyographic study. *Am J Sports Med.* 1991;19:131–137.

67. Witvrouw E, Sneyers C, Lysens R, Victor J, et al. Reflex response time of vastus medialis oblique and vastus lateralis in normal subjects and in subjects with patellofemoral pain syndrome. *J Orthop Sports Phys Ther.* 1994;24:160–165.

68. Thomee R, Renstrom P, Karlsson J, Grimby G. Patellofemoral pain syndrome in young women, II: muscle function in patients and healthy controls. *Scand J Med Sci Sports.* 1995;5:245–251.

69. Werner S. An evaluation of knee extensor and knee flexor torques and EMGs in patients with patellofemoral pain syndrome in comparison with matched controls. *Knee Surg Sports Traumatol Arthrosc.* 1995;3:89–94.

70. Thomee R, Grimby G, Svantesson U, Osterberg U. Quadriceps muscle performance in sitting and standing in young women with patellofemoral pain syndrome and in young healthy women. *Scand J Med Sci Sports.* 1996;6:233–241.

71. Karst GM, Willet GM. Onset timing of electromyographic activity in the vastus medialis oblique and vastus lateralis muscles in subjects with and without patellofemoral pain syndrome. *Phys Ther.* 1995;75:813–823.

72 MacIntyre DL, Robertson DG. Quadriceps muscle activity in women runners with and without patellofemoral pain syndrome. *Arch Phys Med Rehabil.* 1992;73:10–14.

73. Wise HH, Fiebert IM, Kates J. EMG biofeedback as treatment for patellofemoral pain syndrome. *J Orthop Sports Phys Ther.* 1984;6:95–103.

74. Kowall MG, Kolk G, Nuber GW, Cassis JE, et al. Patellar taping in the treatment of patellofemoral pain: a prospective randomized study. *Am J Sports Med.* 1996; 24:61–66.

75. Messier SP, Davis SE, Curl WW, Lowert RB, et al. Etiologic factors associated with patellofemoral pain in runners. *Med Sci Sports Exerc.* 1991;23:1008–1015.

76. Schulthies SS, Francis RS, Fisher AG, Van de Graaff KM. Does the Q angle reflect the force on the patella in the frontal plane? *Phys Ther.* 1995;75:24–30.

77. Horton MG, Hall TL. Quadriceps femoris muscle angle: normal values and relationships with gender and selected skeletal measures. *Phys Ther.* 1989;69:897–901.

78. Kannus P, Niittymaki S. Which factors predict outcome in the nonoperative treatment of patellofemoral pain syndrome? A prospective follow-up study. *Med Sci Sports Exerc.* 1994;26:289–296.

79. Knutson LM, Soderberg GL, Ballantyne BT, Clarke WR. A study of various normalization procedures for within day electromyographic data. *J Electromyogr Kinesiol.* 1994;4:47–60.

80. Redfern MS. Functional muscle: effects on electromyographic output. In: Doderberg GL, ed. *Selected Topics in Surface Electromyography for Use in the Occupational Setting: Expert Perspectives.* Rockville, MD: US Dept of Health and Human Services; 1991:104–120. National Institute for Occupational Safety and Health publication no. 91–100.

81. McConnell JS. Management of patellofemoral problems. *Manual Ther.* 1996;1:60–66.

82. Perez PL, Gossman MR, Lechner D, Stephenson SX, et al. Electromyographic temporal characteristics of the vastus medialis oblique and the vastus lateralis in women with and without patellofemoral pain. In: *Proceedings of the World Confederation for Physical Therapy 13th General Meeting, Washington, DC, June 1995.* Alexandria, VA: American Physical Therapy Association; 1995. Paper no. PO-RR-0239-T.

83. Fitzgerald GK, Karst G, Malone T, Wilk K, et al. Conference. *Phys Ther.* 1997;76:956–966.

84. Grabiner MD, Koh TJ, Miller GF. Fatigue rates of vastus medialis oblique and vastus lateralis during static and dynamic knee extension. *J Orthop Res.* 1991;9:391–397.

85. Shelton GL, Thigpen LK. Rehabilitation of patellofemoral dysfunction: a review of literature. *J Orthop Sports Phys Ther.* 1991;14:243–249.

86. LeVeau BF, Rogers C. Selective training of the vastus medialis muscle using EMG biofeedback. *Phys Ther.* 1980;60:1410–1415.

87. Tepperman PS, Mazliah J, Naumann S, Delmore T. Effect of ankle position on isometric quadriceps strengthening. *Am J Phys Med.* 1986;65:69–74.

88. Wheatley MD, Jahnke WD. Electromyographic study of the superficial thigh and hip muscles in normal individuals. *Arch Phys Med Rehabil.* 1951;32:508–515.

89. Hanten WP, Schulties SS. Exercise effects on electromyographic activity of the vastus medialis oblique and vastus lateralis muscles. *Phys Ther.* 1990;70:561–565.

90. Ventura A, Boschetti GF, Gualtieri D. A surface electromyographic study of vastus medialis and vastus lateralis dominance in knee extension. *J Sport Traumatol Rel Res.* 1994;16:152–160.

91. Skurja M, Perry J, Gronley J, et al. Quadriceps action in straight leg raise versus isolated knee extension. *Phys Ther.* 1980;60:582.

92. Soderberg GL, Cook TM. An electromyographic analysis of quadriceps femoris muscle setting and straight leg raising. *Phys Ther.* 1983;63:1434–1438.

93. Soderberg GL, Minor S, Arnold K, et al. Electromyographic analysis of knee exercise in healthy subjects and in patients with knee pathologies. *Phys Ther.* 1987;67:1691–1696.

94. Ingersoll C, Knight K. Patellar location changes following EMG biofeedback or progressive resistance exercises. *Med Sci Sports Exerc.* 1991;23:1122–1127.

95. Henry J. Conservative treatment of patellofemoral subluxation. *Clin Sports Med.* 1989;8:261–277.

96. Knight KL, Martin JA, Londeree BR. EMG comparison of quadriceps femoris activity during knee extension and straight leg raises. *Am J Phys Med.* 1979; 58:57–69.

97. Montgomery JB, Steadman JR. Rehabilitation of the injured knee. *Clin Sports Med.* 1985;4:333–343.

98. Chesworth BM, Culham EG, Tata GE, Peat M. Validation of outcome measures in patients with patellofemoral syndrome. *J Orthop Sports Phys Ther.* 1989;11:302–308.

99. Stiene HA, Brosky T, Reinking MF, Nyland J, et al. A comparison of closed kinetic chain and isokinetic joint isolation exercise in patients with patellofemoral dysfunction. *J Orthop Sports Phys Ther.* 1996;24:136–141.

100. Rivera JE. Open versus closed kinetic chain rehabilitation of the lower extremity: a functional and biomechanical analysis. *J Sports Rehabil.* 1994;3:154–167.

101. McConnell JS. The management of chondromalacia patellae: a long term solution. *Aust J Physiother.* 1986;32:215–223.

102. McConnell JS. Training the vastus medialis oblique in the management of patellofemoral pain. *Proceedings of the Tenth International Conference of the World Confederation for Physical Therapy, Sydney, Australia, May 1987.*

103. Duarte Cintra AI, Furlani J. Electromyographic study of quadriceps femoris in man. *Electromyogr Clin Neurophysiol.* 1981;21:539–554.

104. Yamashita N. EMG activities in mono and bi-articular thigh muscles in combined hip and knee extension. *Eur J Appl Physiol.* 1988;58:274–277.

105. Grabiner MD, Koh TJ, Von Haffen L. Effect of concomitant hip joint adduction and knee joint extension forces on quadriceps activation. *Eur J Exp Musculoskel Res.* 1992;1:155–160.

106. Andriacchi TP, Andersson GBJ, Ortengren R, Mikosz RP. A study of factors influencing muscle activity about the knee joint. *J Orthop Res.* 1984;1:266–275.

107. Schmidt RA. *Motor Control and Learning: A Behavioral Emphasis*. Champaign, IL: Human Kinetics Books; 1988.

108. Sale D. Neural adaptation to strength training. In: Komi PV, ed. *Strength and Power in Sport*. Oxford, England: Blackwell Scientific Publications; 1992: 249–265.

109. Draper V. Electromyographic biofeedback and recovery of quadriceps femoris muscle function following anterior cruciate ligament reconstruction. *Phys Ther.* 1990;9:11–17.

110. Draper B, Ballard L. Electrical stimulation versus electromyographic biofeedback in the recovery of quadriceps femoris muscle function following anterior cruciate ligament surgery. *Phys Ther.* 1991;71:455–463.

111. Sprenger CK, Carlson K, Wessman HC. Application of electromyographic biofeedback following medial meniscectomy. *Phys Ther.* 1979;59:167–169.

112. King AC, Ahles TA, Martin JE, White R. EMG biofeedback-controlled exercise in chronic arthritic knee pain. *Arch Phys Med Rehabil.* 1984;65:341–343.

113. Lucca JA, Recchiuti SJ. Effect of electromyographic biofeedback on an isometric strengthening program. *Phys Ther.* 1983;63:200–203.

114. Levitt R, Deisinger JA, Remondet Wall J, Ford L, et al. EMG feedback-assisted postoperative rehabilitation of minor arthroscopic knee surgeries. *J Sports Med Phys Fitness.* 1995;35:218–223.

115. Werner S, Knutsson E, Eriksson E. Effect of taping the patella on concentric and eccentric torque and EMG of knee extensor and flexor muscles in patients with patellofemoral pain syndrome. *Knee Surg Sport Traumatol Arthrosc.* 1993;1:169–177.

116. Bohannon RW. Effects of electrical stimulation to the vastus medialis muscle in a patient with chronically dislocating patellae. *Phys Ther.* 1983;63:1445–1447.

117. Werner S, Arvidsson H, Arvidsson I, Eriksson E. Electrical stimulation of vastus medialis and stretching of lateral thigh muscles in patients with patello-femoral symptoms. *Knee Surg Sports Traumatol Arthrosc.* 1993;1:85–92.

118. Kasman G. Use of integrated electromyography for the assessment and treatment of musculoskeletal pain: guidelines for physical medicine practitioners. In: Cram JR, ed. *Clinical EMG for Surface Recordings.* Vol 2. Nevada City, CA: Clinical Resources; 1990: 255–302.

119. De Luca CJ, Merletti R. Surface myoelectric signal cross-talk among muscles of the leg. *Electroencephalogr Clin Neurophysiol.* 1988;69:568–575.

120. Winter DA, Fuglevand AJ, Archer SE. Crosstalk in surface electromyography: theoretical and practical estimates. *J Electromyogr Kinesiol.* 1994;4:15–26.

121. Allington RO, Baxter ML, Koepke GH, Christopher RP. Strengthening techniques of the quadriceps muscles: an electromyographic evaluation. *Phys Ther.* 1966;46:1173–1176.

122. Winter DA. Electromyogram recording, processing, and normalization: procedures and considerations. *J Hum Muscle Perform.* 1991;1:5–15.

123. Yang JF, Winter DA. Electromyographic amplitude normalization methods: improving their sensitivity as diagnostic tools in gait analysis. *Arch Phys Med Rehabil.* 1984;65:517–521.

Appendix 12–A

Surface Electromyographic Application Guide for Patellofemoral Pain Syndrome

The reader is referred to the discussion in Chapter 12 for a review of intervention approaches. The suggestions that follow are derived from those resources. Descriptions and operational definitions are provided to clarify optional practice patterns. The reader is referred to other text materials for additional discussion of surface electromyographic (SEMG) recording technique, clinical assessment, and feedback training strategies described below.[1,2]

CANDIDATES

Implement SEMG for patients
- with patellofemoral pain syndrome (PFPS) with marked quadriceps atrophy, history of subluxation/dislocation, or apparent patellofemoral tracking problems assessed radiographically
- with PFPS who have not responded to other conservative measures within 4 to 6 weeks and who subjectively express a feeling of patellar instability or show evidence of patellar hypermobility on physical examination
- who have undergone knee surgery and have secondary PFPS

Source: Adapted from GS Kasman, JR Cram, and SL Wolf, *Clinical Applications in Surface Electromyography: Chronic Musculoskeletal Pain,* © 1998, Aspen Publishers, Inc.

EVALUATION OBJECTIVES

- to identify generally depressed quadriceps activity
- to identify poorly coordinated quadriceps function—specifically, decreased or ill-timed vastus medialis obliquus (VMO) recruitment relative to vastus lateralis (VL)

SEMG FEEDBACK TRAINING OBJECTIVES

- to increase general quadriceps recruitment
- to restore normal patterns of muscle synergy (increase magnitude, improve timing of VMO recruitment relative to VL)
- to resolve mechanical dysfunction and pain
- to retain and generalize improved motor control to functional contexts
- to resolve or reduce functional limitations and disability

RECORDING SETUP

1. Follow manufacturer's instructions for electrode and skin preparation as well as other requirements for SEMG system operation.
2. Use standard commercial electrodes designed for SEMG recording, 0.5–1.0 cm in diameter, with spacing of active electrode centers 1.5–2.0 cm apart. Place the reference electrode equidistant from each

of the active electrodes (so that a triangle is formed by the three electrodes) or place the reference electrode over a bony prominence such as the fibular head.

3. Confirm optimal electrode placement sites by observation and palpation of the patient's quadriceps during isometric contraction with the knee extended. Apply electrodes during isometric contraction.

    • *VMO*. Identify the superomedial aspect of the patella. Center the distal active electrode about 1.5–2.0 cm proximally, along a line oriented approximately 50 degrees medially oblique to the longitudinal femoral axis. The proximal active electrode should follow along the same line—that is, parallel to muscle fiber direction. These procedures should result in placement of active electrodes visibly over the VMO belly. Modify placements from these recommendations if necessary to account for unusual anthropometric differences. Exercise caution not to place the active electrodes too far in a medial-proximal direction over the hip adductors.

    • *VL*. Identify the superolateral aspect of the patella. Center the distal active electrode about 5.0–7.0 cm proximally, along a line oriented approximately 15 degrees laterally oblique to the longitudinal femoral axis. The proximal active electrode should follow along the same line—that is, parallel to muscle fiber direction. These procedures should result in placement of active electrodes visibly over the distal VL belly. Modify placements from these recommendations if necessary to account for unusual anthropometric differences. Exercise caution not to place the active electrodes too far in a lateral direction over the iliotibial band. Carefully palpate the superior aspect of the iliotibial band if visible demarcation of the VL is unclear. Also exercise caution not to

place the electrodes too far in a proximal-medial direction over the rectus femoris. The desired target region can be confirmed as lying roughly 25% of the distance between the superolateral aspect of the patella and the anterior superior iliac spine.

4. Consider additional sites[1,3] such as the rectus femoris, medial or lateral hamstrings, hip adductor group, tensor fasciae latae, gluteus medius, or gluteus maximus, if PFPS is accompanied by hip muscle weakness or tightness.

EVALUATION PROCEDURES

1. Perform at least five repetitions of each task to assess response consistency. Many more repetitions may be needed to assess SEMG responses with reproduction of symptoms.

2. Select relevant tasks from the following:
    • maximal effort quadriceps setting with the knee extended in supine or long sitting
    • seated maximal and submaximal isometric contractions with the patient's knee in 10 to 15 degrees of flexion and 45 to 60 degrees of flexion
    • seated active range of motion (AROM):
      –repeated trials at progressively increased loads
      –repeated trials at progressively greater velocities
      –during isokinetic testing
    • closed kinetic chain tasks
      –Place a standard bathroom scale under each of the patient's feet to ensure equal weight bearing when such is indicated.
      –Examine both concentric and eccentric movement phases.
      –Include bilateral partial squat, unilateral squat, lunge, step-up, step-down.
    • functional activity analysis of work, home, sports-specific activities that ex-

acerbate symptoms or are performed frequently

3. At a minimum, include one maximal-effort isometric task in the open chain as a standard, and one closed-chain task known to be associated with symptom reproduction.

INTERPRETATION

1. Follow manufacturer's guidelines for display configuration and data management options of SEMG amplitudes. When feasible, a line tracing display of full-wave rectified and overlaid VMO and VL signals, with minimal smoothing, is recommended. Raw visual displays are also appropriate, and bar graph displays may be used for simple analyses. Single-channel devices can be used to compare general quadriceps activity from a symptomatic with an asymptomatic lower extremity, but VMO:VL comparisons will not be very feasible. Graphic printout capability is useful for documentation. Refer to figures in Chapter 12 as well as Figures 12–A–1 and 12–A–2 for representative SEMG tracings of normal and aberrant function.

2. Timing analyses are demanding and require raw or rectified line tracing graphics with a smoothing time constant of 0.1 second or less, SEMG sampling of at least 1000 Hz, frequency bandwidth filter low cutoff of 25 Hz or less, and a high-resolution display with variable sweep speed. The ability to perform off-line manipulation of tracings for calculation of timing variables is desirable.

3. For quantitative assessments, consider discarding the results of the first two repetitions of any task and averaging the results from the three subsequent repetitions. Also, consider establishing baseline response levels for desired SEMG variables when symptoms are absent, and assessing how those scores

change across multiple repetitions of a functional task known to exacerbate symptoms.

4. Select SEMG assessment parameters from the following:
   • Assess amplitude, variance, recruitment slope, decruitment slope of each channel during contraction efforts. SEMG activity should be stable and quiescent before command to contract. Recruitment and decruitment should be prompt and smooth. Activity should return to baseline levels with apparent termination of voluntary contraction.
   • Assess relationship of salient SEMG events to particular range-of-motion arcs. Observe for consistent magnitude elevations or depressions during a painful portion of the AROM arc.
   • Assess left/right peak amplitude symmetry for VMO and VL recordings, respectively. That is, the left and right side of each muscle site should function symmetrically. Satisfactory symmetry is operationally defined as left/right scores within 35% as calculated:
        [(higher side value – lower side value) ÷ higher side value]
   Symmetry assessment assumes an equivalent extrinsic load, left/right AROM excursion, and velocity (for example, pacing regulated by a metronome or isokinetic device). VMO activity may be depressed on the symptomatic side, or both VMO and VL intensities may be altered.
   • Assess nonnormalized VMO:VL peak amplitude ratios. Divide the VMO peak amplitude by the VL peak amplitude during a test task to produce an activity ratio. The left side VMO:VL ratio should be roughly symmetric to the right side ratio, and with the electrode placements as described above, usually approximately 0.8 and greater. However, wide intersubject variation is to be expected with this simple ratio

method (ranging from about 0.5 to 4.0 in asymtomatic persons). Comparisons across subjects cannot be considered appropriate unless a validated database is constructed with the particular circumstances under investigation. A precise ratio range that discriminates normal from aberrant function cannot be stated routinely.

- Assess normalized VMO:VL ratios. Activity from each recording site should generally be normalized for comparison with a healthy population standard. To construct a normalized VMO:VL ratio, perform the following:
 −Instruct the patient to perform a maximally resisted isometric seated knee extension effort at about 45 degrees of flexion. Sustain resistance for 6 seconds. Average the amplitude of VMO and VL activity, respectively, over the middle 2 seconds, and repeat for at least three repetitions. Discard this method if the patient reports pain during the contractions or if scores vary by more than about 15% across repetitions. These scores will serve as a reference for the clinical movement task.
 −Instruct the patient to perform a second task of clinical interest such as a squat to 45 degrees. Average the peak activity of the VMO and the VL over at least three repetitions. Divide the average peak microvolt score for the VMO during the squat by the maximal-effort VMO reference value obtained earlier. Multiply by 100 so that squat activity is expressed as a percentage of seated maximal-effort activity. Repeat the procedure for the VL. Divide the percentage of maximum VMO value by the percentage of maximum VL value to obtain a normalized VMO:VL ratio.
 −Normalized VMO:VL activity ratios should approximate 1.0. Asymmetri-

cally depressed values from a symptomatic side compared with an asymptomatic side are potentially aberrant, as are values less than 0.6.
 −Consider normalization to a submaximal-effort contraction for comparisons across subjects and recording sites if maximal-effort contractions are painful, produce inconsistent responses, or are otherwise suspected of being dysfunctional (see discussion of SEMG limitations in Chapter 12). Normalization methods other than those described above will, however, prove to be more complex and time consuming for the typical clinician to perform.

- Assess VMO:VL timing. Expect coincident tracking of VMO and VL line tracing signals from the same limb recorded through an AROM arc. With use of current commercially available SEMG devices, any difference in recruitment, peak, or decruitment timing that is visibly apparent is potentially significant. Timing deficiencies can be quantified with calculations of average slope, time to peak activity, or time to some percentage of maximum activity that is clinically meaningful. Onset time can be reported as the latency to achieve a microvolt value equivalent to 2 standard deviations above the resting baseline mean. Contraction duration may be noted as the amount of time between onset and baseline recovery (amplitude recovery within 2 standard deviations of the baseline mean).

- Conduct frequency spectral analysis for fatigue assessment. This analysis requires advanced equipment and technique. All SEMG equipment manufacturer's guidelines should be followed explicitly. Observe the median frequency during a standardized isometric contraction of at least 70% of maximum effort (assuming that this can be reliably produced by the patient). Observe the rate of decline in median frequency values (indicative of increased fatigue) during a prolonged effort contraction, comparing left with right sides. To track fatigue during a functional task, obtain SEMG frequency data during a high-level isometric contraction before initiation of functional activity. Then have the patient perform the functional task for a duration expected to induce fatigue or increase symptoms. Repeat the standardized isometric test, extract median frequency values, and compare these values with initial levels for indications of fatigue. Have the patient rest for 1 to 3 minutes, and then repeat the isometric test and frequency analysis. Continue the rest period:frequency test sequence to assess for recovery to initial median frequency values.

- If possible, monitor the patient's thigh for changes in skin temperature, which can be associated with changes in impedance and spurious effects on SEMG frequency and amplitude data.
- Assess analogous scores for SEMG responses from other thigh and hip muscles.

TRAINING PROGRESSIONS FOR COMMON PATIENT PRESENTATIONS

VMO and VL Hypoactivity

Some patients with unilateral symptoms show asymmetrically depressed activity from the involved side VMO and VL during maximal-effort contractions (Figure 12–A–1). Submaximal contractions are also accompanied often by nonselective hypoactivity, although this finding may be variable and sometimes reversed. In these patients, however, VMO and VL activity patterns always follow the same course; there is no evidence of a selective change of VMO func-

tion. A generalized quadriceps impairment is presumed to contribute to patellofemoral dysfunction.

Patients with VMO and VL hypoactivity tend to progress with a carefully graded exercise program. If desired, SEMG feedback can be combined with exercise for general quadriceps muscle uptraining.

1. Follow manufacturer's instructions for feedback display options. Keep the display graphics simple and ensure that the patient can see and hear the feedback clearly. A single feedback channel from either VMO or VL, or more broadly across the quadriceps, is adequate.
2. Instruct the patient to watch or listen to SEMG feedback as he or she exerts a maximal recruitment effort. Encourage repetition of recruitment strategies that produce higher microvolt values.
3. As skill develops, shape quadriceps responses progressively higher. That is, start with simple uptraining goals and, once they are consistently met, challenge the patient by asking for greater-intensity contractions in more demanding contexts. In general:
   - *Incorporate multijoint control.* Start with isolated quadriceps contractions and then have the patient maximize quadriceps activity while simultaneously contracting hip and ankle muscles.
   - *Add background noise and activity as well as cognitive distractor tasks.* Start practice in a quiet, simple environment but challenge skill by adding complexity and unpredictability to the setting.
   - *Randomize training activities.* Begin by calling for many repetitions of one activity, then many repetitions of a different training task, and so forth. Once the patient is oriented to each task, randomize the training sequence. For example, a patient may begin by using SEMG feedback during 20 trials of

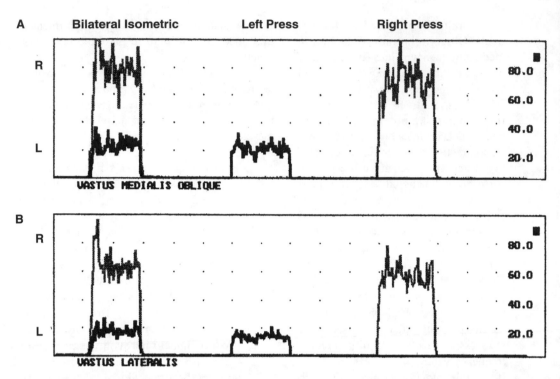

Figure 12–A–1 SEMG Activity of the Left and Right (**A**) Vastus Medialis Obliquus and (**B**) Vastus Lateralis Recorded from a Postsurgical Patient with Chronic Left PFPS. The first set of peaks corresponds to bilateral maximal-effort isometric quadriceps setting with the patient in the supine position. The second and third set of peaks correspond to an equivalent submaximal unilateral leg press task performed on the left and right, respectively. Activity at both recording sites appears proportionately diminished on the left compared with the right. *Source:* Reprinted from GS Kasman, JR Cram, and SL Wolf, *Clinical Applications in Surface Electromyography: Chronic Musculoskeletal Pain*, p 398, © 1998, Aspen Publishers, Inc.

standing weight shift, then 20 trials of partial squat, and finally 20 trials of step-up/step-down. Subsequently, the patient can be instructed to use SEMG feedback during 20 trials of each of the same exercises, but with the task order mixed in a random manner.

• *Withdraw continuous audiovisual feedback.* Start by giving the patient access to SEMG feedback on every trial. Once the patient has demonstrated some degree of competence, hide the feedback every other trial. Alternatively, hide the feedback during physical performance of each trial. After each effort, ask the patient if he or she thinks that the

SEMG goal was met. Once the patient answers, reveal the display (with the previous trial's results) or verbally report the actual results. Discontinuous and delayed feedback, as well as randomization of training tasks, may slow skill acquisition but will likely promote long-term retention.

4. Display SEMG feedback, as relevant, during the following tasks:
• *Isolation of target muscle activity.* Use quadriceps setting or seated active knee extension to orient the patient to quadriceps function and the feedback display. Ensure that the patient understands how the visual or auditory cues

relate to muscle activation and relaxation. If guarding or excessive hamstring activity is suspected, provide SEMG feedback from hamstrings while cueing relaxation of those muscles.

- *Threshold-based uptraining.* Set a threshold microvolt level for the patient to try to exceed. The threshold may be cued by a goal line on a visual display, or onset of an audio signal when the goal is reached. Begin with a threshold value about 10% to 15% above the patient's initial recruitment efforts or one that can be obtained with about 80% to 90% success. Emphasize maximal-effort quadriceps setting at various joint angles.

- *Therapeutic exercises with SEMG feedback and generalization to progressively dynamic movement.* For each training task, progress as appropriate from
  –small to large movement arcs
  –slow to fast speed
  –light to heavy resistance
  Establish adequate symptom control and progressively emphasize closed-chain activities. Select activities relevant to the patient's routine rehabilitation protocol from the following:
  –seated/supine terminal knee extension, full-arc knee extension
  –straight leg raising
  –standing quadriceps setting
  –sit-to-stand, stand-to-sit
  –standing in stride, left/right weight shifting
  –involved side unilateral stance
  –taking one step forward and backward with the involved side, level gait, ramps
  –stationary bike
  –bilateral partial squats
  –stair-stepper
  –front step-ups/step-downs, lateral step-ups/step-downs

  –cross-over and braiding steps, balancing on rocker platforms and rolls
  –partial squats in stride, lunge steps, unilateral squats, jumping, hopping

- *Functional activity performance with SEMG feedback.* Use other relevant work and sports-specific activities that require high-intensity or high-velocity quadriceps activity.

- *Motor copy training.* Some SEMG systems enable a patient to use an SEMG signal from a symptomatic side to match a template created from the asymptomatic side. First, electrodes are placed on the asymptomatic thigh and the patient performs one or a few trials of a dynamic task. The resultant SEMG line tracing is saved and locked onto the display for as many successive sweeps as desired. Next, electrodes are placed in a homologous position on the symptomatic thigh and the patient performs the same task. The patient uses the line tracing signal from the symptomatic side to overlay the template from the asymptomatic side. Thus, the patient uses activity from the asymptomatic side as a guide for coordination of the symptomatic side muscle. For patients with true unilateral problems, the template serves as a normal reference.

- *SEMG-triggered neuromuscular electrical stimulation.* Certain SEMG systems allow for coupling to a neuromuscular electrical stimulator applied over the quadriceps. The paradigm begins with initiation of voluntary quadriceps contraction. SEMG electrodes over the muscle detect the voluntary effort, which is displayed in a routine fashion. When a threshold level of microvolts (set to any desired level by the therapist) is exceeded, a neuromuscular electrical stimulator is triggered to augment quadriceps contraction. SEMG-triggered neuromuscular electrical stimulation can be a powerful tool for neuromuscular reeducation and muscle conditioning. Setup guidelines vary with the particular brand of SEMG device.

5. At the beginning and end of each feedback training session, document peak SEMG microvolt levels, the percentage of trials a threshold value was exceeded, or changes in any SEMG parameter used during the initial evaluation.

6. Integrate SEMG feedback training with indicated physical agents, manual therapies, orthotic devices, and home exercise programs.

7. Consider the potential utility and cost-effectiveness of a home SEMG feedback trainer.

VMO:VL Imbalance

Imbalance of the VMO:VL relationship can be characterized with SEMG in several ways. Patients with unilateral complaints may show decreased VMO activity on the involved side with relative left/right symmetry (or a lesser amount of asymmetry) for the VL. This difference can also be represented by an asymmetrically depressed nonnormalized or normalized VMO:VL ratio. Persons with asymmetric SEMG patterns often seem to have asymmetric patterns of lower extremity alignment and flexibility. The involved side may be observed with greater femoral anteversion, hip medial rotation, iliotibial band tightness, Q angle, or foot pronation.

Symmetry assessment with SEMG is less revealing in patients with bilateral PFPS. Moreover, some patients show bilateral deficits in alignment and flexibility, but complain only of unilateral symptoms. Thus SEMG activity in some patients with unilateral PFPS may be similar when recorded from each limb but different from that displayed by healthy subjects. Activity ratios and timing phenomena should be monitored through functional movements. Problematic range-of-motion arcs and tasks vary across

individuals. Patients with recurrent dislocation or marked hypomobility following surgery or immobilization tend to show the most aberrant SEMG patterns. However, activity can be altered in patients with subtle disease. In a manner analogous to the assessment of patients with low back or shoulder girdle dysfunction, the potential role of muscular imbalance probably varies in different subpopulations. The clinician should not expect to find evidence of VMO insufficiency in all, or even most, patients with nonspecific complaints of anterior knee pain. SEMG feedback training is indicated when aberrant muscle activity patterns are substantiated during examination. Patellofemoral tracking dysfunction and muscle imbalance are then suspected syndrome components. Training focuses on VMO uptraining.

The training progression for VMO:VL imbalance is as follows:

1. Follow guidelines for preliminary setup and patient advancement as described above in the training progression for VMO and VL hypoactivity.

2. Include one feedback channel for the VMO and another for the VL.

3. Instruct the patient to watch or listen to the SEMG feedback as he or she tries to increase recruitment of the VMO relative to the VL. Encourage repetition of recruitment strategies that achieve this goal.

4. Display SEMG feedback, as relevant, during the following tasks:
   • Isolation of target muscle activity. Use seated quadriceps setting and knee extension to demonstrate VMO and VL contributions to knee function. There is no simple maneuver to isolate the VMO from the VL: explain their balancing contribution to control of the patella to the patient.
   • Threshold-based uptraining for VMO:
     −Set a threshold for the VMO and one for the VL at levels consistently

reached during comfortable quadriceps setting trials at about 15% to 25% of maximal effort.

–Instruct the patient to try to increase VMO activity above the VMO threshold and to maintain VL activity below the VL threshold.

–To free the patient to focus visually on the VMO, use an auditory function as an alarm if VL activity exceeds its threshold. Alternatively, set an auditory reward to sound if the baseline VMO:VL ratio is exceeded.

• Therapeutic exercises with SEMG feedback. Use the following to facilitate VMO activity:

–Have the patient perform partial squats combined with hip adductor squeeze by using a semirigid pad between the thighs.

–Consider that, with standard commercial electrode configurations and signal processing, it is not possible to rule out cross-talk from adductor muscles as contributing to the appearance of increased VMO activity.

–Experiment with different foot pronation/supination and hip medial/lateral rotation positions during training tasks. Individual responses may be noted, but there are no known successful training effects for most persons.

• Generalization to progressively dynamic movement. For each task, progress VMO:VL training as appropriate from

–small to large movement arcs

–slow to fast speed

–light to heavy resistance

Select activities that can be performed without exacerbating symptoms, emphasizing closed-chain tasks when possible.

–standing quadriceps setting

–standing in stride, left/right weight shifting

–involved side unilateral stance

–taking one step forward and backward on the involved side, level gait, ramps

–stationary bike

–bilateral partial squats

–sit-to-stand, stand-to-sit

–stair-stepper

–front step-ups/step-downs, lateral step-ups/step-downs

–cross-over and braiding steps, balancing on rocker platforms and rolls

–partial squats in stride, lunge steps, unilateral squats, jumping, hopping, cross-cutting

• Functional activity performance with SEMG feedback. Use other relevant work- and sports-specific activities. Continue training with other movements required to meet the patient's functional activity goals.

• Motor copy training. Use an asymptomatic side VMO as a template for pattern matching with the symptomatic side VMO during any of the above-listed tasks.

• SEMG-triggered neuromuscular electrical stimulation. This procedure is recommended for VMO uptraining if there are no contraindications or precautions (Figure 12–A–2). Set the triggering SEMG threshold so that it is exceeded with the initiation of movement.

5. At the beginning and end of each feedback training session, document peak percentage of left/right asymmetry for VMO and VL activity, respectively; nonnormalized or normalized VMO:VL ratios; or timing variables, each as relevant to SEMG parameters used during the initial evaluation.

6. Integrate SEMG feedback training with indicated physical agents, manual therapies, orthotic devices, taping techniques, and home exercise programs.

7. Consider the potential utility and cost-effectiveness of a home SEMG trainer.

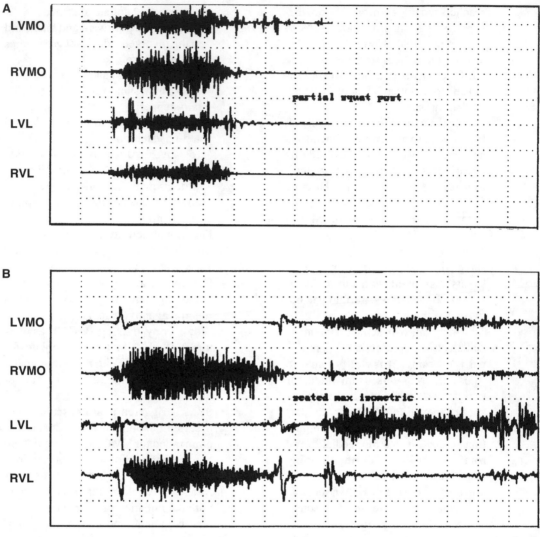

continues

Figure 12–A–2 Effects of SEMG-Triggered Neuromuscular Electrical Stimulation on SEMG Activity of the Left (L) and Right (R) Vastus Medialis Obliquus (VMO) and Vastus Lateralis (VL). (**A**) Activity during partial squat, recorded from the same patient shown in Figure 12–4, after a 20-minute application of SEMG-NMES. (**B** and **C**) Activity from a different patient with chronic patellofemoral pain syndrome, recorded during seated maximal effort isometric quadriceps setting before and after a 20-minute application of SEMG-NMES, respectively. *Source:* Reprinted from GS Kasman, JR Cram, and SL Wolf, *Clinical Applications in Surface Electromyography: Chronic Musculoskeletal Pain*, pp 400–401, © 1998, Aspen Publishers, Inc.

Figure 12–A–2 continued

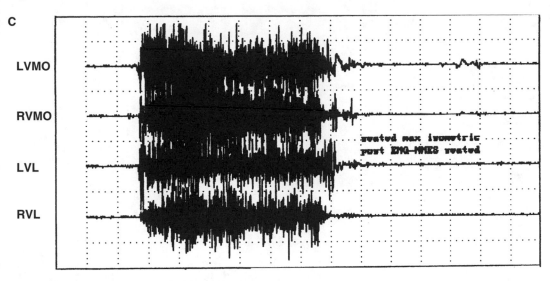

REFERENCES

1. Cram JR, Kasman GS. *An Introduction to Surface Electromyography*. Gaithersburg, MD: Aspen Publishers; 1998.

2. Kasman GS, Cram JR, Wolf SL. *Clinical Applications in Surface Electromyography: Chronic Musculoskeletal Pain*. Gaithersburg, MD: Aspen Publishers; 1998.

3. Basmajian JV, Blumentsein R. Electrode placement in electromyographic biofeedback. In: Basmajian JV, ed. *Biofeedback: Principles and Practice for Clinicians*. 3rd ed. Baltimore: Williams & Wilkins; 1989:369–382.

CHAPTER 13

Biomechanical Management of Patellofemoral Pain and Dysfunction with Foot Orthotic Devices

INTRODUCTION

For many years, anecdotal evidence has linked abnormal foot pronation with knee pain. As early as 1888, Royal Whitman noted a correlation between leg and knee pain and flatfoot.[1] In the 1930s, Ober used a Thomas heel as part of his conservative treatment of patellofemoral dislocations.[2] During the height of the "running boom" in the 1970s and early 1980s, many articles appeared relating the effects of foot dysfunction and lower extremity injuries.[3-26] Most of these articles cited the knee as one of the most common sites of running injuries.[3-25] In 1987, Nicholas and Marino theorized a human linkage system in which foot dysfunction affected all lower extremity function.[27] Initial research was conducted to elucidate the biomechanics of running and to develop shoe gear that could minimize the stress of running.[28-37]

This chapter investigates both the documented and speculative correlation between foot pathomechanics and knee joint function. Although much anecdotal evidence is available, few good long-term scientific studies exist to support the use of foot orthotics in the treatment of knee pain. Even investigators who support the use of orthotics have a difficult time explaining the mechanism of action of foot orthotics. Nevertheless, throughout the course of medical history many anecdotal methods of treatment have eventually been proven to have a rational scientific basis.

It is hoped that this chapter will challenge readers to open their mind to an approach to patellofemoral pain that complements other modalities outlined elsewhere in this book.

PRACTICAL BIOMECHANICS OF THE LOWER EXTREMITY

When the foot is on the ground in a closed kinetic chain (CKC), it is the interface between the support surface and the leg above. As motion occurs above and below, the foot must react and adapt to an ever-changing environment. It must alternately act as a rigid lever to support and propel the body above, and a mobile adapter to the terrain below.[38-42] In a CKC, the foot reacts much like the foundation of a building during an earthquake; it must support all above while adapting to what occurs below.[41] At all times it must absorb shock and attenuate ground reactive forces.[38-41] To complicate matters, all of this must occur within a set time frame or pathology can ensue.[38-41]

Normal Biomechanics of the Lower Extremity

The inability of the foot to perform properly the tasks outlined above can lead to compensation in the foot itself or in the limb above. This compensation is postulated to be the basis for many foot and lower extremity injuries.[3-7, 9-11,14,16-18,21,25,26,38-41,43,44] In the foot, compensation occurs through the subtalar joint (STJ) and midtarsal joint (MTJ).[38–42,45] Manter demonstrated that the axis of the STJ is a pronatory/supinatory axis.[45] The axis runs from the posterolateral aspect of the calcaneus to the dorsomedial aspect of the talar head, deviating 42 degrees on the transverse plane and 16 degrees on the sagittal plane (Figure 13–1).[45,46] He also stated that obligatory motion in the MTJ must occur in response to STJ pronation/supination in a CKC. The function of the STJ is both shock absorption and torque conversion.[42,47,48] It attenuates ground reactive forces and converts transverse plane leg motion (internal/external rotation) into frontal plane foot motion (inversion/eversion). In gait, the STJ moves from pronation to supination in a strict phasic manner. These motions are described below.

Pronation

The ability of the foot (STJ) to unlock itself and adapt to terrain is associated with pronation (Figure 13–2). Pronation is a triplane motion whereby the talus adducts, moves anteriorly, and

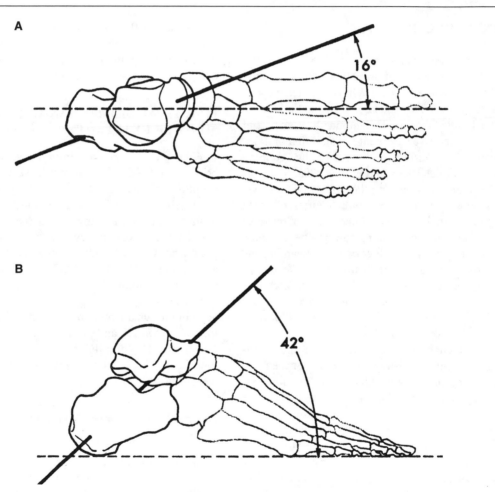

Figure 13–1 The Axis of the Subtalar Joint as Described by Manter. (**A**) The joint deviates from the longitudinal axis of the foot by 16 degrees. (**B**) Manter found a deviation of 42 degrees from the vertical axis. *Source:* Reprinted with permission from R Mann and VT Inman, *Journal of Bone and Joint Surgery*, Vol 46A, pp 469–481, Copyright © 1964 by The Journal of Bone and Joint Surgery, Inc.

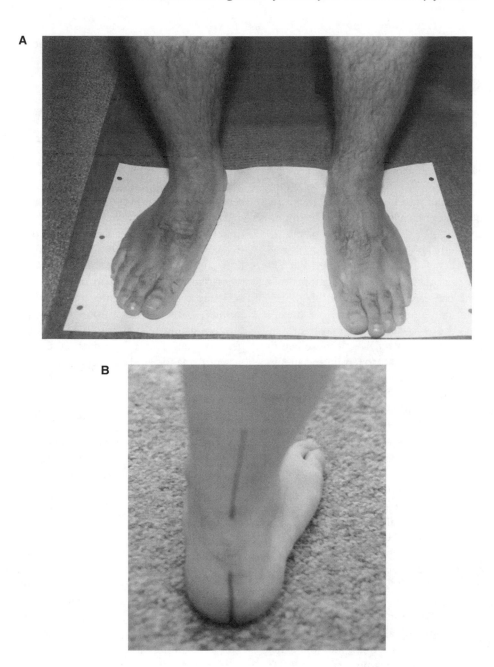

Figure 13–2 Pronation. In closed kinetic chain (CKC) pronation, the arch of the foot "collapses" toward the support surface as the subtalar joint (STJ) and midtarsal joint (MTJ) unlock. In CKC pronation, the talus adducts, plantarflexes, and moves anteriorly on the calcaneus. The calcaneus everts in response to these motions. In the leg above, the tibia must internally rotate and anteriorly migrate in order to maintain ankle joint congruency. **(A)** Note the "bulge" on the medial aspect of the foot below the malleolus. This is the medially displaced (adducted) talar head. **(B)** Note the "too many toes sign" associated with excessive pronation. In both figures one may also visualize the increased internal tibial rotation.

plantarflexes in respect to the calcaneus, which everts in CKC.[49] STJ pronation is initiated when body weight is applied to the foot. This creates a valgus thrust due to the unbalanced alignment of the tibia and calcaneus.[42] The combination of calcaneal eversion and talar adduction produced by this valgus force alters the supportive position of the sustentaculum tali and allows the talus to plantarflex and move anteriorly in respect to the calcaneus.[47] The tibia, which rides on the talus, must then internally rotate and anteriorly displace in order to maintain ankle joint congruence (Figure 13–3).[50] There is approximately 1/2 degree of internal tibial rotation for every degree of calcaneal eversion.[48] Manter reported that STJ pronation is accompanied by obligatory MTJ motion that causes an unlocking of this joint.[45] The medial column of the foot is left unsupported and drops toward the support surface. This causes the foot to act like "a loose bag of bones," allowing it to adapt to terrain and attenuate shock throughout the foot and lower extremity. Inadequate, excessive, or asynchronous pronation (abnormal pronation) prevents the foot from performing properly and may lead to injury.

Supination

Supination is as important to normal foot function as pronation (Figure 13–4). Supination is associated with the ability of the STJ and MTJ to "lock" the foot. The foot becomes rigid, which enables it to support the limb and body above and provides a stable platform over which they can pass.[38–41] CKC supination is a triplane motion where the talus abducts, moves posteriorly, and dorsiflexes while the calcaneus inverts.[38,40] Because tibial motion must follow talar motion to a certain extent, the tibia externally rotates and displaces posteriorly.[38,40] STJ supination is initiated by (1) external rotation in the leg at the end of midstance that is created by the resistive force of the ground as the forefoot contacts the support surface, and (2) the torque created as the contralateral limb advances forward.[38–42] Supination allows the foot to "fix" itself to the support surface, providing support for the limb while ultimately allowing the body to

propel itself forward. Inadequate, excessive, or improperly timed supination (abnormal supination) can lead to injury.

Normal Versus Abnormal Compensation

Compensation is defined as a change of structure, position, or function of one part of the body in an attempt to adjust to a deviation of structure, position, or function of another part.[38] In some cases, this compensation may be required (normal compensation). For example, the foot adapts to accommodate for changing terrain or adjusts to adapt to trunk or lower limb motion to maintain equilibrium. Abnormal compensation is when the foot is forced to adapt to abnormal structure or function in the trunk or lower extremity. Postural or structural abnormalities in the foot or lower extremity (eg, forefoot varus, genu valgum, femoral antetorsion) create a persistent demand for abnormal compensation that may result in pain.[38]

Hypermobility and Excessive Rigidity

In normal function, joint stability is a condition of near balance where joints move only within their normal planes of motion, and motion is minimal.[38] A joint that exhibits significant motion, or motion in a direction that is contrary to its normal plane of motion is considered to be unstable.[38] *Hypermobility* is defined as instability, or the presence of any significant motion in a joint during a time when there should be no motion.[38] Hypermobility in a joint leads to momentary subluxation (partial dislocation) and subsequent trauma to the joint. An individual may develop abnormal compensation to avoid this excessive motion and trauma. Abnormal pronation may be the cause (or effect) of hypermobility in the STJ or MTJ. It may also be caused by abnormal compensation as a result of abnormal structure, position, or function in the trunk or lower extremity (eg, secondary to genu valgum, leg length asymmetry, femoral antetorsion or anteversion) or secondary to pathology within the foot itself (eg, rearfoot or forefoot varus or valgus).

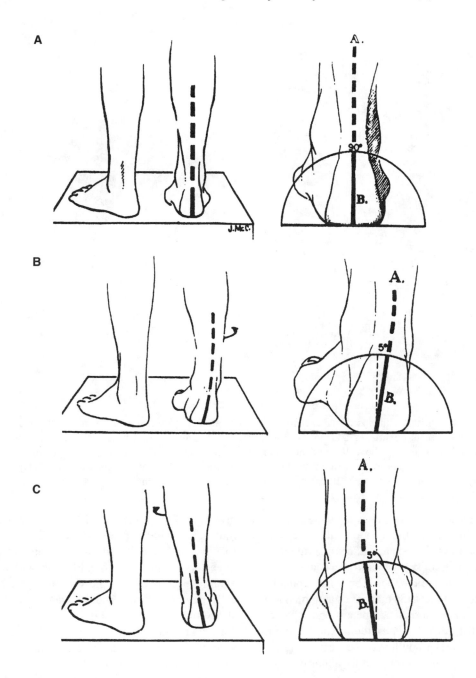

Figure 13–3 The Calcaneal Stance Position in the Neutral, Supinated, and Pronated Foot. (**A**) The bisection of the calcaneus (line B), and its relationship to the bisection of the lower leg (line A) in the neutral STJ position. There is a 0-degree angle with both lines parallel. (**B**) The foot supinated 5 degrees at the STJ. The calcaneus is inverted, lines A and B form a 5-degree angle, and the tibia (lower leg) is externally rotated. (**C**) The foot pronated 5 degrees. The calcaneus is everted, lines A and B form a 5-degree angle, and the tibia (lower leg) is internally rotated. *Source:* Reprinted with permission from JE Di Giovanni and SD Smith, Normal Biomechanics of the Adult Rearfoot: A Radiographic Analysis, *Journal of the American Podiatric Association*, Vol 66, No 11, p 814, © 1976, American Podiatric Medical Association.

A

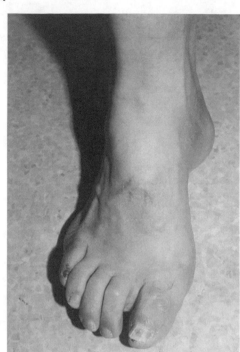

B

Figure 13–4 Supination. In closed kinetic chain (CKC) supination, the arch "rises up" from the support surface. (**A**) The talus abducts, dorsiflexes, and moves posteriorly on the calcaneus. (**B**) The calcaneus inverts in response to these motions. In the leg above, the tibia must rotate externally and migrate posteriorly to maintain ankle joint congruency. In **A** one can see the extreme height of the arch and the excessive gripping of the digits typified by excessive supination. In both **A** and **B**, one may visualize the increased external tibial rotation.

Excessive rigidity occurs when there is an absence of normal motion in a joint at a time when that motion should occur.[41] Excessive rigidity in the lower extremity is generally related to abnormal supination of the foot. Abnormal supination may occur in the same manner as abnormal pronation, or as abnormal compensation for pathology in the trunk, lower extremity, or the foot itself. Both hypermobility and excessive rigidity can be a product of, or lead to, abnormal compensation.

Normal Biomechanics of the Foot and Kinematics of Gait

The gait cycle in humans is divided into two phases and multiple stages (Figures 13–5 through 13–7). The *stance phase* of gait is comprised of five stages: heel contact, foot flat, midstance, heel-off, and toe-off (Figure 13–6).[38–41,51–53] The *swing phase* is subdivided into three stages: acceleration, midswing, and deceleration (Figure 13–7). The walking cycle typically begins with the heel contact stage in the stance phase of gait. In this stage, the calcaneus contacts the ground slightly inverted (2 to 3 degrees in walking, 4 to 6 degrees in running) due to supination of the STJ.[52] As body weight progresses forward over the foot, the STJ and MTJ pronate. This causes a rapid unlocking of these joints and allows the metatarsal segments to loosen (foot-flat stage). The contralateral limb now enters the swing phase. Forward motion of this limb causes resupination of the STJ and MTJ in the stance limb as the foot enters midstance.[38,51] Supination continues throughout

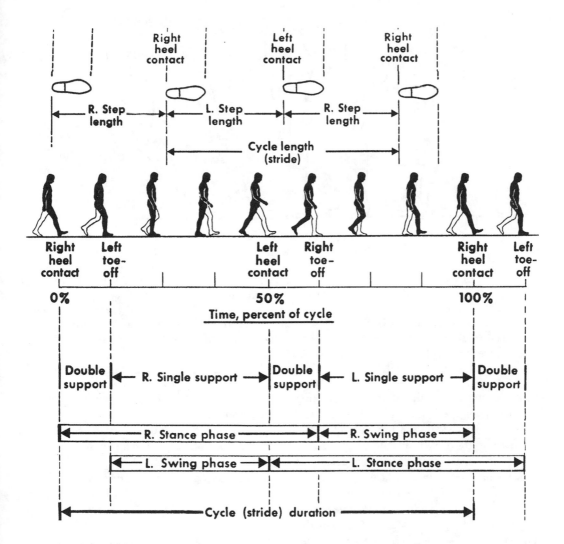

Figure 13–5 The Human Gait Cycle. The gait cycle is characterized by two phases: the stance phase and swing phase. While one leg is in the stance or support phase, the contralateral leg is in the swing phase. In the walking gait cycle, there may be single or double limb support at various times, but at no time are both limbs off the ground. The stance phase begins with heel contact of one limb, and ends with heel contact of the contralateral limb. A stride is measured from heel contact of one limb to a second heel contact in the same limb. *Source:* Reprinted with permission from VT Inman, HJ Ralston, and F Todd, *Human Walking*, p 26, © 1981, Williams & Wilkins.

midstance, locking the STJ and MTJ and tightening the metatarsal segments. This supination is a result of rapid STJ inversion, as the heel is lifted (heel-off stage) because of the angle that the gastrocsoleus muscle forms with the STJ as it inserts into the calcaneus. The rigidity provided by supination provides a stable platform for the first metatarsal and hallux during the toe-off stage. Supination occurs throughout this stage, into and throughout all three swing phase stages until the limb reenters the stance phase at heel contact.[52] Weight transfer and equilibrium are required in the last two stages of stance. This is accomplished by supination.

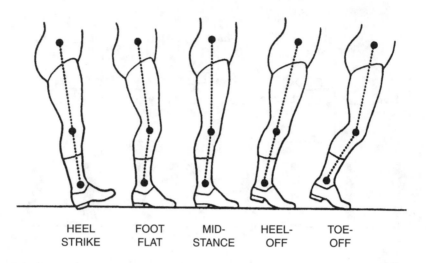

|HEEL STRIKE|FOOT FLAT|MID- STANCE|HEEL- OFF|TOE- OFF|

Figure 13–6 The Stance Phase of the Human Gait Cycle (Walking). The stance phase is divided into five stages: heel contact, foot flat, midstance, heel-off, and toe-off. The foot is supinated at heel contact. Pronation occurs during foot flat to early midstance (to attenuate shock, adapt to terrain, and convert lower leg torque). Resupination occurs in midstance to late stance and continues until toe-off (to provide a stable platform for support and propulsion for the body above). *Source:* Reprinted with permission from KK Wu, *Foot Orthoses: Principles and Clinical Applications*, p 40, © 1990, Williams & Wilkins.

The running gait cycle differs from walking in some major areas (Figures 13–8 and 13–9).[11,26,28,31–34,52] The range of motion required in all lower extremity joints is increased in running (in most cases, it almost doubles).[31,52] The stance phase in running lasts about half as long as in walking.[28,31,33,52] The ground reactive force in running is about 2 to 3 times body weight (in walking, it is about 70% of body-weight).[26,31,32,34,52] Abnormal foot mechanics lead to injury more often in running than in walking. This occurs due to the increased range of motion and shock attenuation required during running, and the decreased time during which these tasks must be accomplished.[3–7, 10–19,21–26,29,32–36,43,44,52]

Pathomechanics of Gait

As described above, there is a normal pattern and sequence that typifies normal human loco-motion. Any disruption of this pattern can lead to dysfunction. There are three major causes of a pathomechanical gait: (1) the failure of a normal event to occur; (2) improper timing of that event;

or (3) an increased or decreased magnitude of that event. Any factor that prevents, retards, or changes the magnitude of normal STJ or MTJ pronation/supination during gait may lead to abnormal biomechanics.[41] Abnormal foot biomechanics during gait may, in turn, cause disorders posturally and/or structurally in the foot, lower leg, or trunk.[27,38,41]

FACTORS THAT ALTER NORMAL BIOMECHANICS AND KINEMATICS OF GAIT

Criteria for Normal Foot and Lower Leg Function

Root et al[38] defined the normal foot and leg alignment during static stance as follows (Figure 13–10):

1. The distal 1/3 of the leg is vertical to the support surface.
2. The knee, ankle, and STJ lie in the transverse plane parallel to the support surface.

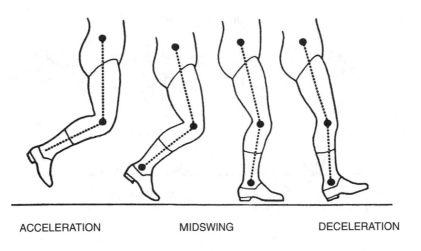

ACCELERATION   MIDSWING   DECELERATION

Figure 13–7 The Swing Phase of the Human Gait Cycle (Walking). The swing phase of gait is divided into three stages: acceleration, midswing, and deceleration. The acceleration stage marks the end of double limb support. In midswing, the accelerating limb clears the ground and then enters the deceleration stage to prepare for heel contact. The foot remains supinated throughout all phases. *Source:* Reprinted with permission from KK Wu, *Foot Orthoses: Principles and Clinical Applications*, p 40, © 1990, Williams & Wilkins.

3. The STJ is in its neutral position (ie, neither pronated nor supinated).
4. Bisection of the posterior surface of the calcaneus is vertical to the support surface.
5. The plantar forefoot plane parallels the plantar rearfoot plane, and both are parallel to the support surface.

In 1953, Hicks showed that the first and fifth metatarsals had triplanar axes of motion, and were therefore capable of independent and more complex movement than the lesser metatarsals (Figure 13–11).[54] Motion in the lesser metatarsals can only occur in one plane (dorsiflexion/plantarflexion).

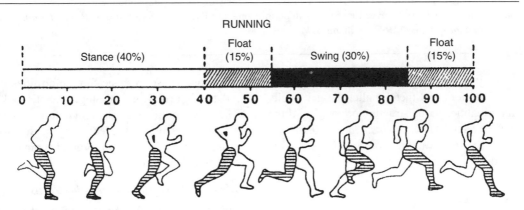

RUNNING

| Stance (40%) | Float (15%) | Swing (30%) | Float (15%) |

0   10   20   30   40   50   60   70   80   90   100

Figure 13–8 The Human Gait Cycle (Running). In the running cycle, the stance phase is reduced in comparison to walking (it comprises 60% of the walking cycle, but only 40% of the running cycle). There is an airborne (float) phase in running where both legs are off the support surface. This never occurs in the walking cycle. *Source:* Reprinted with permission from KK Wu, *Foot Orthoses: Principles and Clinical Applications*, p 44, © 1990, Williams & Wilkins.

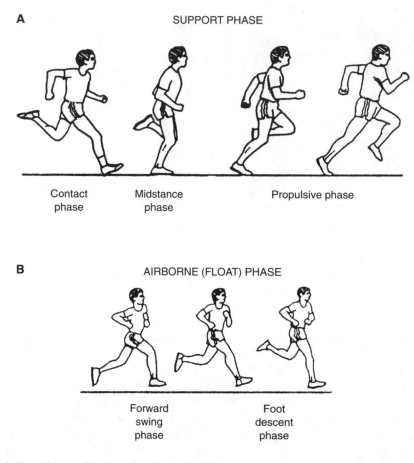

Figure 13–9 Two Phases of the Running Cycle. (**A**) Within the support phase, there are three phases: the contact phase (the foot is supinated), the midstance phase (the foot pronates), and the propulsive phase (the foot resupinates). (**B**) The airborne (float) phase consists of the forward swing phase and the foot descent phase (the foot remains supinated). *Source:* Reprinted with permission from KK Wu, *Foot Orthoses: Principles and Clinical Applications*, p 44, © 1990, Williams & Wilkins.

Many factors can alter the normal biomechanics of the foot and thereby alter the gait cycle. Abnormalities in the structure or position of the foot are referred to as *intrinsic factors. Extrinsic factors* are abnormalities or conditions outside the foot.[41]

Intrinsic Factors

Abnormal development of the STJ or MTJ in a child can lead to structural foot deformities in adulthood. These intrinsic foot deformities can lead to abnormal or pathologic function. The five most common intrinsic foot deformities are: calcaneal varus, calcaneal valgus, forefoot varus, forefoot valgus, and forefoot supinatus (a positional deformity).

Calcaneal Varus (Subtalar Joint Varus)

In utero, the posterior aspect of the calcaneus lies in varus to the body of the bone (Figure 13–12).[55–57] As the child develops, a derotation

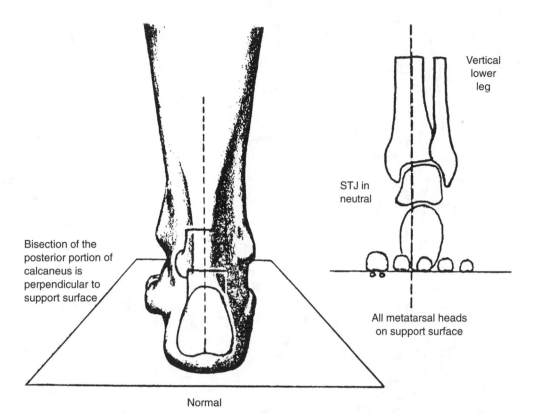

Bisection of the posterior portion of calcaneus is perpendicular to support surface

Vertical lower leg

STJ in neutral

All metatarsal heads on support surface

Normal

Figure 13–10 Biomechanical Ideal. Root and colleagues defined these criteria for normal foot and lower leg alignment. *Source:* Copyright © 1971, Thomas Sgarlato.

occurs that allows the posterior aspect of the calcaneus to align with the corpus calcaneum (about 3 to 4 degrees). If this rotation does not occur by the time the child has been walking for about 3 months, a condition called *calcaneal varus* is said to occur. It is defined as a fixed position of inversion of the posterior aspect of the calcaneus.[40,57] When significant calcaneal varus occurs in a child or adult, it can lead to compensation in the STJ. The STJ will pronate until the posterior aspect of the calcaneus is vertical to the support surface (Figure 13–13).[56,57] Compensation for this deformity can affect the knee, because STJ pronation is generally accompanied by obligatory excessive internal rotation of the lower leg.[38,40,42,53] This excessive rotation must be absorbed by the knee, hip, or low back; in susceptible individuals, the rotation may lead to pathology in those areas.[53,56,58] The frontal plane component of STJ compensation can cause increased valgus stress on the knee.[18,56,59,60]

Calcaneal Valgus (Subtalar Joint Valgus)

Although much more rare than subtalar varus, subtalar valgus is a genetic foot deformity (not ontogenic) that occurs because the lateral aspect of the talus is developmentally shorter than the medial aspect (RO Schuster, unpublished lecture notes, 1971–1975) (Figure 13–14). This creates a fixed position of eversion in the subtalar joint. The deformity leads to a congenital flatfoot (pes planovalgus) and causes the forefoot to compensate abnormally by supination. Knee pain is linked to the flattened arch and forefoot compensation that occur in this disorder. The situation is

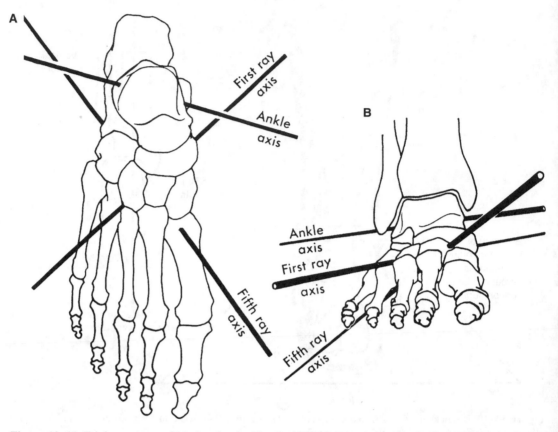

Figure 13–11 Triplanar Axes of Motion for the First and Fifth Metatarsals. (**A**) shows the dorsoplantar foot view, and (**B**) shows the anterior/posterior foot view. The first and fifth rays have an independent triplanar motion. The lesser metatarsals (2, 3, and 4) move primarily in one plane (dorsiflexion, plantarflexion). In the "biomechanical ideal," all metatarsals must function on the same plane and be parallel to the support surface with the STJ in neutral position. *Source:* Reprinted with permission from HL DuVreis, *Surgery of the Foot*, 2nd ed, p 27, © 1965, CV Mosby Company.

similar to that seen in forefoot varus or valgus (described below).

Forefoot Varus

In utero, the plantar aspect of the foot is in varus throughout much of its development (Figure 13–15).[55] The head and neck of the talus are similarly positioned in varus. Normal ontogenic development of the talar head and neck requires a gradual valgus torsion of the talar head (ie, the angle between the neck of the talus and the longitudinal axis of the foot decreases).[55,57] The final position of the neck of the talus determines

the forefoot to rearfoot relationship. This generally ends with the forefoot parallel to the ground and perpendicular to the bisection of the posterior portion of the calcaneus in adult stance (Figure 13–16).[57] A failure to rotate causes a fixed position of inversion of the midtarsal joint (and therefore the forefoot) to a neutral subtalar joint in static stance (Figure 13–17). The condition where the plantar surface of the forefoot is inverted to the plantar surface of the rearfoot is called *forefoot varus*.[38,40,56–58] The STJ and MTJ must pronate in order to allow the medial aspect of the forefoot to drop to the support surface. At

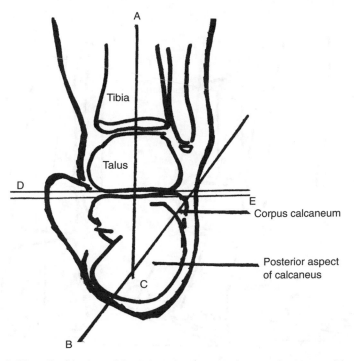

Figure 13–12 The In Utero Positioning of the Calcaneus. In utero, the posterior aspect of the calcaneus is held in varus to the body of the bone. Line A/C represents a line bisecting the body of the talus and corpus calcaneum. Line B/C represents a line bisecting the posterior aspect of the calcaneus. The angle formed by ACB shows the varus alignment of the posterior portion of the calcaneus. Note that Lines D and E are parallel; this shows that the STJ is in neutral position. Similar lines could be drawn showing that the ankle is also in neutral position.

the same time, the calcaneus must evert to accompany this motion.[38,40,56-58] Some investigators believe that knee pathology may arise because the abnormal STJ pronation required during midstance (when the knee is moving toward terminal extension) can cause a delay in the external tibial rotation.[18,38,40,56,60]

Forefoot Supinatus

Forefoot supinatus is a triplane, reducible deformity where the forefoot is adducted, plantarflexed, and slightly inverted with restricted motion at the MTJ.[38] It is difficult to differentiate this condition from forefoot varus (a uniplanar, fixed, osseous deformity).[38] Some clinicians choose to treat the two conditions differently. This author chooses to treat both deformities the same way because they may both cause

similar pathology, and in the adult it is often difficult to fully reduce the supinatus. Implications for knee pathology in the adult and adolescent are similar to those of forefoot varus.[38,58]

Forefoot Valgus

Although forefoot valgus may sometimes be ontogenic in origin, it most commonly occurs as compensation for other foot or superstructural problems.[56] It may encompass the entire forefoot (global) or be limited to plantarflexion of the first metatarsal (local). It may exist as a rigid or flexible deformity.[56,57,61] When the condition is rigid or progressive, the clinician should rule out neuromuscular disease or cerebral palsy.[38,40,61] When the entire forefoot is held in a fixed position of eversion to the rearfoot, the condition is termed *forefoot valgus*.[38,40,56,61] When only the

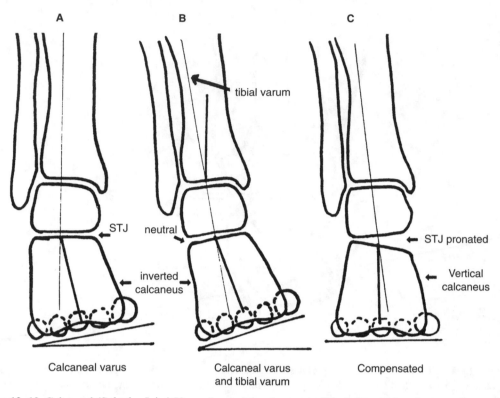

A   **B**   **C**

tibial varum

STJ   neutral

inverted calcaneus

STJ pronated

Vertical calcaneus

Calcaneal varus

Calcaneal varus and tibial varum

Compensated

Figure 13–13 Calcaneal (Subtalar Joint) Varus. In utero development of the calcaneus has the posterior portion of the bone in varus to the body of the bone. Ontogenically, the bone must "derotate." (**A**) Failure to do so causes a residual deformity with the heel bone inverted to the support surface with the STJ in neutral position in stance. (**B**) When combined with other deformities such as tibial varum, this abnormal position may be accentuated. (**C**) When STJ varus exists in the adult foot, the STJ must compensate in order to allow the forefoot to contact the support surface. STJ compensation is accomplished by foot pronation. Abnormal pronation may affect the limb above adversely. *Source:* Reprinted from Tiberio D, Pathomechanics of Structural Foot Deformities, *Journal of Physical Therapy*, 1988, Vol 68, No 12, p 1843, with permission of the American Physical Therapy Association.

first ray is plantarflexed and everted to the rearfoot, and the second to fifth metatarsals remain on the same plane, it is termed a *plantarflexed first ray* (Figure 13–18).[38,40,56,61] Both deformities compensate similarly and may lead to pathology. When the deformities are fixed and rigid, these foot types prevent or delay pronation due to increased supination of the STJ and, thus, compromise the ability of the knee to handle shock.[38,56] Increased STJ supination at midstance denies the internal tibial rotation needed to allow normal knee flexion. Absent or delayed knee flexion at midstance impairs the

knee's ability to handle the ground reactive forces generated in gait, and this causes a varus stress on the tibiofemoral joint.[34,38,56] The increased external rotation of the lower leg created by this abnormal supination may also be a factor in the development of other lateral knee disorders such as the iliotibial band friction syndrome.[6,11,38,56]

Lower Extremity Malalignment

Abnormal position or structure in the leg may cause abnormal foot compensation. The

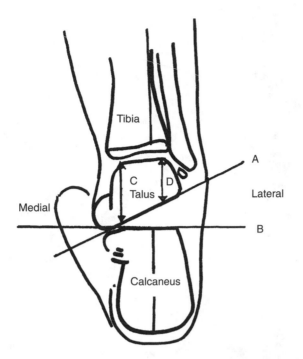

Figure 13–14 Calcaneal (Subtalar Joint) Valgus. In utero, the lateral aspect of the talus (line D) develops shorter than the medial aspect (line C). If unresolved, this difference in height causes an obliquity in the STJ (line A to line B) in stance when the bisection of the posterior portion of the calcaneus is perpendicular to the support surface. Compensation must occur to stabilize the STJ and allow the foot to function on the support surface. This compensation occurs in the midtarsal and forefoot, causing the foot to be congenitally flat. The congenital flatfoot may adversely affect the limb above.

most common lower leg malalignments are torsional abnormalities (femoral or tibial), angular deformities (varus/valgus about the hip, knee, or ankle joints), leg length asymmetry, and positional malalignments (due to tight hip, knee, or lower leg muscles; capsules; or ligaments).[38,40,62–64] Uncompensated torsional abnormalities in the lower extremity may lead to aberrations in gait such as intoeing (due to internal femoral or tibial torsion) or outtoeing (due to external femoral or tibial torsion).[62,63] Compensation for torsional deformities can occur via foot adduction/abduction and/or STJ pronation. James and Lutter both cite torsional abnormalities and the attendant compensatory STJ pronation as a major cause of knee problems in athletes.[6,18,63]

Angulation deformities (varus/valgus) about the hip, knee, or ankle joints may be compensated for by abnormal foot pronation or supination.[38–41,62] Lutter reported that "miserable malalignment syndrome" with pronation creates a valgus stress on the knee and accounts for 7% of all knee injuries.[18] Paulos et al cited genu valgum, internal femoral torsion, and abnormal foot mechanics as malalignments of the extremity that could lead to patellar malalignment and pain due to the "law of valgus."[65] Blake et al described theoretical mechanisms whereby coxa vara/valga; genu varum/valgum; and pathomechanics of the STJ and MTJ may all adversely affect normal knee function.[66]

Asymmetry of leg lengths may be compensated for by various mechanisms. A commonly

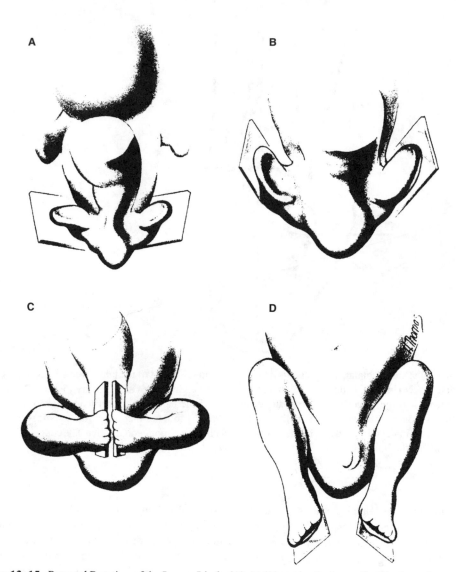

Figure 13–15 Prenatal Rotation of the Lower Limb. (**A**) At 4½ weeks, the lower limb buds are in extreme varus, minimal foot development is seen. (**B**) By 5½ weeks, the limb is more developed, in less varus, and foot development is still minimal. (**C**) At 8 weeks, limb varus lessens and foot development is seen. Note that the plantar aspects of the feet are aligned on parallel planes in extreme varus. (**D**) By 12 weeks, the lower limb develops more fully, and the varus reduces significantly. The varus placement of the foot also reduces significantly. At birth, both the lower limb and foot should have little to no varus rotation. *Source:* Reprinted with permission from WL Jaffe, PJ Gannon, and JT Laitman, Paleontology, Embryology, and Anatomy of the Foot, in *Disorders of the Foot and Ankle: Medical and Surgical Management*, MH Jahss, ed, p 12, © 1991, WB Saunders.

seen mechanism is STJ pronation on the longer side (thus lowering the arch and shortening the side) and STJ supination on the shorter side (raising the arch and lengthening this side).[64]

According to Lutter: "Secondary knee valgus may result from leg length discrepancy in which the longer leg pronates and produces increased valgus as a compensatory mechanism."[18(p687)] He

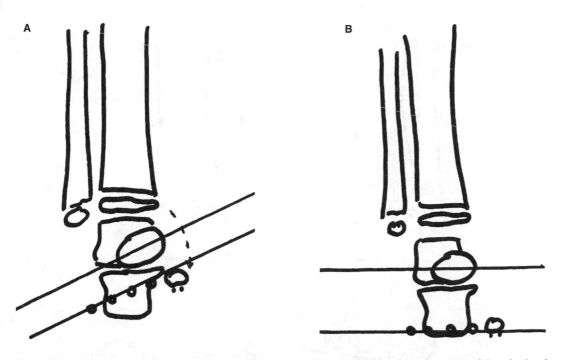

Figure 13–16 Ontogenic Derotation of the Talar Head and Neck. (**A**) The in utero alignment of the talar head and neck to the body of the bone. Note that the talar head is held in varus to the body, and the forefoot (which is aligned to the talar head) is also held at varus. (**B**) In normal ontogenic development, the talar head and neck must rotate in relation to the body. The forefoot follows this motion, allowing the forefoot to position itself parallel to the support surface. The adult criteria for biomechanical normalcy is then fulfilled (ie, the forefoot is perpendicular to a bisection of the posterior aspect of the calcaneus with the STJ in neutral position). This rotation should occur in utero. If it persists in the walking infant or adult, it is termed *forefoot varus*, and compensation must occur.

reported that this increased valgus could lead to knee injury in runners. Positional malalignments due to tight soft tissues about the lower extremity joints may act in a manner similar to structural malalignments and also cause abnormal foot compensation. Positional deformities may also affect knee function.[38,40,66]

Shoes

Improper shoe gear is often cited as a cause of athletic injuries in the lower extremity (Figure 13–19).[6,11,18,22–26,28,29,33–37,44,67,68] Nearly all of the scientific research done to define what constitutes a "good" shoe has been conducted on athletic shoe gear or children's shoes. Currently it is necessary to extrapolate the criteria for accept-

able nonathletic adult shoe gear from this research. Athletic shoes should possess certain qualities in order to prevent injury and enhance performance. They must provide stability and attenuate shock while remaining flexible and durable, and yet provide proper traction.[69–71] Frederick noted that it is difficult to design the "ideal" running shoe due to dichotomies inherent in the above criteria that often require compromise in making performance shoes.[69]

Shock attenuation is primarily a function of the materials that comprise the midsole. Paradoxically, midsole materials that are too hard or soft may increase the risk of injury. Most athletic shoe midsoles are made of ethylene vinyl acetate (EVA), polyurethane (PU) foam, nonfoam viscoelastics, air systems, or combinations of the

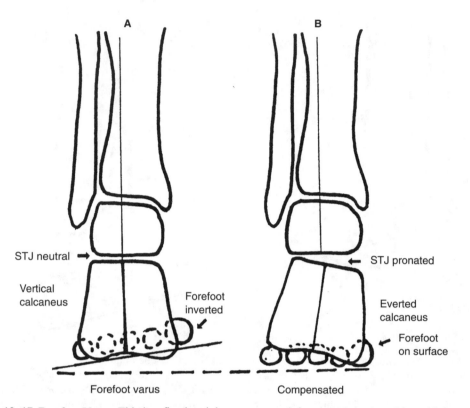

A

B

STJ neutral →

Vertical
calcaneus

Forefoot
inverted

← STJ pronated

Everted
calcaneus

Forefoot
on surface

Forefoot varus

Compensated

Figure 13–17 Forefoot Varus. This is a fixed, uniplanar, osseous deformity where the midtarsal joint and fore-foot are held in inversion to the rearfoot when the STJ is in neutral position. (**A**) The plantar surface of the forefoot is inverted to the plantar surface of the rearfoot, with the bisection of the posterior portion of the calcaneus remaining perpendicular to the support surface. (**B**) In order for the forefoot to contact the support surface, compensatory pronation through the STJ and MTJ must occur. This allows the forefoot to contact the ground, but causes the calcaneus to evert. Compensation in the foot and lower leg may be a cause of patellofemoral dysfunction. *Source:* Reprinted from Tiberio D, Pathomechanics of Structural Foot Deformities, *Journal of Physical Therapy*, 1988, Vol 68, No 12, p 1844, with permission of the American Physical Therapy Association.

above. An example of a design dichotomy is that increased cushioning creates increased instability.[69] A balance must be struck between these two parameters in order to create the "ideal" shoe.

Flexibility is linked to the thickness and composition of midsole material, and the stabilizing elements in the heel, midsole, forefoot, and upper part of the shoe.[69,70] Unfortunately, more durable outsoles are generally more inflexible and/or lacking in traction.[69–71] Removable arch supports, reinforced uppers (with stabilizers or banding), and variable lacing (via extra eyelets

and/or ring systems) are used to enhance the shoe's ability to resist pronation and decrease injury. Because the midsole or cushioning materials wear out more rapidly than the rest of the shoe, athletic shoes should be discarded after 3 to 6 months of regular use, regardless or how they look.[70]

THE KNEE IN GAIT, NORMAL FUNCTION, AND DYSFUNCTION

At heel contact, the knee is usually fully extended. It then rapidly flexes about 15 to 20 de-

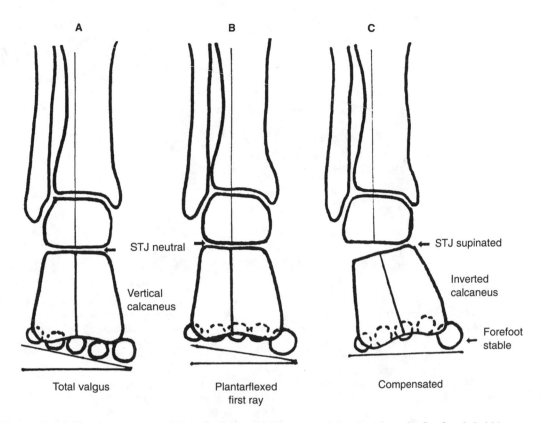

Figure 13–18 Forefoot Valgus. This is a fixed, uniplanar, osseous deformity where the forefoot is held in eversion to the rearfoot with the STJ in neutral position. (**A**) Total forefoot valgus is when the entire plantar surface of the forefoot is everted to the plantar surface of the rearfoot while the bisection of the posterior aspect of the calcaneus remains perpendicular to the support surface. (**B**) Plantarflexed first ray occurs when only the first ray is plantarflexed and inverted to the rearfoot, but the lesser rays (2–5) remain on the same plane and perpendicular to the rearfoot. (**C**) When fixed and rigid, compensation for either deformity leads to STJ supination with calcaneal inversion. Compensation for this deformity can also lead to knee dysfunction. *Source:* Reprinted from Tiberio D, Pathomechanics of Structural Foot Deformities, *Journal of Physical Therapy,* 1988, Vol 68, No 12, p 1845, with permission of the American Physical Therapy Association.

grees toward the end of the contact phase.[51,60] During midstance the knee reextends and continues to extend throughout the heel-off stage into toe-off. It must then flex again to allow the foot to clear the support surface.[38,51,60] In the swing phase, the knee initially flexes rapidly until midswing when it begins to extend. Extension continues throughout the deceleration stage until full extension is reached and the heel contacts the ground again.[51,60] Knee flexion is always accompanied by internal tibial rotation, and extension is accompanied by external tibial rotation.[51,60]

Many factors outside the knee may exacerbate a patella's tendency to displace laterally. Excessive STJ pronation causes excessive internal tibial torsion, forward excursion of the tibia, and varus at the knee.[59] When these motions occur during the midstance of gait or beyond, knee flexion must occur to maintain knee and ankle congruency.[42,53,56,60,63,72–74] Injury to the knee may occur due to the attempt of the lower leg to ex-

The upper part of the shoe should enhance its stability. This is accomplished through banding or reinforcement in the midfoot, stabilizer bands or straps in the lacing system, or the use of variable lacing.

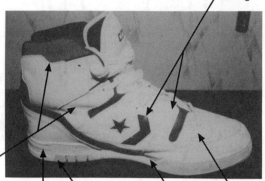

Heel counters that are noncompressible, higher-cut shoes, and ankle straps enhance the shoe's stability.

Carbon rubber outsoles are more durable.

Heel "cradles" or reinforced heels provide enhanced medial and lateral motion support.

Flexibility in the forefoot is an important consideration. The shoe should bend or "break" easily at the ball of the foot.

Midsoles made of polyurethane or ethylene vinyl acetate are good shock attenuating materials. The addition of air bags or gel pads does little to enhance cushioning.

Figure 13–19 The Anatomy of a Performance Athletic Shoe. Certain characteristics make an athletic shoe more desirable and can enhance performance. Athletic shoes must provide stability, cushioning (shock attenuation), and traction, while remaining flexible and durable. Shoe design dichotomies make it impossible for a shoe to be excellent in all of these categories, thus the ideal shoe is a compromise. Fit and comfort should be the primary concern when an athlete chooses a performance shoe.

tend while the tibia is still internally rotated, in varus, and anteriorly inclined. Tiberio postulates that internal tibial rotation occurring during the time when external rotation is required creates "a biomechanical dilemma" for the knee.[60] Unless this dilemma is solved by some type of compensation, it may lead to increased stress on the articulations of the knee. We know that this dilemma exists, but the mechanism of compensation and the reaction of the knee to this stress are still theoretical.

RESEARCH

Research Linking Foot Pathomechanics and Knee Disorders

As early as the turn of the twentieth century, orthopaedists and podiatrists acknowledged the effectiveness of foot orthotic devices in controlling foot and lower extremity pain. Whitman[1] and Ober[2] both recognized the effect of foot pronation on the knee and used devices to control it in their management. In the early 1970s, Schuster[3] and Subotnick[4] (both podiatrists) and Sheehan[5] (a sports medicine physician) suggested the use of foot orthotics to control knee pain associated with running. Most of their observations were anecdotal, but their philosophy influenced some progressive orthopaedists. In the early 1980s, a growing body of literature espoused the use of foot orthotics as a method of preventing selected running injuries, including overuse injuries of the knee.[6,7,11,13,18,19,63] According to James: "Foot function and its influence on the knee and patellar mechanics [is] another frequently ignored relationship."[63(p216)] DeHaven et al noted that the "squinting patellae" associated with lower extremity malalignment could frequently be improved by limiting pronation.[8] Lutter wrote extensively on the link between foot pathomechanics and knee problems in runners, stating: "Medial knee injuries come from hyperpronation and lateral injuries come from persistently supinated cavo-varus feet."[18(p691)]

Unfortunately, all of these authors presented purely clinical data with little or no scientific substantiation. Stacoff et al, working on athletic shoe design, reported that certain lower extremity injuries were associated with an excessive rate (amount per unit time) or maximal angle of pronation.[35] Other researchers suggested that anatomically defined ankle and subtalar joint motions might be used to predict athletic injuries.[75]

Research Quantifying Foot Motion, Pronation, and Lower Leg Biomechanics

In 1979, Bates and colleagues were among the earliest researchers to attempt to quantify lower extremity function in runners.[28] They filmed 11 college-aged runners and measured the variability of certain motions in the lower extremity. Although they were unable to find any differences that were statistically significant, they noted that the range of variability suggested the need to find average or representative values. These values could then be used to detect the subtle differ-

ences known to exist. In a second article, the same authors attempted to link running injuries to excessive foot pronation.[7] They treated runners with rigid foot orthotics and found that 78% were able to return to activity with reduced symptoms. They then randomly selected six orthotic wearers and filmed them while running barefoot, in running shoes, and in the same shoes with orthotics. They noted that "both the period of pronation and the amount of maximum pronation were significantly reduced."[7(p338)] They concluded that modification of foot dysfunction could be used successfully to treat certain types of running injuries. In their series of 65 injured runners, 18 (12%) had knee pain (12 with nonspecific pain; 6 with "chondromalacia").[7]

Rodgers and LeVeau studied 29 orthotic-wearing runners.[76] They measured six variables and found only two to be statistically significant (a reduced maximal angle and reduced time of pronation). They concluded that although their study supports the findings of Bates et al, their results "do not conclusively prove or disprove the effectiveness of FOD [foot orthotic devices]."[76(p89)] Of their subjects, 41% cited knee pain as the reason for wearing orthotics. Clarke et al,[77] Cavanagh et al,[78] and Smith et al[79] all found significant decreases in pronatory measurements using soft or semirigid orthotics in biomechanics laboratories.

During the early 1980s, researchers tried to solve the enigma of the role of pronation in lower extremity injury. Despite much research, controversy still existed. Results varied, and few researchers completely agreed on their findings. The major pitfall seemed to be the difficulty in determining exact subtalar and talocrural (ankle) joint motions. This was because of the complexity of motion in these joints, and the methods by which the motion data were obtained. Until the mid-1980s, most research was performed using two-dimensional (2-D) walking or running analysis.[80] Due to the widespread acceptance of Inman's oblique hinge theory of STJ motion,[51] researchers believed that calcaneal eversion was an acceptable 2-D parameter to indicate the degree of pronation.[29,81] More recent three-dimensional (3-D) analysis has shown that some of the earlier 2-D data concerning foot motion, pronation, and lower extremity joint kinematics were flawed.[75,80,81] In particular, investigators found discrepancies when they analyzed 3-D data using the Inman model of STJ motion, which raised doubts about the theory's viability.[75] These findings have had a profound effect on researchers' ability to explain or predict lower leg and knee motion in relation to STJ motion. Furthermore, researchers reported differences in calcaneal inversion/eversion angle and the timing of certain phasic activities when comparing 2-D and 3-D data.[75,80,81] More importantly, 3-D analysis has shown that forefoot stability may be as important as rearfoot stability in maintaining normal foot and lower leg function.[75] Early researchers assumed that controlling rearfoot motion would stabilize the entire foot and lower leg, but 3-D analysis shows that this is probably not true. Discrepancies in the data obtained by these two methods of research can be explained when one realizes that 2-D analysis measures motion around reference points outside the body while 3-D analysis measures motion of one body segment to another (a more precise indicator).[80] Moreover, early researchers used flexible or semiflexible orthotic devices designed primarily to control rearfoot motion. If forefoot stability is as important as 3-D analysis suggests, orthotics designed in this manner would be incapable of controlling the forefoot, and therefore incapable of completely controlling foot and lower leg function.

Most of the research done since the mid-1980s has used 3-D analysis. In 1990, Novick and Kelley found that rigid orthotics that aligned both the rearfoot and forefoot showed significant statistical changes in eight measured 3-D parameters.[82] Among their findings, they noted reduction in the calcaneal eversion angle and velocity, and decreased total rearfoot motion. The magnitude of varus tibial angular acceleration in the leg was likewise reduced. This finding is important, because many authors have postulated that foot-related knee dysfunction is linked to an increased amount of varus, and that the attendant rotation of the tibia at the knee level is secondary to abnormal pronation.[3,4,6,10,14,16,18,19,53,58–60,66,75,83,84]

Knutzen and Bates found that rearfoot motion during the contact phase of running was "a major contributing kinetic factor to knee rotation."[53(p395)] They studied 12 runners using photoelectric cells, a force plate, an electrogoniometer, and an electrodynogram. They tried to correlate certain kinetic variables (such as ground reactive force, fore-aft force, and mediolateral force) in the foot-to-knee rotation. They found that increased time of lateral heel contact with the ground, and increased time of peak lateral heel pressure were accompanied by decreased internal knee rotation. The clinical significance of these findings is that they link knee rotation to foot motion. Many authors have noted that asynchronous pronation/supination in the foot is a predisposing factor in knee dysfunction due to increased internal rotation of the knee.[4,7,10,18,19,58,60,66,67,73,83–85] It is possible that orthotics designed to keep the foot supinated (ie, on the lateral border of the foot) for a longer period of time can help to reestablish the proper timing of pronation/supination, diminish the internal rotation of the knee, and theoretically reduce knee injury.

Other researchers have shown relationships between force platform data and knee joint motion.[34,85–87] The vertical contact force was shown to be related to the angle of the knee joint at heel contact.[85] Anatomically impaired knees showed abnormal fore-aft and mediolateral values in the foot.[86] Stauffer et al noted a decreased rate and magnitude of vertical load at heel contact, smaller and delayed fore-aft forces, and delayed mediolateral shift with increased lateral forces in patients with diseased knee joints.[87] An obvious question is that if alterations in knee mechanics can alter foot mechanical parameters measured by force plates, could not alterations in foot mechanics have a similar effect on the knee?

Eng and Pierrynowski found that flexible orthotics that are "balanced" in the rearfoot and forefoot can effect 1 to 3 degrees of change in the frontal and transverse motions of the talocrural (ankle) joint and STJ in selected subjects.[88] They noted that frontal plane knee motion is also altered. They found that, paradoxically, knee motion is decreased with orthotics while walking, but increased while running. They reasoned that, although orthotics are thought to control knee pain by reducing frontal plane motion, "perhaps it is not so much a reduction of motion but an alteration of the loading of the patellofemoral joints that can result in a reduction of pain."[88(p843)] The same researchers had previously found that "in addition to an exercise program, the use of soft orthoses is an effective means of treatment for patients with patellofemoral pain syndrome."[89(p68)]

Research and Theory Regarding the Use of Foot Orthotic Devices To Control Patellofemoral Pain

The Quadriceps (Q) Angle and Foot Pronation

Many authors have suggested that reduction of certain types of patellofemoral pain may be associated with reduction in the Q angle (see Chapter 3). In 1979, Steadman found "an arch pad plus a small medial heel wedge can be effective in maintaining the Q angle at a smaller degree and derotating the femur and patella."[9(p375)] James stated that in patients with "miserable malalignment" there was "a patella which inclined toward the midline" and "an increased Q angle."[63(p215)] He suggested that, although foot orthotics were not a panacea for knee pain, "they could provide a good result based on correct analysis of leg-heel forefoot alignment, proper casting technique, and precise fabrication."[63(p236)] Lutter analyzed 3500 runners and found that only 10% were biomechanically normal.[18] See Chapter 1 for controversy regarding the term *normal*. He noted that a high percentage of patients with "runner's knee" had higher Q angles and abnormal foot pronation.[18] He claimed that excessive foot pronation in running increased both the Q angle and the load on the

patella. He believed that abnormal pronation resulted in increased valgus stress on the knee. Of the injured runners he studied, 7% had "miserable malalignment"—a combination of internal femoral torsion, external tibial torsion, and foot pronation. He recommended using foot orthotic devices to control this and other maladies of the knee. Moss et al studied 14 female runners with anterior knee pain and compared them to 15 healthy runners. These authors found two anthropometric variables that could be used to predict runners who may have a predisposition to patellofemoral pain: the Q angle and body weight.[85] Their predictions were 89% accurate. They noted further that although decreased values in the velocity of maximal pronation "may have been a contributing factor in the development of patellofemoral stress syndrome,"[85(p68)] leg strength was not.

The above anecdotal observations provide evidence that control of pronation with foot orthotics may decrease knee valgus, reduce the Q angle, and ameliorate certain knee disorders. There is some factual research to support these claims.

The Q Angle and Lower Extremity Mechanics

In 1987, Olerud and Rosendahl reported that for every 1 degree of rearfoot supination (measured as calcaneal eversion) there was 0.44 degrees of external tibial rotation.[48] Reiley refers to this research in stating: "It is possible to decrease the 'Q' angle by decreasing foot pronation. For every 1 degree increase in foot supination, there is a .44 degree decrease in the 'Q' angle."[90(p4)] He states: "It is probably this relationship between foot pronation and the 'Q' angle that accounts for the observation that 75% of runners' knee problems involve an abnormal foot."[90(p4)]

D'Amico and Rubin found that foot orthotics reduced the Q angle an average of 6 degrees in a 21-patient study.[59] They suggested that this foot-knee relationship might be an indication for the use of foot orthotics in treatment of patellar malalignment syndromes.

Other researchers have noted the intimate link between foot and leg mechanics, although they have not specifically related these changes to Q angle changes. Inman said there was a one-to-one relationship between talar adduction and internal tibial rotation.[74] McCulloch et al stated, "from initial contact to midstance, foot pronation and tibial internal rotation of equivalent amounts occur simultaneously with a predictable amount of stance phase knee flexion."[91(p3)]

Discussion

From the above research, it might seem that a reduction of the Q angle via foot orthotics would be a rational method of treatment for patellofemoral disorders. The problem with this theory is that increased STJ pronation with its attendant internal tibial rotation should *not* produce an increased Q angle under normal circumstances. The Q angle should decrease with CKC pronation due to internal tibial rotation, and it should increase with supination and external tibial rotation. Many authors have tried to explain this dichotomy.[59,60,65,92] Larson[92] and Paulos et al[65] both erroneously stated that the Q angle decreased in pronation of the foot due to external rotation of the tibia as the knee extended. We know that pronation is accompanied by internal tibial rotation, so this explanation cannot be substantiated mechanically. In 1986, D'Amico and Rubin postulated that, although internal tibial rotation did occur secondary to foot pronation, "the femur internally rotates with greater excursion than the tibia, causing the patella to move plantarly and laterally [with] . . . a concomitant increase in the quadriceps angle accompanying pronation."[59(p339)] In 1987, Tiberio stated that pronation beyond midstance in gait created a "biomechanical dilemma" for the knee; normal mechanics dictate that the tibiofemoral joint extend during midstance, which cannot occur while the tibia is internally rotated on the femur.[60] He agreed with D'Amico and Rubin, stating that this dilemma might be solved by the femur compensating for excessive pronation by increased internal rotation over the tibia. (In CKC, the foot is fixed to the ground; the femur and torso above are the only other areas where compensatory motion might occur.)

In summary, investigators have reported some anecdotal and scientific evidence regarding the role of the Q angle in patellofemoral syndrome. Furthermore, changes in Q angle can be linked to foot pronation. However, the exact mechanism by which this interrelationship creates injury is still unknown.

Research on Transverse/Frontal Plane Knee Motion and Lower Extremity Mechanics

Recent research may explain why some investigators have implicated transverse plane motion more than frontal plane motion. Transverse plane motion is internal and external tibial rotation. Frontal plane motion is adduction/abduction rotation of the tibia. Tomaro et al studied overuse injuries of the lower extremity and found that the *subtalar joint ratio* of the patient determines whether an injury occurs due to transverse plane or frontal plane motion.[93] They found that higher than normal STJ ratios lead to more transverse plane motion, while lower ratios favor frontal plane motion. They have shown that it is not merely increased STJ motion (pronation) that is important, but also the type of STJ motion (ie, the STJ ratio). In some cases, pronation favors transverse plane motion, and in others it favors frontal plane motion.

Many authors have provided ratios relating foot pronation/supination to internal/external tibial motion, but few have attempted to quantify this motion. Knutzen and Bates indirectly measured knee joint rotation in walking and running and found a maximum rotation of 14.21 degrees (± 6.2 degrees).[53] Eng and Pierrynowski found 4.9 degrees of frontal plane and 5.1 degrees of transverse plane motion during the propulsive phase of walking.[88] (If a measuring device is only accurate to around 1 degree, it is not reasonable to report results down to one-hundredth, or even a tenth, of a degree.) Both teams believed that the use of foot orthotics could control some of this motion. Beckett et al found increased rotational knee motion due to pronation may cause noncontact anterior cruciate ligament injuries in the knee.[94] Among other findings, they noted that the anterior cruciate ligament injuries group had significantly higher navicular drop scores (a measure of the amount of pronation). They postulated that pronation and the attendant internal tibial rotation caused a repetitive preloading of the anterior cruciate ligament, thereby weakening it and predisposing this group to injury. This finding has been supported by Woodford-Rogers et al[95] but refuted by Smith et al.[96]

Foot Orthotic Devices and Knee Pain: Current Concepts and Research

In 1989, Eng and Pierrynowski studied 20 female subjects who were diagnosed with patellofemoral pain and exhibited foot deformity (subtalar varus and forefoot varus).[89] Ten subjects were given isometric quadriceps and straight-leg exercises (the control group); a second group of 10 subjects (the treatment group) did the same exercises but also wore full-length, flexible orthotics designed to control rearfoot and forefoot pathology. The authors noted: "Although both groups demonstrated a significant reduction in reported pain, the treatment group demonstrated greater reduction than the control group."[89(p68)] Reduction of pain was consistent in all parameters measured: walking, running, stair ascent, stair descent, sitting, and squatting. The two groups were studied for 8 weeks; means and standard deviations were calculated for the descriptive characteristics, and independent T tests were used to compare the variables between the two groups. The authors accepted significance at the .05 level. They reported: "We are confident that the orthotic was responsible for the observed differences between the treatment and control groups."[89(p68)] They theorized that orthotic devices controlled the transverse and frontal plane rotation of the tibia on the femur, and thus more evenly distributed patellofemoral joint reactive forces.

In 1988, Donatelli et al studied 53 patients (20 males and 33 females) in a retrospective study on the effectiveness of foot orthotics.[97] Of the patients, 53% were treated with orthotics alone; the other 47% were treated by various physical modalities in conjunction with the orthotics. Of the subjects, 31% complained of knee pain and 95% had a forefoot varus deformity (average 8.4 degrees). The information obtained by the questionnaires was subjected to chi-square analysis, and the criteria for significance selected for the study was $p < 0.05$. Orthotic intervention was successful in relieving pain in 96% of all surveyed patients; 90% of patients treated with orthotics alone reported pain relief; 70% were able to return to their previous activity (running, tennis, walking, etc) with orthotics that supported approximately 60% of their measured foot deformity. The authors noted that the success of orthotic therapy depended on the criteria used for prescribing orthotics and improving the techniques used to biomechanically evaluate the foot.

Other, less-controlled studies have reported similar findings in using orthotics. Bates et al found that 78% of runners treated with orthotics had reduced symptoms (18% had knee pain).[7] Eggold reported that in 146 runners treated with orthotics, over 75% noted pain relief of 70% or more.[14] Pretorius et al treated 48 runners with knee pain and found that 77% recovered completely with a change in running shoes, or shoe change and orthotics.[21] Newell and Bramwell examined 329 runners with knee pain over an 11-month period of time.[16] They reported that 270 of these runners (most of whom had failed to respond to other methods of treatment) were given orthotics, posting a 76% cure rate. Blake and Denton reported on a 1-year follow-up of 180 injured athletes who used orthotics.[98] They gave 51 athletes (28%) orthotics for a variety of knee disorders (medial meniscal disease, Osgood Schlatter's condition, patellar tendinitis, osteoarthritis, iliotibial band syndrome, lateral meniscus disease, medial quadriceps muscle injury, and "chondromalacia"). Of these 51 patients, 70% responded that wearing orthotics had "definitely" helped their condition, and 19% reported that orthotics helped "somewhat." In two separate articles, Lutter found that 35% of the runners he examined had knee pain, and 78% of these injuries were foot related.[18,19] He wrote, "Not all runners' knee problems can be treated with an orthosis," but "utilization of an orthoses can be an important adjunct in managing pronation problems."[99(p113)]

FOOT ORTHOTIC DEVICES

Definition

One of the best definitions of foot orthotic devices is from Bordelon: "An orthotic device is an orthopedic appliance or apparatus used to support, align, prevent or correct deformities or to improve the function of the movable parts of the foot."[61(p37)] According to this definition, many devices might be considered orthotics including arch supports, foot inlays, shoe innersoles, heel cups or cushions, and felt pads. For the purposes of this discussion, a foot orthotic device is defined as *a shoe insert fabricated over a cast so that the neutral STJ and MTJ positions are consistently maintained.*

Casting and Fabrication of Foot Orthotic Devices

According to Root and colleagues, the best method of capturing the normal contours of the foot is via a neutral-position cast.[83] Casting is done with the STJ in its neutral position (ie, neither pronated or supinated). Unfortunately, Root's concept of a neutral STJ position is pure theory. Many authors have tried scientifically to determine a norm. There has been little consensus regarding a true neutral STJ. Thus, we are left with theory and unscientific methodology in determining this position. Many methods have been proposed to determine the neutral position of the STJ. A simple, yet very effective method was described by Schuster (unpublished lecture notes, 1971–1975) and illustrated by Brody.[11] The clinician palpates the talar head both medially and laterally just anterior to the malleoli (in the area of the sinus tarsi) (Figure 13–20). The

STJ is then maximally inverted and everted. When equal talar head pressure is felt on both the medial and lateral sides of the sinus tarsi, the neutral STJ position has been found. Measurement of rearfoot to leg, and rearfoot to forefoot relationships are established using a goniometer (or similar measuring device) (Figure 13–21). A rearfoot varus measurement of 2 to 3 degrees is common and may even be acceptable, but any significant degree of forefoot deviation (varus or valgus) should be accounted for in the fabrication of the orthotic.[11,38–41,83,97] The values obtained via measurement are recorded and incorporated into the orthotic device by posts or "shims" that help the device maintain neutral position. A cast of the foot is taken using fast-drying plaster of Paris strips with the STJ in its neutral position (Figure 13–22). A positive model is obtained from this negative impression by pouring liquid plaster into the foot mold. After the positive model is smoothed and shaped, it is used as a form or "last" over which the orthotic shell is made. The material selected for the shell is pressed over the positive model under pressure so that the exact contour of the patient's foot is captured. The shell is then shaped and formed so that it will fit into a shoe. If needed, posts are added in the rearfoot and forefoot from the measurements obtained in the steps above (Figure 13–23). In essence, posts help the foot maintain neutral position by bringing the ground up to the foot (Figure 13–24).

Functions

Wu outlined 12 functions required of foot orthotic devices[52] (comments in parentheses are this author's).

1. to provide maximal and even distribution of weight-bearing stress over the sole of the foot
2. to reduce the stress and strain on the foot, ankle, knee, hip, and spine by properly controlling the inversion and eversion of the STJ, and supination and pronation of the MTJ, and by absorbing some of the ground reactive force

A

B

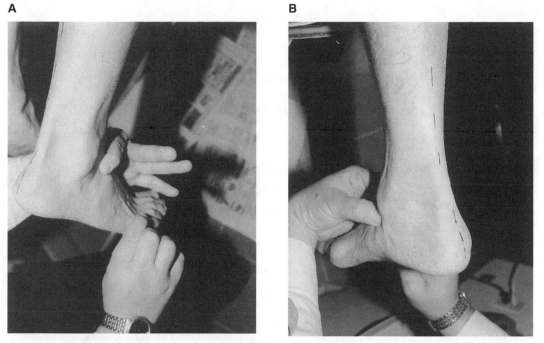

Figure 13–20 Locating the Neutral Subtalar Joint (STJ) Position. **(A)** Lateral view, **(B)** medial view. The examiner places a thumb and forefinger on either side of the STJ in the sinus tarsi. The joint is then maximally inverted and everted while the examiner palpates the talar head with the thumb and forefinger. When equal pressure is felt by each finger, the neutral subtalar position is found.

3. to provide relief for sensitive and painful areas of the sole such as atrophic, scarred, calloused, or ulcerated areas
4. to support the longitudinal arch (important) and transverse arch (unimportant)
5. to relieve metatarsalgia
6. to control the amount, degree, and rate of pronation during walking and running
7. to help to control abnormal foot pronation (this is the most important function)
8. to help the foot accommodate for missing parts caused by congenital abnormalities or amputation (or for deformities caused by arthritis or other disfiguring diseases)
9. to supplement the support provided by ankle foot orthotics
10. to aid in equalization of leg-length discrepancies
11. to limit the motions and weight-bearing stresses of symptomatic foot joints

12. to decrease the pressure or irritation due to external sources (shoe gear) or internal sources (bony abnormalities)

Wu noted that certain properties make an orthotic device more desirable[52] (comments in parentheses are this author's).

- It provides good support, pain relief, and biomechanical correction for the foot (and also the ankle and lower leg).
- It has no harmful effect on other parts of the body.
- It is aesthetically pleasing to gain the patient's acceptance.
- It has proper fit and contour for comfortable wear.
- It is lightweight but durable (moderate bulk to fit most shoes except for high heels).
- It is reasonably priced.

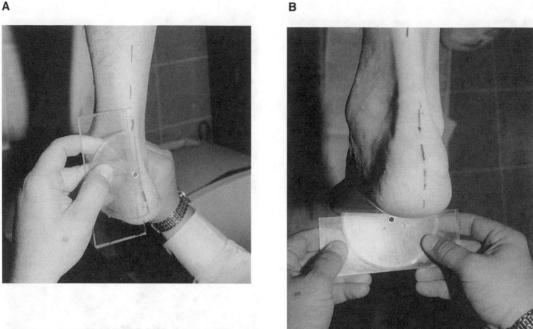

Figure 13–21 Determination of Rearfoot Positioning. (**A**) The rearfoot-to-leg and (**B**) rearfoot-to-forefoot relationships are measured using a goniometer or tractograph. These measurements are recorded and used to calculate the rearfoot and forefoot varus/valgus values, which can later be used to determine the amount of posting to be added to the orthotic shell. Note the reference lines that bisect the long axis of the tibia and the posterior aspect of the calcaneus. They are used as the landmarks for determining the amount of angular deviation in the rearfoot and forefoot.

- It is easy to fabricate and fit (and easy to adjust).
- It is easy to maintain and service.
- It is easy to mold to the foot with short setting time (for orthotics made from a cast, this pertains to the materials used in casting).
- It is constructed from materials that are breathable and moisture retardant (a moot point because orthotics can be covered or treated with materials to achieve this goal).
- It is radiolucent (unimportant in most cases).
- It is resistant to environmental factors such as water, oil, urine, temperature changes, and ultraviolet light.

CLASSIFICATION OF FOOT ORTHOTIC DEVICES

Devices that change the biomechanical function of the foot can be classified in many ways. The two most common methods are (1) classification by orthotic function (arch supportive devices, accommodative orthotics, and functional orthotics), and (2) classification according to materials used in construction (flexible, semiflexible, semirigid, and rigid materials). To design an orthotic device properly, the clinician must have a clear idea of the tasks the device is to perform, knowledge of the properties of the materials used in construction, and knowledge of the method of construction.

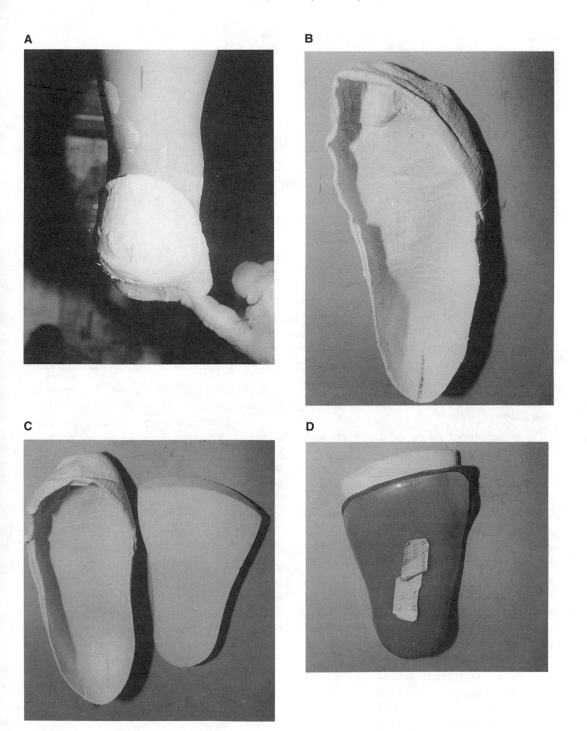

Figure 13–22 Steps in Orthotic Fabrication. (**A**) A cast is taken with the foot held in neutral STJ position. (**B**) The negative impression obtained is filled with plaster to obtain a positive foot model. (**C**) The model is shaped and smoothed so it can be used as a form or "last," over which the orthotic shell can be pressed to obtain exact foot contour. (**D**) The shell is then smoothed, shaped, and altered to fit shoe gear. Posts are added in the final stage.

A

B

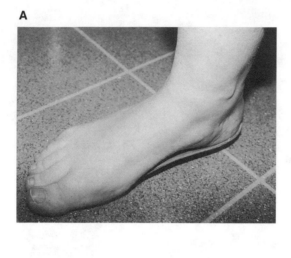
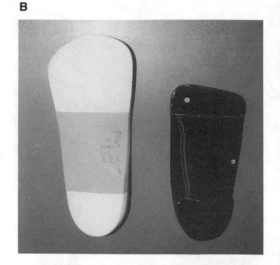

Figure 13–23 Posts or "Shims" Added to Orthotics Device. (**A**) The orthotic shell that was molded and shaped to fit the shoe is "corrected" via the addition of posts that act like "shims" to hold the foot in the proper relationship to itself and to the ground. (**B**) Two types of rearfoot and forefoot posted devices are shown: extended forefoot posting (left) and shorter metatarsal-length posting (right).

Classification of Orthotics by Function

Arch Supportive Devices

The most rudimentary device used to support the foot is the arch support. This device is generally constructed from flexible or semiflexible materials and may be generic (constructed over a common last or form) or specific (constructed over the individual's foot) (Figure 13–25). In either case, the support limits the collapse of the arch by placing materials in "bulk" under the longitudinal arch of the foot. These materials present a physical barrier to "arch collapse." *Navicular drop* is the measure of arch collapse during weight bearing (Figure 13–26).[100] Schuster found that in pronated feet, the tarsal navicular would drop toward the support surface during weight bearing (unpublished lecture notes, 1971–1975). He calculated that the navicular drop in a pronated foot was 5 to 10 mm more than the normal foot. Brody and others have used this test to verify abnormal pronation.[100,101] The navicular drop is defined as the difference between the original navicular height (measured from the support surface with the STJ

in neutral position) to the height of the navicular in relaxed stance.[100] Brody found that a 10-mm drop was average in normal feet and considered a drop of 15 mm or more to be abnormal (excessive pronation).[101] Mueller et al stated: "A navicular drop of greater than . . . 10 mm is considered abnormal and may be a contributing factor to foot pathology that the clinician should address."[100(p202)]

Arch supports address this concern. Placing enough "bulk" or support material under the longitudinal arch physically prevents the navicular from dropping toward the ground. However, devices like these are a crude and inefficient way of preventing abnormal pronation. They function only by limiting arch collapse and do little to control abnormal rearfoot and forefoot motion commonly seen in mechanically unstable feet. The inefficiency of arch supportive devices stems from their method of construction and the materials used in construction. Arch supports are formed statically over a form or last with an arch of known height and shape or dynamically over an individual's foot, with materials that try to maintain their basic shape. Most over-the-

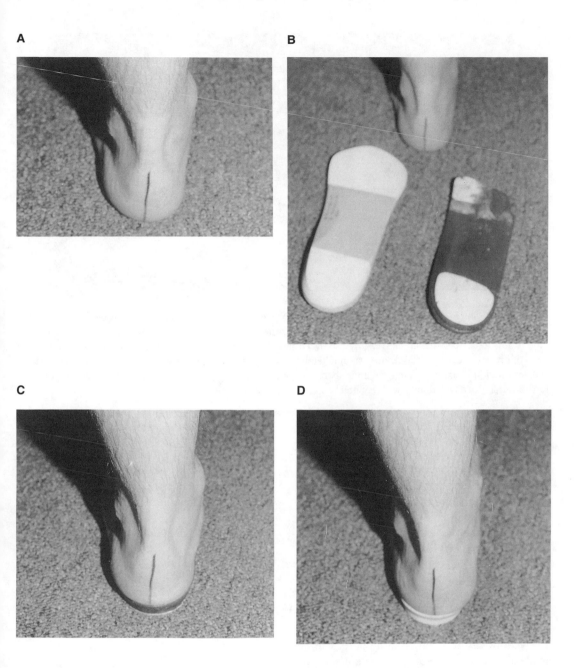

Figure 13–24 The Effect of Posted Orthotics in Maintaining Neutral STJ Position. (**A**) The patient is in a relaxed calcaneal stance position. Note the everted position of the calcaneus to the support surface (as indicated by the reference line on the calcaneus). (**B**) The same patient is shown with two orthotics: the orthotic on the left is posted in the rearfoot and has an extended forefoot post. The device on the right is rearfoot posted with a metatarsal-length forefoot post. (**C**) The patient is standing in the metatarsal-length device. Note the minimal change in the heel eversion. (**D**) The patient is in the extended-forefoot (sulcus) length device. Note the superior calcaneal alignment. The alignment change is primarily due to the sulcus-length forefoot post.

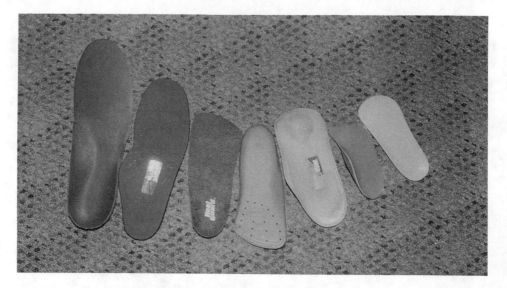

Figure 13–25 Arch Supportive Devices. Various commercially available arch supportive devices are shown above. They are generally constructed of flexible or semiflexible materials pressed over a generic form or last. This results in devices that are universally useful but not as therapeutically effective as custom-made arch supports or orthotics. Commercial devices are not "arch specific," lack proper posting or biomechanical correction, and are often too flexible to properly limit abnormal foot motion. They may be useful in individuals with mild foot deformity or as a temporary device before a custom-made orthotic is fabricated.

counter supports are formed statically from flexible materials. They are not specific to the patient's arch, and, therefore, they allow excessive navicular drop. Moreover, because flexible materials are used in their construction, they are incapable of maintaining shape and "bottom out" or become distorted, which allows additional drop. Supports like Spenco (Spenco Company, Waco, Texas), Lynco (Apex Products, Hackensack, New Jersey), or Dr. Scholl's (Schering-Plough, Memphis, Tennessee) are examples of over-the-counter devices made in this fashion.

Dynamically molded arch supports can be made directly over the foot or over a cast of the foot. They are generally fabricated from flexible or semiflexible materials. They are more effective than commercially available supports by virtue of their more precise arch contour, and they therefore prevent navicular drop, but they still distort under weight bearing and do little to control abnormal rearfoot and forefoot motion. Clinicians can make dynamically molded sup-

ports from materials like styrene butadiene rubber (SBR), moldable foams (plastazote), or heat-sensitive plastics (orthoplast). These devices make an excellent temporary or beginning support. Many clinicians use them to "wean" patients into more supportive devices.

The advantages of arch support devices are as follows:

- readily available or easily made
- low in cost
- will fit most shoes
- good temporary or beginner device
- good shock attenuation

Disadvantages of arch support devices include the following:

- poor fit and comfort
- poor patient acceptance
- limited effectiveness
- limited sizes (applies to over-the-counter devices)
- limited materials for construction

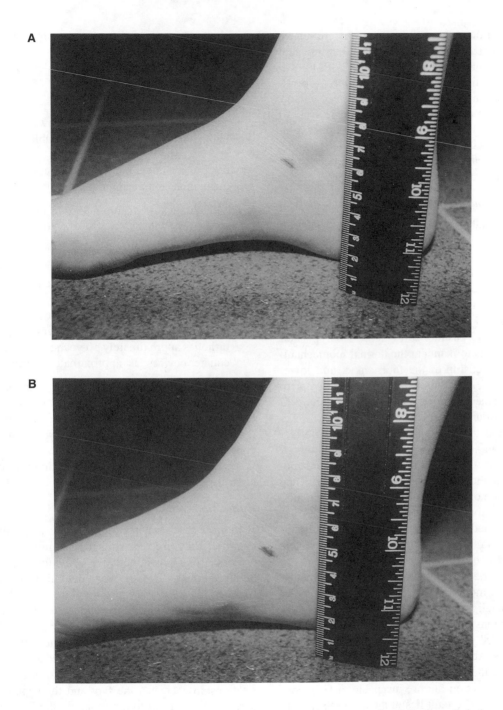

Figure 13–26 Navicular Drop. Navicular drop is a measure of the amount of arch "collapse" during weight bearing. It is defined as the difference between the navicular height with the foot in subtalar neutral position and the navicular height with the foot in relaxed position. (**A**) The foot is shown in neutral position. Note the navicular height (as measured to the top of the pen mark over the navicular) of about 6.4 cm. (**B**) The same foot is shown in relaxed stance. Note the navicular height of about 4.9 cm. The net change of 1.5 cm or 15 mm is considered abnormal or excessive pronation.

Some of these disadvantages can be eliminated or minimized by dynamically molding the support, but clinicians must have the skill, knowledge, and time to construct the support properly.

Arch supports may be the device of choice, depending on the type of injury, the severity of the foot or lower leg deformity, and patient compliance. As already noted, these devices may be an excellent initial treatment option because of their wide availability and modest cost.

Accommodative Orthotics

Although arch supports do not fit the definition of orthotic device presented above (a shoe insert fabricated over a cast so that the neutral STJ and MTJ positions are consistently maintained), accommodative supports are true orthotics. They are commonly constructed of semiflexible or semirigid materials molded over a neutral STJ position cast (Figure 13–27). Their function is to maintain the normal biomechanical relationship of the foot, ankle, and lower leg.[38–41,83] Accommodative devices attempt to control the velocity and degree of excessive STJ motion during the stance phase of gait.[102] Accommodative orthotics are usually more effective than arch supports at controlling abnormal foot function because of the method of construction and the materials used in construction. They are made over a neutral STJ cast of the patient's foot, so the arch contour is precise. They are constructed from semiflexible or semirigid materials, so they resist "bottoming out" or distortion. When indicated, posts can be added to the orthotic device to control abnormal rearfoot or forefoot motion. The effects of ankle and lower leg malalignment such as tibia varum/valgum, or torsions of the tibia or femur on the foot are controlled more effectively by accommodative devices. Accommodative orthotics are so named because they can accommodate for foot or lower leg dysfunction but are incapable of fully controlling it. The fault lies in the materials used to construct the devices. Semiflexible and semirigid materials distort less than flexible materials; however, under repetitive or excessive loading or torque, distortion or deformation occurs, and the ability to resist abnormal motion is di-

minished. The use of more rigid materials in construction obviates this problem.

The advantages of accommodative orthotics are as follows:

- effective in athletes and adults
- excel when maximal control is unwanted
- high patient compliance, comfortable
- attenuate shock well
- contour well over bony prominences
- maintain adequate angular control

Disadvantages of accommodative orthotics include the following:

- require casting for fabrication
- bulkier than more rigid orthotics
- less effective in maximal motion control
- costly
- adjustments require skilled professional
- last approximately 3 to 5 years (rigid orthotics approximately 10 years; over-the-counter devices last approximately 1 year)

Accommodative orthotics bridge the gap between flexible arch supportive devices and more rigid orthotics. When biomechanical correction is required and shock attenuation is also a prime concern (as is the case in most sports activities), this is the best type of device to use for long-term control.

Functional Orthotics

In most cases, when podiatrists use the term *orthotic*, they are referring to the functional orthotic. Like accommodative orthotics, functional orthotics are made over a neutral-position STJ cast; however, because they are generally fabricated from semirigid or rigid materials, they undergo less deformation even under maximal loads in weight bearing. They are termed "functional" because their purpose is to reduce dysfunction by reestablishing the normal angular relationships between the foot and the support surface, the rearfoot to forefoot, and the foot to the lower leg (Figure 13–28).[38–41] Although all of the supportive devices described in this chapter are capable of supporting the longitudinal arch (by controlling navicular drop), functional devices are the most effective.[102] This is attribut-

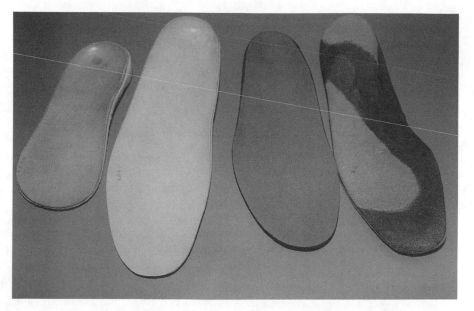

Figure 13–27 Accommodative Orthotic Devices. These devices are generally fabricated from semiflexible or semirigid materials molded over a neutral STJ cast. Devices above are (right to left): sulcus-length leather, full-length leather, full-length soft plastazote, and full-length hard or black zote.

able to the increased rigidity of the shell that enhances support of the arch, as well as the increased efficiency of any post added to the device.

Functional devices are commonly used when maximal biomechanical control is essential. For example, they are used with children where functional control allows more normal foot development. Bordelon states: "Since there is no scientific evidence that shoes do correct the flatfoot deformity, and since the only studies that have statistically shown correction on a conservative basis are those of Bleck and Bordelon, the author utilizes a custom-moulded insert of polypropylene [ie, a functional orthotic]."[61(p70)] Bordelon found that orthotics were capable of improving flatfoot conditions in young patients both clinically and radiographically, with an average rate of correction of 5 degrees per year.[61] This class of orthotic is helpful in controlling severe biomechanical dysfunction in adults as well as children.

Advantages of functional orthotics include the following:

- extremely stable
- maximal biomechanical control
- lightweight
- minimal bulk (fit shoes well)
- very durable (last 10 years or more)

Disadvantages of functional orthotics include the following:

- must be fabricated over a cast
- difficult to adjust (special equipment and skill)
- often uncomfortable (low compliance)
- poor shock attenuation
- expensive

Orthotics differ from arch supports in function. Arch supports hold up the arch by virtue of bulk alone. They allow the navicular to drop and then attempt to "push" it back up using a "bulk" filler under the longitudinal arch. Orthotics, on the other hand, support the arch by precise contour, less deformation (they retard navicular drop), and they attempt to reposition the foot joints (especially the STJ and MTJ). In normal

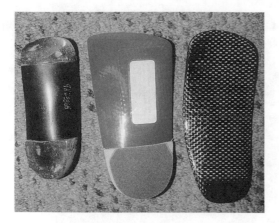

Figure 13–28 Functional Orthotics. Functional orthotics are usually made of semirigid or rigid materials over a neutral-position STJ cast. The orthotics shown above are (left to right): a rohadur orthotic with rearfoot and forefoot posted, a fiberglass orthotic with an extrinsic rearfoot and intrinsic forefoot post, and an unposted orthotic made of TL-61. Functional devices are best used when maximal biomechanical control is essential and shock attenuation is not required.

---

function, the bones and joints of the foot articulate in such a fashion that arch contour is maintained by bone-to-bone contact (like an arched bridge that relies on stone-to-stone contact). According to DuVries: "The arch is maintained by several mechanisms. The bones are so shaped as to present curved articulating surfaces to one another. . . . Such an arch does not break down."[103(p32)] Properly designed orthotics are capable of restoring this bone-to-bone contact and therefore do not have to rely as much on bulk to retard arch collapse. This helps to explain why orthotics are capable of controlling some types of dysfunction when arch supports fail. Arch supports act like a "truss" to support a collapsing arch, whereas orthotics act as "arch formers," restoring the normal joint relationships and retarding abnormal compensation.

Classification of Orthotics by Materials Used

The materials used in construction of orthotics impart certain physical properties that can af-

fect the way the device performs. Clinicians who provide orthotic therapy should have a reasonable knowledge of orthotic materials and their properties. Orthotics can be classified according to the properties imparted to them by the materials used in fabrication.

Flexible Materials

Flexible materials are used in orthotic construction because they provide cushioning, reduce friction (shearing forces), attenuate ground reactive forces, and provide support for the foot and arch.[104] Open- or closed-cell (microcellular) foam rubber or foam polymers are widely used flexible materials.[52] Open-cell foams have intercommunicating air pockets that allow for increased heat dissipation and evaporation.[102] Closed-cell foams have noncommunicating air chambers and therefore make these foams better insulators. Flexible materials do not stand up well under high loads (they "bottom out" or deform), and they are not durable. Because of this, devices made of these materials generally require bulk to support the foot and function like arch supports rather than orthotics. These materials are commonly used in prefabricated, over-the-counter supports, but they can also be dynamically molded to a patient's arch under pressure and/or heat.

The following flexible materials are used in the construction of orthotics:

- Plastazote—is a cross-linked polyethylene, closed-cell foam (CL-PE). It is one of the most commonly used flexible materials. It is manufactured in four densities, and a combination of densities enhances durability and makes a more supportive device.[105] Plastazote is heat moldable, easily contoured, and lightweight; it provides adequate shock absorption; and it is easily adjusted. Aliplast, Pelite, and Evazote are types of plastazote.[52,105]
- Rubber—can be a closed-cell foam rubber (Spenco), or sponge rubber (Lynco). It is frequently used in over-the-counter arch supports and widely available. Devices

made of rubber are usually preformed since it is not easily heat moldable or adjustable. Rubber devices are commonly covered with fabric to reduce foot friction over the rubber.[105] Rubber retains its shape better, is more durable, and reduces shearing and ground reactive forces better than plastazote, but it is much heavier and harder to adjust.

- Polyurethane foam—is an open- or closed-cell foam made of polyester resins. The open-cell variety is called Poron or PPT (Langer Biomechanics, Deer Park, New York). Ovaflex and Vylite are other forms of polyurethane foam. Polyurethane foams are elastic, resist deformation better than most other flexible materials, and attenuate shock well. Like the rubber foams, they are commonly preformed and heavy; however, polyurethane foam is easier to adjust and the open-celled foam "breathes" easier.[105]
- Styrene butadiene rubber (SBR)—is a co-polymer or rubber that is extremely moldable under pressure and/or heat. It is durable and lightweight, attenuates shock well, and contours and adjusts easily.[102] Neoprene, a polychloroprene, is similar to SBR, but less heat moldable and more durable.[105] Both materials are used extensively in flexible or semiflexible devices.

Flexible devices are an excellent choice when shock attenuation and/or reduction of shearing force is essential. Because of their flexibility, these devices act primarily as arch supports and therefore precise fit and design (casting) is not required. Flexible devices are comfortable, lightweight, and inexpensive; they are easily fabricated, contoured, and adjusted. Inexpensive, prefabricated over-the-counter devices are readily available in stores.

However, as a group, flexible devices provide little functional control; the materials distort or "bottom out" under heavy or repetitive loads. They also tend to be more bulky and less durable than other materials used in the construction of orthotics.

Flexible devices are best used as a temporary or transitional device before casted orthotics, or in disorders primarily related to arch dysfunction (eg, with patients with minimal foot or superstructural deformity). Conditions such as plantar fasciitis or tendinitis of the lower leg often respond well to flexible devices. These devices are also extremely effective in protecting bony prominences and guarding against ulcerations on the plantar aspect of the foot (especially in patients with diabetes).

Semiflexible Materials

Historically, orthotics made from materials in this category have been constructed of leather-covered cork, leather-covered rubber butter (a mixture of latex and cork dust), laminated leather, or rubber (RO Schuster, unpublished lecture notes, 1971–1975). The leather is shaped over a last or cast of a foot and is then united to a shell of cork (or other similar material) that is used to "bulk" up the arch. The device is then shaped and contoured, and posts are added when indicated. Rigid or semirigid materials can occasionally be used in the fabrication of semiflexible orthotics. When thin enough, these materials exhibit semiflexible properties. When laminated, flexible materials can be made to perform in a semiflexible manner.[52] Semiflexible materials are hybrids and can exhibit properties that are similar to flexible or rigid materials. They resist deformation better, are more durable, and generally less bulky than flexible materials. They lack the overall stiffness, memory, and durability, and they are more bulky than rigid materials.

Semiflexible materials are commonly used in orthotic fabrication.[102] Orthotics in this category are constructed over a neutral-position cast, but over-the-counter devices can be prefabricated or molded dynamically or by heat. Because precise arch contour is a key to control, casted devices are more biomechanically correct and, therefore, work better.

The following materials can be used to make semiflexible devices:

- Cork—Cork can be heat moldable or non–heat moldable.[102] Heat-moldable cork can be pressed over a positive cast and used as a shell for orthotics. Non–heat-moldable cork must be bonded to leather or other materials that have been preshaped. Cork combined with a rubber binder (Korex) enhances its ability to attenuate shock while reducing its tendency to crack.[104] Cork is easily molded and shaped, and it is moderate in bulk and weight. It is easily adjustable, resists deformation adequately, and is generally comfortable. Birkocork is a heat-moldable type of cork; Korex is non–heat moldable.
- Hard plastazote (hard zote)—This high-density plastazote (high-density CL-PE), also called "black zote," is the most dense form of plastazote.[104] It resists deformation almost as well as cork and has similar properties.
- Polyethylene (HMW)—This is the high molecular weight form of polyethylene (a lightweight thermoplastic). Used in thin sheets, it acts as a semiflexible material (similar to hard zote). Thicker sheets are semirigid. Under repeated stress, this material can crack or fatigue.[102] Ortholen and Subortholen are examples of this material.
- Polypropylene—This is a polyolefin similar to plastazote, but it is more dense, and deforms less. It is a butadiene polymer and, like polyethylene, it performs differently in varied thickness.[52] Thin sheets are semiflexible. Polypropylene is the lightest of the major plastics.[104]
- Acrylics and composites—These materials can perform in a semiflexible manner when thin, but they are more prone to fracture or fatigue in this form (the properties of acrylics and composites are described below in the discussion of rigid materials).

As a group, semiflexible orthotics incorporate the best features of flexible devices while minimizing their weaknesses. Orthotics made from these materials generally perform in an accommodative fashion. When casted, they precisely contour the arch and foot and are usually ex-tremely comfortable. They attenuate ground reactive forces well (although not as well as flexible devices), and they resist deformation better than flexible devices. They are more stable and more durable than flexible devices, and adjust just as easily.

However, in order for this material to function as an accommodative orthotic, it must be fabricated over a neutral-position cast. Semiflexible materials perform well as accommodative devices, but they are a poor choice when functional control is needed. They are usually bulkier, heavier, and much less durable than semirigid or rigid orthotics.

Orthotics made from semiflexible materials are among the best for use in athletic patients, especially sports that involve running or jumping, or those that require shock attenuation (RO Schuster, unpublished lecture notes, 1971–1975). They are flexible enough to allow the motions necessary for sport, yet they still provide accommodative control and attenuate ground reactive forces. Semiflexible orthotics are extremely effective in controlling patellofemoral dysfunction, plantar fasciitis, and "shin splint syndrome."

Semirigid Materials

Thermoplastics, acrylics, composites, and/or combinations of flexible materials with more rigid materials are the common starting materials used in the fabrication of semirigid orthotics.[104] The materials are firm to rigid in durometer rating. Semirigid materials resist deformation well and are very durable; however, they are only somewhat flexible and only adequate for shock attenuation.[104] These materials are somewhat adjustable and lightweight; they contour adequately and are less bulky than flexible or semiflexible materials. Semirigid materials can be designed precisely to achieve specific biomechanical goals.[104] When fabricated from a neutral-position cast, devices made from these materials perform as functional orthotics. When prefabricated or dynamically molded, they perform more like accommodative devices.

The following materials can be used to construct semirigid devices:

- Thermoplastics—These materials are rigid in a cool state but moldable when heated.[52] The temperature at which the plastic becomes pliant (the plastic point) varies. Low-temperature materials are capable of being dynamically molded to a patient's foot (for use as a temporary or office-fabricated orthotic). The most commonly used low-temperature thermoplastics are the plastazotes, which when laminated or joined to more rigid materials can perform in a semirigid manner.[52] Polyvinyl chloride (PVC) sheets have a low plastic point and are also used in fabrication of semirigid orthotics.[52,105] High-temperature thermoplastics include polyethylene (HMW) and polypropylene (discussed above). When heat molded or vacuum molded over a neutral-position cast in the proper thickness, these materials can be used to make semirigid orthotics.[52,105]

- Composites—Materials such as fiberglass or carbon graphite can be combined with other materials to make sturdy orthotic shells. Depending on the combination of materials used and the thickness of these materials, they can be semirigid or rigid. TL-61 is a composite with an acrylic core sandwiched between two layers of carbon graphite. It is extremely lightweight, durable, thin, nondeforming, and easily adjusted and contoured.[52] Unfortunately, it attenuates shock poorly, is brittle, and is often uncomfortable.[104] Fiberglass, especially when impregnated with acrylic resin, can be molded over a neutral cast to produce a semirigid or rigid orthotic with properties similar to those of TL-61.[102]

When fabricated over a neutral cast, orthotics made from semirigid materials are among the best at achieving functional control while still allowing for shock attenuation not possible with rigid materials. They improve weight transfer, support and stabilize foot deformities, and can help relieve abnormal pressure.[104] They are easily contoured, moderate to lightweight with minimal bulk, and usually comfortable.

However, to be maximally effective, they must be made over a neutral-position cast. The materials are hard and often have rough surfaces that must be smoothed well and/or covered with soft materials to ensure comfort and compliance. They are more difficult to adjust and generally more uncomfortable than devices made of more flexible materials. When shock attenuation is a prime concern, semirigid orthotics may not be the best choice.

The best use for semirigid orthotics is for athletes or individuals who require significant functional control along with some shock attenuation. In addition, these devices are effective in situations where minimal bulk without loss of functional control is a goal. Semirigid materials are an excellent choice when it is necessary to control flexible foot deformities and their sequelae, and a rigid orthotic cannot be used. They are equally effective in controlling structural foot deformities (such as bunions, hammertoes, flatfoot, and metatarsalgia), and postural symptoms (such as foot-related patellofemoral disorders, and hip or low back pain syndromes).

Rigid Materials

Rigid orthotics are usually constructed from hard, high-temperature thermoplastics, acrylics, or steel.[52] Orthotics made from these materials function best when made over a neutral-position cast; they then perform as functional orthotics and are more comfortable.[104] These materials offer maximal resistance to deformation; they are stable, durable, and lightweight with minimal bulk. On the other hand, they provide almost no shock attenuation, they are inflexible, and they are often uncomfortable and more difficult to fabricate and adjust than other types of orthotics. Still, rigid materials are superior when functional control is absolutely essential.

The following materials can be used to construct rigid orthotic devices:

- Stainless steel—Some of the earliest orthotics constructed were made from stainless steel (eg, Whitman steel plate).[1,102] Stainless steel (an alloy of nickel and chromium steel) is used in 16 or 18 gauge and hammered over a cast or last to cold-form an orthotic device.[104] This material makes a device that is extremely durable, supportive, and resistant to deformation. However, fabrication is difficult and must be done by a master craftsman, and steel devices are often uncomfortable, heavy, and difficult to wear and adjust. This material has fallen out of favor recently because of newer materials that have many of the same properties and are easier to work with.[104]

- Acrylics—Acrylics are thermoplastic materials made of polymerized methyl methacrylate or acronitriles.[102,104] These materials are heated and then pressed or vacuum molded over a neutral-position cast to produce an orthotic shell.[52,102,104] Acrylic devices are rigid, supportive, durable, lightweight, and easy to fabricate. Sophisticated equipment is required to fabricate and adjust the device.[104] Devices made of rohadur (a type of acrylic) were commonly used until the material was suspected of being carcinogenic and taken off the market.[102] Acrylics are available under the names Acridur and Flexidur.
- Thermoplastics—Polypropylene and polyethylene perform like rigid materials when used in thick sheets. In this form, they are heavier, bulkier, and more prone to stress failure than other rigid materials; otherwise, their properties are similar.
- Composites—Fiberglass and graphite composites are among the newer materials being used to fabricate rigid orthotics. Depending on the composition and thickness, these materials may be better than all the other materials in this category. They are lightweight, durable, thin, easy to contour, and as comfortable as any rigid material. However, they are more costly and require special equipment for fabrication.

When maximal control is required, orthotics made from rigid materials are superior to all others. They are especially suited for providing control of STJ and MTJ function, improving weight transfer, stabilizing flexible foot deformities, and limiting excessive motion.[104] Rigid orthotics are preferred for pediatric deformities and/or developmental foot pathology.[61] In the adult, rigid materials may be used to limit progressive foot deformities such as bunions and hammertoes.[38,104] When reduction of bulk is essential, rigid orthotics are the best option.

On the other hand, rigid orthotics provide minimal shock attenuation, may increase pressure over bony prominences, and can crack or fracture under excessive loads (which may limit their use in the athletic patient).[11,104] Fabrication of rigid orthotics requires sophisticated machinery and skilled technicians, and these devices should be made over a neutral-position cast.[104] These materials are often uncomfortable and difficult to adjust.

When control of the STJ and MTJ is essential and shock attenuation is of minimal importance, rigid devices are an excellent choice. They are also useful as an everyday device for functional control, but more flexible materials should be used for sports. They are especially suited for control of developmental pediatric or adolescent foot deformities, or in adults with lower leg, knee, hip, or low back problems that have been recalcitrant to other treatment.

Materials Used for Computer-Generated Orthotics

A new trend in orthotic construction is a semirigid or rigid orthotic device made from a computer-generated model.[102] The clinician uses a specifically designed scanner in the office to generate an image of the plantar surface of an individual's foot. These data are transmitted to a laboratory and fed into a computer that is capable of reconstructing the image and then directing a mill to fashion an orthotic device from the acquired data. Solid blocks of polypropylene or polyethylene are milled to fashion semirigid or rigid orthotics in this manner. Computer-aided technology eliminates the need for in-office casting, fabrication and preparation of a positive model from the negative cast, fabrication of the shell by pressing materials over the positive model, and finishing or shaping the final device. All of these steps are done by the computer or the mill. It is purported that this allows properly equipped laboratories to cut costs and reduce turnaround time in orthotic production. Unfortunately, at this time, there are some severe limitations. The initial setup costs for this technology are high for both the user and the laboratory; therefore, this technology is not widely available. The choice of materials that are capable of being computer milled is limited, and orthotics made in this manner are not as precise as casted devices. The final product is often uncomfortable and commonly needs adjustment. With refined technique, wider availability, improved materials, and decreased costs, this technology may be the wave of the future.

THE DESIGN OF ORTHOTIC DEVICES

Length and Shape

Clinicians must take into account many factors when designing an orthotic device. The length and shape of the device are just as important as the materials used in fabrication. Proper orthotic function requires the device to be specific for foot type; injury profile; activity level; and the age, weight, and shoe style of the patient. The vast majority of orthotics are made in three lengths: metatarsal head length, sulcus length, and full length (Figure 13–29).[52,104]

Metatarsal-Length Orthotics

Metatarsal-length devices extend from the posterior aspect of the heel proximally to the metatarsal heads (Figure 13–30).[52,104] This length is preferred for orthotics made from rigid or semirigid materials that cannot be extended under the metatarsal heads because of their rigidity or inflexibility. Metatarsal-length devices work primarily by controlling rearfoot motion and navicular drop (arch collapse).[58] They are less effective in controlling the foot at toe-off through the forefoot than orthotics posted further forward.[58,84]

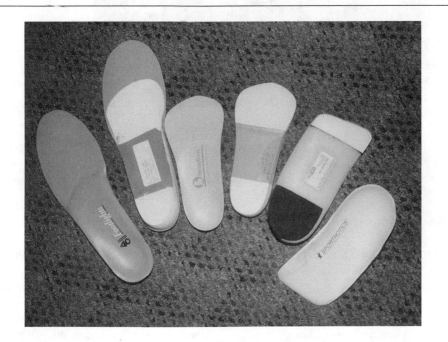

Figure 13–29 Orthotic Lengths. Shown above are the three most common orthotic lengths. On the left is a full-length device (note that the forefoot post ends at sulcus length). In the middle is a sulcus-length orthotic device (also with sulcus-length posts). On the right is a metatarsal-length device (posted in the metatarsal area only). All orthotics are posted extrinsically in the rearfoot and forefoot.

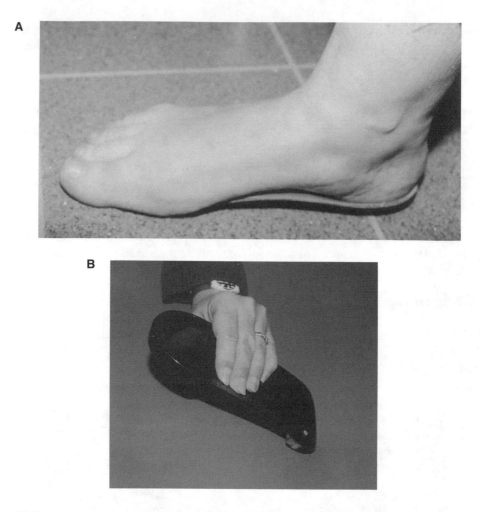

Figure 13–30 Metatarsal Length Orthotics. (**A**) These devices extend from the posterior portion of the heel and end proximally to the metatarsal heads. (**B**) The shell is usually made of semirigid or rigid material that will not bend when force is applied. These devices are somewhat less effective in controlling push-off through the forefoot than orthotics posted further forward and, therefore, less effective in controlling the biomechanics of sports.

Sulcus-Length Orthotics

These orthotics extend from the posterior aspect of the heel and continue under the metatarsal heads, ending at the sulcus or web space of the toes (Figure 13–31).[52] Orthotics made from flexible or semiflexible materials are commonly designed in this length. Semirigid or rigid materials can be extended to this length by adding softer materials that run under the metatarsal heads. When posts of flexible or semiflexible materials are incorporated into a device and extended under the metatarsals at the sulcus level, increased efficiency (especially in the control of forefoot motion) is seen.[3,4,44,58,84] *Sulcus-length orthotics represent the state of the art for control of patellofemoral disorders or in athletes.* Schuster maintains that orthotics that are posted at sulcus length increase the efficiency of the orthotic control by 53% (unpublished lecture notes, 1971–1975). Newton and Durkin noted that in athletes "with a high degree of forefoot

A

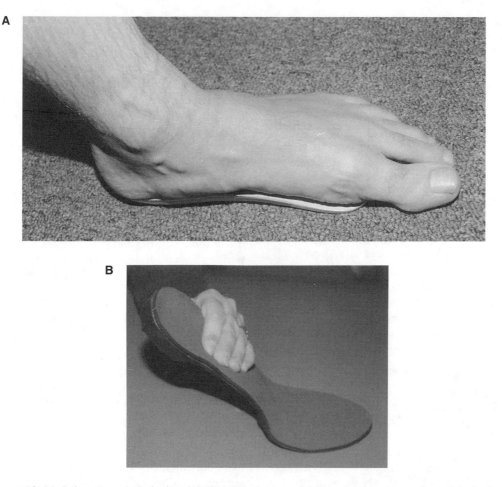

B

Figure 13–31 Sulcus-Length Orthotics. **(A)** These devices extend from the posterior portion of the heel, continue under the metatarsal heads, and end at the sulcus or web space of the toes. The shell can be made of semiflexible, semirigid, or rigid materials. Top covers of flexible or semiflexible materials can be added to increase the length, and posts of semiflexible or semirigid materials can be used to extend the orthotic to sulcus length. **(B)** The orthotic bends or "breaks" at the sulcus level while maintaining its shape at the rearfoot, arch, and forefoot areas; yet it still flexes easily through the toe area. This type of orthetic is excellent for patellofemoral disorders, especially those seen secondary to sports activities. Increased bulk and weight are the main drawbacks.

---

deformity, functional control may be compromised once the heel is lifted from the ground. . . . Thus forefoot functional control is crucial. . . . The long sulcus length forefoot post has proven very successful in controlling these individuals in their athletic activities."[84(p215)] Recent 3-D studies have shown that forefoot stability may play an integral role in rearfoot stability.[29,75] These studies indicate that instability in

the forefoot at push-off may create instability in the rearfoot. This concept runs contrary to the accepted biomechanical theory that a stable rearfoot creates a stable forefoot, and may explain the increased efficiency noted by many clinicians with extended sulcus-length posting. In their retrospective study, Donatelli et al noted: "Forefoot varus was, in the authors' opinion, the major cause of abnormal pronation during the stance phase of gait."[97(p210)] Properly posted, sulcus-length devices are far superior in controlling this deformity.[58,84]

Full-Length Orthotics

The full-length orthotic extends from the posterior aspect of the heel to beyond the end of the toes.[52] In most cases, an orthotic shell made from rigid, semirigid, or semiflexible materials ending at metatarsal or sulcus length is extended forward using top covers made of flexible or semiflexible materials. Full-length devices are especially effective in providing accommodation for abnormal loading patterns in the forefoot or toe area.[104] When posted at sulcus level, full-length devices control foot motion from heel contact to toe-off, just like sulcus-length devices posted in the same manner. The extended length of the device creates extra bulk, which makes the orthotic harder to fit into shoe gear.[104]

Other Factors Influencing Orthotics Design

Foot Type

Excessively pronated feet are often erroneously referred to as "flatfeet." Although flatfeet may look clinically similar to pronated feet, these are two different conditions. A flatfoot is flat both on and off weight bearing, whereas pronated feet are flat only on weight bearing. Flatfeet may function normally in some cases, but pronated feet are always biomechanically compromised. Orthotics made for flatfeet or pronated feet must control and support the medial column of the foot and prevent excessive STJ or MTJ motion.[38–41,83] Orthotics designed for supinated or "cavus" feet must attenuate ground-reactive forces and help to increase rearfoot motion.[38–41,83] Pronation generally requires a more rigid, functional control, whereas supination requires more flexible, accommodative control. Changing the length and shape of the device has little effect on pronated or supinated feet and is only considered when these conditions are combined with other foot deformities (eg, forefoot varus/valgus).

Injury Profile

The patient's injury profile may influence the design of the orthotic. In orthotics used for foot-related patellofemoral dysfunction, the important feature is the device's ability to control arch collapse and rearfoot and forefoot motion. Although any abnormal foot deformity may adversely affect patellofemoral mechanics, forefoot varus appears to be the most destructive. Aggressive control is suggested.[3,4,29,44,53,56,58,60,84,97] Orthotics of all lengths have shown some efficacy in reducing foot-related knee dysfunction. In patellofemoral disorders, orthotics made from semiflexible or semirigid materials with extended forefoot posting (sulcus-length posting) appear to be more effective.[3,44,58,60,84]

Activity Level, Age, Weight, and Shoe Style

In general, the more active a patient is, the less rigid the device should be.[58,84,104] Younger patients may be placed in more rigid materials, while older patients require more flexible materials.[61,104] Heavier patients generally require more rigid orthotics or laminated or reinforced flexible materials to prevent arch deformation.[102,104] Shoe style may be important to the patient, but orthotics should be designed to control abnormal motion and should never be altered to fit a particular shoe if it compromises the efficiency of the device. This is especially true of orthotics designed to fit women's high heels or men's tightly fitted shoes.

SUCCESSFUL USE OF ORTHOTICS IN PATIENTS WITH KNEE DYSFUNCTION

There are several keys to managing knee disorders successfully via foot orthotic devices. Not every foot-related knee problem requires the use of an orthotic. Patellofemoral pain can be managed in many ways. Many individuals can be adequately managed by knee exercises, change of shoe gear, arch paddings, strappings, or over-the-counter arch supports. When treatment is unsuccessful, or when the clinician sees significant forefoot pathology, custom-made orthotics may be indicated. In order to ameliorate patellofemoral dysfunction, custom devices must be designed to reduce excessive rearfoot motion at heel contact, prevent navicular drop during midstance, and control abnormal forefoot motion at propulsion. The best choice may be a functional or accommodative device made of semiflexible or semirigid materials fabricated over a neutral-position cast with corrective posting in the rearfoot and forefoot (Figure 13–32). Extended forefoot posting (ie, posting that extends under the metatarsals to the toe sulcus) may be superior in controlling knee-to-foot alignment and reducing patellofemoral dysfunction.

Most patients suffering from foot-related knee pain have one of the following foot deformities: forefoot varus, flexible forefoot valgus, or forefoot supinatus. Schuster noted forefoot varus deformity of 3 to 4 degrees or more in patellofemoral disorders, while Donatelli et al found an average of 8.4 degrees.[3,97] Compensation for the above deformities is generally via abnormal pronation, which creates a "flatfoot" appearance of the foot. Patients with rearfoot pathology with no other associated foot or lower extremity pathology are less likely to experience knee dysfunction. These patients often respond very well to commercially available arch supports and/or change in shoe gear. This is especially true when the magnitude of the rearfoot deformity is minimal (rearfoot varus of 6 to 8 degrees or less).

Management of Patients with Patellofemoral Pain

It is wise to begin with a "temporary orthotic" (arch support) for patients complaining of patellofemoral pain. The device can be a dynamically molded styrene butadiene rubber (SBR) arch support. SBR blanks are readily available through many supply houses. They are usually 1/8 inch in thickness and shaped in such a manner that they can mold up to become arch supports when the heat and pressure of the foot is applied to them within a shoe (Figure 13–33). The addition of an extra 1/4 inch of SBR into the longitudinal arch gives it a thickness of 3/8 inch in the longitudinal arch, which is needed to control the navicular drop. The added material is skived (smoothed) so that all edges are tapered. The device is then placed into the patient's shoe and used for walking and running for about 2 weeks, which allows the device to conform to the individual's arch. After using the appliance for 2 weeks, the patient is reevaluated; any improvement in knee pain is noted. If the symptoms are significantly improved, another 1/8 inch of SBR is added to the longitudinal arch. This restores the bulk that is compacted in the molding process. It is recontoured and used as the final arch support. One can use other molding materials or over-the-counter supports, as long as the arch is properly supported. Patients with little or no response are more thoroughly examined to determine the degree and location of any biomechanical deformity. Patients with significant deformity are casted in neutral position and fitted for a properly designed custom orthotic. If there is minimal observable biomechanical pathology and minimal response to a temporary device, the patient is reexamined to be certain that the etiology of the pain is mechanical.

Common Causes of Failed Orthotic Therapy

Inability To Control "Navicular Drop" (Arch Contour)

The ability of a device to contour precisely to an individual's arch is very important in increasing the efficiency of biomechanical control of the device. If the arch is not adequately contoured, the navicular will "drop" until it meets resistance from the device. As previously noted, navicular drop can be used as an indicator of excessive pronation. Over-the-counter arches or poorly fabricated, custom-made orthotics often fail to control knee pathology because they allow abnormal pronation to continue.

Poor Selection of Material Used for Fabrication of Orthotics

Even when arch contour is precisely maintained, improper selection of materials to construct the orthotic may allow excessive deforma-

tion of the device and thereby fail to limit abnormal foot motion. This is especially true in obese patients or in individuals engaged in rigorous activity or sports. In running, loads of 2 to 3 times body weight are common at the foot level and are transmitted to the orthotic.[26,31–34] This can cause the device to deform or "bottom out" if the materials are improperly selected, which allows increased navicular drop and leads to abnormal pronation. Devices that fail to provide adequate medial column support of the foot are

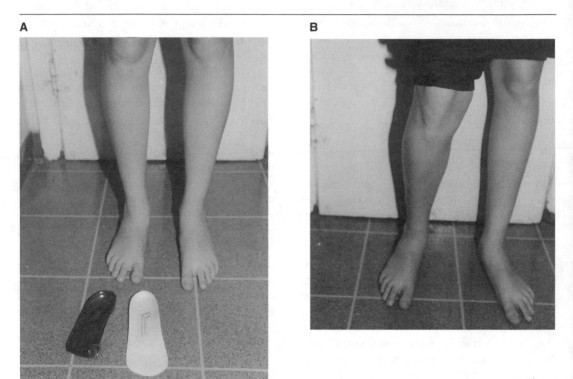

A

B

continues

Figure 13–32 Comparison of Orthotics. (**A**) A patient with "miserable malalignment" syndrome (ie, internal femoral torsion, external tibial torsion, and abnormal foot pronation) is given two types of orthotics: a rigid metatarsal-length orthotic posted both rearfoot and forefoot (left) and a semirigid orthotic posted at the rearfoot with sulcus-length posting at the forefoot (right). (**B**) The patient, who is wearing no orthotic, flexes the knee approximately 30 degrees. Note, that if an imaginary "plumb line" were dropped from the center of the patella to the support surface, it would fall medial to the first metatarsal joint. (**C**) The same patient stands on the metatarsal-length device with the knee bent at 30 degrees. The imaginary "plumb line" from the center of the patella to the support surface would now fall close to or over the first metatarsal joint. (**D**) The patient stands in the sulcus-length device with the knee bent 30 degrees. The same imaginary "plumb line" is now centered between the first and second metatarsal (ie, proper alignment). This shows that correction of knee joint position is affected most profoundly by how far the forefoot post extends, and not the rigidity of the orthotic shell or the amount of rearfoot posting. It shows the efficacy of extended- (sulcus-) length forefoot posting on foot-related knee dysfunction.

Figure 13–32 continued

C

D

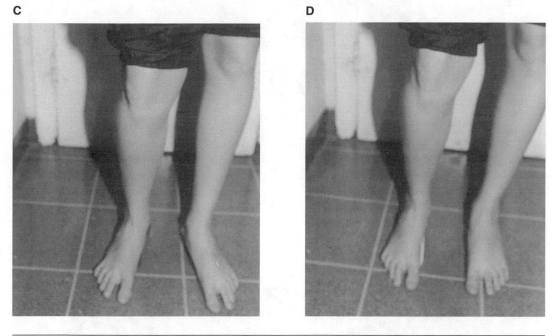

50% to 60% less effective in controlling patellofemoral pain (RO Schuster, unpublished lecture notes, 1971–1975).

Poor Stabilization of the Heel

For an orthotic device to perform properly, it must be able to "cup" or surround the calcaneus, preventing it from "rolling" excessively either medially or laterally. To stabilize the heel successfully, precise contour and proper posting is required. In most cases, this requires the orthotic to be fabricated from a neutral-position cast. Some clinicians believe that this can be achieved by molding heat-moldable materials directly to the patient's foot and contouring the material to the heel by hand.[18,19,61,99] This can be successful in some instances, but contouring may be inad-

equate and allow excessive rearfoot motion that can adversely affect the knee.

CONCLUSION

This chapter has familiarized the reader with the use of foot orthotic devices as a treatment alternative for patellofemoral pain. Despite any controversy that may exist, there is ample anecdotal and some scientific evidence to support claims about the effectiveness of orthotics. Given the current emphasis on cost control and outcomes studies in the managed care environment, the clinician who treats knee disorders needs every weapon the armamentarium can hold. Orthotic management adds another effective tool to combat the troublesome knee.

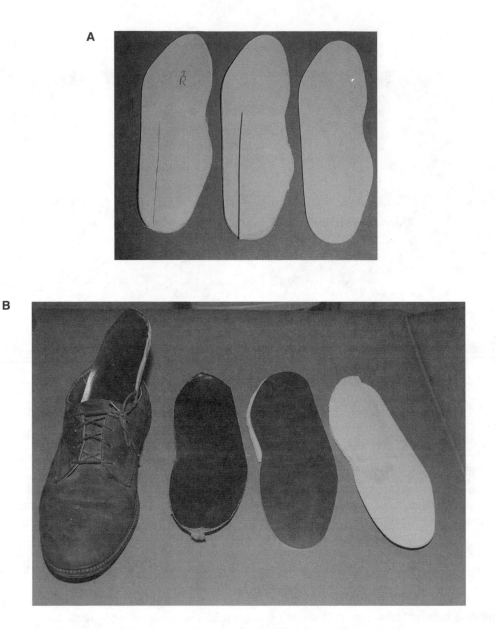

Figure 13–33 Fabrication of a Temporary Orthotic. (**A**) The steps in fabrication of a temporary styrene butadiene rubber (SBR) flexible arch support. From right to left: the SBR blank (1/8 inch thick); 1/4 inch of SBR is added to the blank in longitudinal arch; the SBR is "skived" (smoothed) on all edges. (**B**) The blank is placed in a shoe and the patient walks and runs on it for 2 weeks. The material form fits to the arch under pressure to form a "temporary customized" arch support. A final layer of 1/8 inch SBR is added into the long arch to finish the device. This type of support can be used as an inexpensive starter device to help to determine the need for more expensive, custom-made orthotics.

REFERENCES

1. Whitman R. Observations of forty-five cases of flatfoot with particular reference to etiology and treatment. *Boston Med Surg J*. 1888;118:598.

2. Ober FR. Recurrent dislocation of the patella. *Am J Surg*. 1939;43:497–500.

3. Schuster RO. Podiatry and the foot of the athlete. In: Altman M, ed. *Modern Therapeutic Approaches to Foot Problems*. Mt Kisco, NY: Futura Publishing Co; 1973:79–84.

4. Subotnick SI. Orthotic foot control and the overuse syndrome. *Arch Pod Med Foot Surg*. 1975;2(B):207–213.

5. Sheehan G. An overview of overuse injuries in distance runners. *Ann NY Acad Sci*. 1977;301:877–880.

6. James SL, Bates BT, Osternig LR. Injuries to runners. *Am J Sports Med*. 1978;6:40–50.

7. Bates BT, Osternig LR, Mason B, James SL. Foot orthotic devices to modify selected aspects of lower extremity mechanics. *Am J Sports Med*. 1979;7:338–342.

8. DeHaven KE, Dolan WA, Mayer PJ. Chondromalacia patella in athletes: clinical presentation and conservative management. *Am J Sports Med*. 1979;7:3–11.

9. Steadman JR. Non-operative measures for patellofemoral problems. *Am J Sports Med*. 1979;7:374–375.

10. Buchbinder MR, Napora NJ, Biggs EW. The relationship of abnormal pronation to chondromalacia of the patella in distance runners. *J Am Podiatry Assoc*. 1979;69:159–161.

11. Brody DM. Running injuries. *Ciba Clin Symp*. 1980;32(4):1–36.

12. Pagliano J, Jackson D. The ultimate study of running injuries. *Runner's World*. November 1980:42–50.

13. Clement DB, Taunton JE, Smart GW, McNicol KL. A survey of overuse running injuries. *Phys Sports Med*. 1981;9(5):47–58.

14. Eggold JF. Orthotics in the prevention of runner's overuse injuries. *Phys Sports Med*. 1981;9(3):125–131.

15. Gudas CJ. Patterns of lower extremity injury in 224 runners. *J Exerc Sports Med*. 1982;16:50–59.

16. Newell SG, Bramwell ST. Overuse injuries to the knee in runners. *Phys Sports Med*. 1984;12(3):81–92.

17. Cox JS. Patellofemoral problems in runners. *Clin Sports Med*. 1985:4:699–715.

18. Lutter LD. The knee and running. *Clin Sports Med*. 1985;4:685–697.

19. Lutter LD. Orthopedic management of runners. In: Bateman JE, Trott AW, eds. *The Foot and Ankle*. New York: Thieme-Stratton Co; 1980:155–158.

20. Kujala VM, Kvist M, Osterman K. Knee injuries in athletes: review of exertion injuries and retrospective study of outpatient sports clinic material. *Sports Med*. 1986;3:447–460.

21. Pretorius DM, Noakes TD, Irving G, Allerton K. Runners' knee: what is it and how effective is conservative management. *Phys Sports Med*. 1986;14(12):71–81.

22. Jacobs SJ, Berson BL. Injuries to runners: a study of entrants to a 10,000 meter race. *Am J Sports Med*. 1986;14:151–155.

23. Marti B. Benefits and risks of running among women: an epidemiological study. *Int J Sports Med*. 1988;9:92–98.

24. *Nike Sports Research Review: Common Running Injuries*. Beaverton, OR: Nike; March–April 1989.

25. Stanish WD. Overuse injuries in athletes: a perspective. *J Med Sci Sports Exerc*. 1984;16:1–7.

26. Subotnick SI. The biomechanics of running: implications for the prevention of foot injuries. *Sports Med*. 1985;2:144–153.

27. Nicholas JA, Marino M. The relationship of injuries in the leg, foot and ankle to proximal thigh strength in athletes. *Foot Ankle*. 1987;7:218–228.

28. Bates BT, Osternig LR, Mason BR, James SL. Functional variability of the lower extremity during the supports phase of running. *J Med Sci Sports Exerc*. 1979;11:328–331.

29. *Nike Sports Research Review: Rearfoot Stability*. Beaverton, OR: Nike; November–December 1989.

30. *Nike Sports Research Review: Women in Sports*. Beaverton, OR: Nike; March–April 1990.

31. Mann RA, Hagy JL. Running, jogging, and walking: a comparative electromyographic and biomechanical study. In: Bateman JE, Trott AW, eds. *The Foot and Ankle*. New York: Thieme-Stratton Co; 1980:167–175.

32. Scranton PE, Hootman BD, McMaster JH. Forces under the foot: a study of walking, jogging, and sprinting, force under normal and abnormal feet. In: Bateman JE, Trott AW, eds. *The Foot and Ankle*. New York: Thieme-Stratton Co; 1980:186–194.

33. Scranton PE, Rutkowski R, Brown TD. Support phase kinematics of the foot. In: Bateman JE, Trott AW, eds. *The Foot and Ankle*. New York: Thieme-Stratton Co; 1980:195–205.

34. Cavanagh PR, LaFortune MA. Ground reactive forces in distance running. *J Biomech*. 1980;13:397–406.

35. Stacoff A, Denoth J, Kaelin X, Stuessi E. Running injuries and shoe construction: some possible relationships. *Int J Sport Biomech*. 1988;4:342–357.

36. Clarke E, LaFortune MA, Williams KR, Cavanagh PR. The relationship between center of pressure location and rearfoot movement in distance running. *J Med Sci Sports Exerc.* 1980;12:138.

37. Bates BR, James SL, Osternig LR. Evaluation of within runner variability and subject condition interaction when evaluating running shoes. *J Med Sci Sports Exerc.* 1980;12:138.

38. Root ML, Orien WP, Weed JH. *Normal and Abnormal Function of the Foot.* Los Angeles: Clinical Biomechanics Corp; 1977.

39. Wernick J, Langer S. *A Practical Manual for a Basic Approach to Biomechanics.* Hicksville, NY: Edigan Press; 1972;1:10–23.

40. Sgarlato TE. *A Compendium of Podiatric Biomechanics.* San Francisco: California College of Podiatric Medicine; 1971:79–108,171–180.

41. Langer S, Polchaninoff M, Hoerner EF, Wernick J. *A Practical Manual of Clinical Electrodynography.* 2nd ed. Deer Park, NY: MMI Press; 1989:4–14.

42. Perry J. Anatomy and biomechanics of the hindfoot. *Clin Orthop Rel Res.* 1983;177:9–15.

43. Nigg BM. Biomechanical load analysis and sports injuries of the lower extremity. *Sports Med.* 1985;3:367–379.

44. Levy AM, Fuerst ML. *Sports Injury Handbook: Professional Advice for Amateur Athletes.* New York: John Wiley & Sons; 1993:106–133.

45. Manter JT. Movements of the subtalar and transverse tarsal joints. *Anat Rec.* 1944;80:397.

46. Mann RA, Inman VT. Phasic activity of intrinsic muscles of the foot. *J Bone Joint Surg.* 1964;46A:469–481.

47. Borelli AH, Smith SD. Surgical considerations in the treatment of pes planus. *J Am Podiatr Med Assoc.* 1988;6:305–309.

48. Olerud C, Rosendahl Y. Torsion transmitting properties of the hindfoot. *Clin Orthop Rel Res.* 1987;214:285–295.

49. DiGiovanni JE, Smith SD. Normal biomechanics of the adult rearfoot: a radiographic analysis. *J Am Podiatry Assoc.* 1976;66:812–824.

50. D'Amico JC. The postural complex, I. *J Am Podiatry Assoc.* 1976;66:568.

51. Inman VT, Ralston HJ, Todd F. *Human Walking.* Baltimore: Williams & Wilkins; 1981:1–62.

52. Wu K. *Foot Orthoses: Principles and Clinical Applications.* Baltimore: Williams & Wilkins; 1990:39–44.

53. Knutzen KM, Bates BT. Use of kinetic support phase parameters in the prediction of knee movement. *J Am Podiatr Med Assoc.* 1988;78:389–395.

54. Hicks JH. The mechanics of the foot, I: The joints. *J Anat.* 1953;87:345–357.

55. Barither D. Prenatal development of the foot and ankle. *J Am Podiatr Med Assoc.* 1995;85:753–764.

56. Tiberio D. Pathomechanics of structural foot deformities. *J Phys Ther.* 1988;68:1840–1849.

57. Kolker L. A biomechanical analysis of flatfoot surgery. In: Altman M, ed. *Modern Therapeutic Approaches to Foot Problems.* Mt. Kisco, NY: Futura Publishing Co; 1973:25–311.

58. McNerney JE. Considerations in the use of foot orthoses for patellofemoral disorders. Presented at the Challenge of the Patella Seminar. New York: Columbia Presbyterian Medical Center; 1994.

59. D'Amico JC, Rubin M. The influence of foot orthoses on the quadriceps angle. *J Am Podiatry Assoc.* 1986; 76:337–340.

60. Tiberio D. The effect of excessive subtalar joint pronation on patellofemoral mechanics: a theoretical model. *J Orthop Sports Phys Ther.* 1985;9:160–165.

61. Bordelon RL. *Surgical and Conservative Foot Care.* Thorofare, NJ: Slack Inc; 1992:37–45, 68–73.

62. McDonough MW. Angular and axial deformities of the legs of children. *Clin Podiatry.* 1984;1:601–620.

63. James SL. Chondromalacia of the patella in the adolescent. In: Kennedy JC, ed. *The Injured Adolescent Knee.* Baltimore: Williams & Wilkins; 1979:205–251.

64. Baylis WJ, Rzonca EC. Functional and structural limb length discrepancies evaluation and treatment. *Clin Podiatr Med Surg.* 1988;5:509–519.

65. Paulos L, Rusche K, Johnson C, Noyes FR. Patellar malalignment: a treatment rationale. *J Phys Ther.* 1980;60:1624–1632.

66. Blake RL, Burns DP, Colson JP. Etiology of atraumatic medial knee pain. *J Am Podiatry Assoc.* 1981;71:580–583.

67. Lysens RJ, de Weerdt W, Nieuboer A. Factors associated with injury proneness. *Sports Med.* 1991;12:281–288.

68. Becker NL. Specific running injuries and complaints related to excessive loads: medical criteria of the running shoe. In: Segesser B, Pforringer W, eds. *The Shoe in Sport.* Chicago: Year Book Medical Publishers; 1989:16–25.

69. Frederick EC. The running shoe dilemmas and dichotomies in design. In: Segesser B, Pforringer W, eds. *The Shoe in Sport.* Chicago: Year Book Medical Publishers; 1989:26–35.

70. McNerney JE. Coming up with the shoe that matches the sport. *NY Times.* February 18, 1991.

71. McNerney JE. How golf shoes work . . . and how to choose a pair that works for you. *Golf Illustrated.* June 1990:78–82.

72. Brown LP, Yavorsky P. Locomotor biomechanics and pathomechanics: a review. *J Orthop Sports Phys Ther.* 1987;9:3–10.

73. Donatelli R. Abnormal biomechanics of the foot and ankle. *J Orthop Sports Phys Ther.* 1987;9:11–16.

74. Inman VT. *The Joints of the Ankle.* Baltimore: Williams & Wilkins; 1976:56–67.

75. Engsberg JR, Andrews JG. Kinematic analysis of the talocalcaneal/talocrural joint during running support. *Med Sci Sports Exerc.* 1987;19:275–283.

76. Rodgers MM, LeVeau BP. Effectiveness of foot orthotic designs used to modify pronation in runners. *J Orthop Sports Phys Ther.* 1982;4:86–90.

77. Clarke TE, Frederick EC, Hlavac HF. Effects of a soft orthotic on rearfoot movement in running. *Pod Sports Med.* 1983;1:20–23.

78. Cavanagh PR, Clarke TE, Williams K, Kalenak A. An evaluation of the effects of orthotics force distribution and rearfoot motion during running. Presented at American Orthopedic Society for Sports Medicine Seminar; June 1978; Lake Placid, NY.

79. Smith LS, Clarke TE, Hamill CL, Santopietro F. The effects of soft and semi-rigid orthoses upon rearfoot movement in running. *J Am Podiatr Med Assoc.* 1986; 76:227–233.

80. *Nike Sport Research Review: Three-Dimensional Kinematics.* Beaverton, OR: Nike; April–July 1991.

81. Soutas-Little RW, Beavis GC, Verstraets MC, Markus TL. Analysis of foot motion during running using a joint coordinate system. *Med Sci Sports Exerc.* 1987;19:285–293.

82. Novick A, Kelley DL. Position and movement changes of the foot with orthotic intervention during the loading response of gait. *J Orthop Sports Phys Ther.* 1990; 11:301–311.

83. Root ML, Orien WP, Weed JH, Hughes RJ. *Biomechanical Examination of the Foot.* Vol 1. Los Angeles: Clinical Biomechanics Corp; 1971.

84. Newton J, Durkin JF. *Running to the Top of the Mountain.* Chicago: J & J Winning Edge Press; 1988;118–132.

85. Moss RL, DeVita P, Dawson ML. A biomechanical analysis of patellofemoral stress syndrome. *J Ath Train.* 1992;27:64–69.

86. Balakrishnan S, Thornton-Trump AB. Reaction parameter variation with gait changes. *Proceedings of the Special Conference of the Canadian Society for Biomechanics.* Ottawa, Canada: Organization Committee, Canadian Society of Biomechanics; 1980:100.

87. Stauffer RN, Chad EY, Gyory AN. Biomechanical gait analysis of the diseased knee joint. *Clin Orthop Rel Res.* 1977;126:246.

88. Eng JJ, Pierrynowski MR. The effects of soft foot orthotics on three dimensional lower limb kinematics during walking and running. *J Phys Ther.* 1994;74:45–53.

89. Eng JJ, Pierrynowski MR. Evaluation of soft foot orthoses in the treatment of patellofemoral pain syndrome. *J Phys Ther.* 1993;73:62–70.

90. Reiley MA. *Guidelines for Prescribing Foot Orthotics.* Thorofare, NJ: Slack Inc; 1995;3–5.

91. McCulloch MV, Brunt D, Vander Linden D. The effects of foot orthoses and gait velocity on lower limb kinematics and temporal events of stance. *J Orthop Sports Phys Ther.* 1993;17:2–10.

92. Larson RL. Subluxation-dislocation of the patella. In: Kennedy JC, ed. *The Injured Adolescent Knee.* Baltimore: Williams & Wilkins; 1979:161–204.

93. Tomaro JE, Burdett RG, Chadrad AM. Subtalar joint motion and the relationship to lower extremity overuse injuries. *J Am Podiatr Med Assoc.* 1996;86:427–432.

94. Beckett ME, Massie DL, Bowers KD, Stoll DA. Incidence of hyperpronation in the ACL injured knee: a clinical perspective. *J Ath Train.* 1992;27:58–62.

95. Woodford-Rogers B, Cyphert L, Denegar CR. Risk factors for anterior cruciate ligament injury in high school and college athletes. *J Ath Train.* 1994;29:343–346.

96. Smith J, Szczerba JE, Arnold BL, et al. Role of hyperpronation as a possible risk factor for anterior cruciate ligament injuries. *J Ath Train.* 1997;32:25–28.

97. Donatelli R, Hurlburt C, Conaway D, St. Pierre R. Biomechanical foot orthotics: a retrospective study. *J Orthop Sports Phys Ther.* 1988;10:205–212.

98. Blake RL, Denton JA. Functional orthoses for athletic injuries: a retrospective study. *J Am Podiatr Med Assoc.* 1985;75:359–362.

99. Lutter LO. Foot-related knee problems in the long distance runner. *Foot Ankle.* 1980;1:112–116.

100. Mueller MJ, Host JV, Norton BJ. Navicular drop as a composite measure of excessive pronation. *J Am Podiatr Med Assoc.* 1993;93:198–202.

101. Brody DM. Techniques in evaluation and treatment of the injured runner. *Orthop Clin North Am.* 1982; 13:541.

102. Levitz SJ, Whiteside LS, Fitzgerald TA. Biomechanical foot therapy. *Clin Podiatr Med Surg.* 1988;5:721–736.

103. DuVries HL. *Surgery of the Foot.* 2nd ed. St Louis, MO: CV Mosby Co; 1965;32.

104. Schwartz RS. Foot orthoses and materials. In: Jahss MH, ed. *Disorders of the Foot and Ankle.* Philadelphia: WB Saunders Co; 1991:2866–2878.

105. Jones LS, Caselli M. The foam zone. *Biomech Mag.* 1996;3:73–77.

CHAPTER 14

Surgery

There should be no distinction between the terms *conservative* and *surgical* when it comes to treatment of the patella. Treatment should always be conservative—be it surgical or not.

—RPG

Patellar pathology is underdiagnosed and overoperated.

–Old Chinese proverb

The timing of surgery and the choice of procedures for surgery involving the patella remain controversial. In 1959, Cotta[1] in Germany performed a literature review and found 139 procedures pertaining to the patella. This was before *any* of today's commonly used procedures had been described. Whenever there are many operations for one problem, it is a strong indication that none of the operations approaches perfection. In regard to the patella, "the clinical problem" can actually be a combination of many different problems. This only makes decision making and comparison of surgical reports in the literature that much more difficult. The surgeon must determine exactly what condition he or she is operating on. Categories include chronic malalignment, acute dislocations, chondral lesions, and combinations of these conditions.

INDICATIONS

The common platitude is that surgery is indicated when nonoperative treatment has failed. In principle, this is true. However, this orthopaedic cliché should be amended to read "appropriate" nonoperative treatment. As noted in the previous chapters, there is more to nonoperative treatment than attaching weights to the ankle or placing the

As noted in the Introduction of this book, this discussion does not include the surgical treatment of patellar fractures or tendinous disruptions. Special thanks go to Dr Philippe Cartier for assistance with Figures 14–1 and 14–7.

patient in an exercise machine (the "electric chair").

Having said this, how long does one place a patient on a physical therapy program before proposing surgery? There is no definitive answer to this question. In my opinion, the severity of the pathology plays a role. For example, some patients may have no more than mild tilt of the patella that is easily reducible (ie, the examiner can easily lift the lateral border of the patella to make the patella horizontal). In others, the patella is severely tilted and subluxed ("hanging off the lateral condyle") and cannot be manually corrected. In the former case, I would expect a nonoperative regimen to be successful. In the latter, I might, in very select cases, bypass physical therapy and propose surgery. The duration of symptoms and prior treatments also have to be considered. A patient with 1 week of pain following an initiation to in-line skating and another patient with long-standing symptoms who has already been through many treatment regimens will be seen in a very different light. Each case must be individualized.

On average, I start with a regimen of 3 times a week for 4 weeks. As a rule, I like to see progress with the nonoperative regimen in order to justify persevering with physical therapy after the initial sessions have been completed. If there is no progress, the clinician must make a judgment as to whether the patient is noncompliant or whether the pathology is beyond nonoperative treatment. Finally, before proposing surgery, the surgeon should be reasonably certain that a particular operation will address the problem.

Carson has suggested that electrical stimulation of the vastus medialis obliquus (VMO) can be used to check the effectiveness of physical therapy: if electrical stimulation of the VMO leads to untilting and centering of the patella, then physical therapy should be continued. If not, physical therapy may be a waste of time.[2] I am not convinced that he is correct, because imperceptible changes in patellar positioning can make a clinical difference. This is evidenced by patients who feel better when taping is applied even though no change in patella positioning can be demonstrated.

There should be no such thing as a nonconservative approach to the patella. By the time surgery is recommended, it should be viewed as the conservative approach.

In summary, indications for surgery include intractable pathology anticipated to be refractory to nonoperative treatment (rare), or failure of appropriate nonoperative therapy. The patient should be judged likely to be compliant with the postoperative regimen. The surgeon should have a clear understanding of the pathology that he or she is treating and should feel comfortable that the operations in his/her armamentarium will adequately address the pathology.

INFORMED CONSENT

When operating on a patient for pain (as opposed to instability), obtaining an informed consent is even more complex and time consuming than in other areas of orthopaedic surgery. Not only is there a mechanical problem, but there may be a biological problem. In some patients, the pain is not purely related to malalignment. Thus, even after the malalignment is corrected, pain persists. Reflex sympathetic dystrophy (RSD) is the only biological condition for which we have a name, cause, and treatment. The other biological causes remain undiscovered and therefore unnamed. I call them RSD-like conditions for lack of a better term.

The surgeon who proposes surgery has to project a confident, optimistic picture (what patient wants a tentative surgeon?). Nevertheless, the surgeon must undertake the delicate balancing act of projecting this image while informing the patient of this biological aspect over which the surgeon has no control. The patient may also turn out to have inflammatory arthritis, a neuropathy, or referred pain that is not initially apparent, and surgical realignment of the patella will not improve these conditions.

GENERAL PRINCIPLES

There are two fundamentally different surgical approaches to the malaligned patella:

1. Perform a "simple" operation and move on to more complex operations if the first does not work.
2. Address all the pathology from the start, even if this involves a complex operation.

Which approach to choose depends on how simple the "simple" operation is and how complex the alternative is. Simplicity and complexity are very much in the eye of the beholder, and this subjectivity accounts for the continued controversy over which approach to choose. My personal preference is for the second approach, and I will return to this subject at the end of the chapter.

Generally speaking, the goal of surgery is to address one or more of the following conditions:

- tilt
- medial deficiency
- medial-lateral displacement
- lateralized tibial tuberosity
- patellar height
- trochlear dysplasia
- painful chondral lesions

Surgical procedures have been arbitrarily divided into proximal and distal procedures. All seek to somehow transform a tilted and/or lateral-tracking patella into a less tilted, centrally tracking patella. *Proximal realignments* involve surgical manipulation of the lateral retinaculum, the medial retinaculum, the vastus lateralis, the vastus medialis obliquus, or any combination thereof. Like balancing a marionette, it is a question of tightening certain "strings" and giving others more slack. The term *distal realignment* denotes (by convention) a transfer of the tibial tuberosity. Certain procedures do not fall into either category (eg, prosthetic resurfacing of the patella or trochlea).

As noted in Chapter 1, there is still confusion and controversy with respect to nomenclature. To some surgeons, a lateral release is not considered a realignment or a reconstruction (as in, "We will perform a lateral release and then go to a formal reconstruction if this does not work."). To others (including myself), any procedure that changes the position, tracking, or articular contact area of the patella qualifies as a reconstruction and a realignment. The difference in philosophy stems from the fact that some surgeons consider the lateral release to be a small procedure to be done arthroscopically, and "reconstructions" are done with a formal skin incision. The problem with this nomenclature is that it can lead the surgeon to think of the lateral release as a minor, relatively risk-free procedure to be done nearly on a casual basis, while other procedures are major and therefore require more planning, more discussion with the patient, and more concerns with respect to complications. In my experience, such a distinction between the lateral release and other procedures is not warranted.

SPECIFIC PROCEDURES*

The Lateral Retinacular Release

Overview

The lateral retinacular release has been an integral part of almost all realignment procedures

---

*Procedures designed to address chronic malalignment, acute events, and arthritic lesions are not listed in the separate chapters of this book. There is considerable overlap between these conditions, and, accordingly, they are all discussed in this chapter.

and since the 1970s has often been carried out as an isolated operation. In fact, the isolated lateral retinacular release is now probably the most commonly performed realignment procedure. It is such a technically simple procedure that one has to wonder why it was not popularized sooner. I believe the answer to this question is quite simple: until the 1970s, orthopaedists concentrated on the unstable patella that slipped out of the trochlea. The focus was on the subluxating or dislocating patella, not on the painful tilted patella. Patients who underwent surgery felt the patella slip and/or had episodes of frank dislocation requiring reduction by a doctor. As early as 1974, Merchant and Mercer[3] from California published a report on the lateral release for just those cases. At the time most surgeons believed that a more significant reconstruction was required for unstable patellae. Ficat from southwestern France was the first to popularize the concept of the tilted patella, which could be perfectly centered in the trochlea yet malaligned by virtue of tilting in the axial plane.[4] He also popularized the concept of operating on the painful tilted patella. In the nonoperated knee, this tilt is always lateral, (ie, the lateral border of the patella dips down while the medial border is raised—like an airplane turning). Tilting of the patella is always associated with increased tightness of the lateral retinaculum.

Ficat hypothesized that tilting of the patella caused excessive pressure on the lateral facet of the patella, thus leading to the "excessive lateral pressure syndrome." It stands to reason that the treatment for this syndrome is simple release of the lateral retinaculum, which technically means surgical separation of the lateral retinaculum from the lateral border of the patella. When done through a large incision, this procedure is as quick as closing a scissors. When done through a small incision or arthroscopically, it is more challenging but still relatively simple relative to other procedures. Its simplicity has certainly contributed to its meteoric success.

Some patients seem to have excessive play about the patella in both the medial and lateral direction, the so-called hypermobile patella. Can the lateral retinaculum in such cases be tight?

Perhaps not in the absolute sense but, relative to the medial retinaculum, the answer is yes.

Alternate Mechanism of Action

Fulkerson and Grossling have noted that patients with patellar pain can have fibrosis of the nerves within the lateral retinaculum.[5] Perhaps this is part of the pain source. Whether this fibrosis is the primary problem or merely secondary to chronic contracture of the lateral retinaculum is a matter of conjecture. In any case, division of the lateral retinaculum can have a denervating effect on the patella, and some have suggested that this plays a significant role in the pain relief obtained after a lateral release.[6] Failure to obtain pain relief or—worse yet—aggravation of the pain could be due to the creation of a neuroma during the procedure.[6] There is a precedent for denervating the knee to obtain pain relief when the sensory nerves are believed to be the source of the pain.[7]

Indications

The lateral release can be carried out as an isolated procedure or in combination with other procedures. There is little controversy with respect to combining the lateral release with other procedures. For example, when performing a medial plication or a distal realignment, a lateral release is usually carried out. The controversy begins when one discusses the lateral release as the only form of surgical realignment. In favor of this approach is the fact that the procedure is relatively straightforward (no special instructional course required), it can often be done in an ambulatory surgery setting, and there are indeed articles in the orthopaedic literature supporting it. Against it are the fact that, although it is simple, it still involves a trip to the operating room and an anesthetic, it still requires a full course of physical therapy, it can still lead to significant complications, and there are equally numerous articles to suggest that the isolated lateral release does not work well in all patients with patellar pathology. Even if it does work well, will it hold up in the long run? As of this writing, a number of serious scholars of the patella such as Dejour,[8] Dupont, and Cartier (all in Ficat's country of origin) no longer perform isolated lateral releases.

This controversy is related to the question of whether tightness of the lateral retinaculum is the primary pathology or whether this tightness is simply secondary to the chronically displaced and/or tilted patella. If one believes the former premise, it is reasonable to section the lateral retinaculum and expect the condition to be cured. If one believes the latter scenario, then it is logical to assume that in time the lateral retinaculum will tighten up. On top of this, one has to look at other parameters about the knee that can cause patellar pain and/or instability. In the presence of such parameters, can the isolated lateral release suffice? Opinions remain divided.

Another possibility is that the isolated release may be indicated for certain patients. In a study carried out by Shea and Fulkerson, patients who had tilt but no clinical or radiological subluxation did well following the isolated lateral release.[9] These patients did not have a sense of instability, and the patella was centered in the trochlea on computed tomography (CT) images carried out in the early degrees of flexion. On the other hand, patients who demonstrated features of instability either clinically or radiographically did not do well with the isolated lateral release. The authors' conclusion was that the isolated lateral release is indicated for patients whose only pathology is patellar tilt. This approach to decision making appears to be a step in the right direction, as no procedure works for every patient. The downside to this approach is that making the determination of tilt versus lateral displacement is not always straightforward: even a subluxating patella can appear well centered on computerized imaging.

Contraindications

Patients with no malalignment cannot be expected to gain much from this basic realignment procedure. In Shea and Fulkerson's study,[9] only one of eight patients without any form of tilt or lateral displacement on CT scanning had a good result. At the other extreme, extensive chondral lesions are likely to remain painful after a lateral retinacular release. Lateral displacement and dislocation of the patella remain more controversial as indications for the lateral retinacular release.

Surgical Technique and Variations

Many variations of the lateral retinacular release have been described. Deep to the lateral retinaculum lies the synovium of the joint—the smooth, moist layer that secretes synovial fluid. In performing a lateral release, some surgeons choose to leave the synovium unopened, and others choose to release the synovium along with the retinaculum. The lateral retinaculum is usually released from approximately the superior pole of the patella. It can be taken proximally along the lower fibers of the vastus lateralis (VL) but not into the vastus. Distally, it is taken to a variable distance. At the very least, the release is carried out to the level of the inferior pole, but it can be carried out all the way to the tibial tuberosity.[10] All of these variations qualify as a lateral release. Exactly how far the release should go is also a subject of controversy. A "turn up" sign has been described, whereby the lateral release is carried out to the point where the patella can be "turned up" 90 degrees.[11] This sign was recommended to guard against an insufficient release, but in some patients this amount of release is excessive.

The lateral release is said to be an open release when an incision is made at the lateral border of the patella. The incision is usually near the superior pole of the patella so as to directly visualize the superolateral geniculate vessels, which are located transversely across the incision, approximately at the level of the superior pole of the patella just deep to the retinaculum. These vessels are responsible for one of the more common perioperative complications of this procedure—a hemarthrosis (blood in the joint). The risk of a hemarthrosis can probably be decreased by direct visualization and cauterization of the vessels. However, a hemarthrosis can occur even with this approach. Presumably, vessels can go into spasm at the time of surgery, only to open

up and bleed in the postoperative period. For this reason, it is not unreasonable to put a drain in the knee. The incision can be closed with a subcuticular closure (so-called plastic surgery), which will avoid the "railroad track" look. However, the incision may spread in time, as incisions about the knee are wont to do. According to traditional teaching, the horizontal incision can give better cosmesis, and it remains an acceptable surgical approach.[12] However, the incision may need to be longer to give adequate visualization proximally and distally. Moreover, a study that specifically compared the cosmesis of long transverse incisions and long parapatellar incisions found triple the number of cosmetically good results in the parapatellar group.[13] (*Note*: Generally speaking, there is still controversy as to whether vertical skin incisions should be midline, medial parapatellar, or lateral parapatellar. Medial incisions allow proximal medial and lateral soft tissue procedures through a relatively small incision, but lateral incisions present less of a problem with skin anesthesia and neuromas and may be less vulnerable to trauma.[14])

The lateral release is said to be an arthroscopic release when it is effected via one or more of the arthroscopy portals. These arthroscopic releases can be done from inside out or outside in. When done from outside in, a hooked instrument is passed between the skin and the retinaculum. For example, a small hook at the end of a long, thin instrument is passed from the anterolateral portal up to the proximal portion of the retinaculum. The hook is pushed into the joint and pulled distally, thus cutting the retinaculum from approximately the superior to the inferior pole of the patella. This can be done with a metallic hook or with cautery. When done with cautery, the overlying skin is at risk for being burned—a risk that can be decreased by injecting fluid between the skin and the retinaculum. When done from inside out, the same hooked instrument is inserted into the joint and pushed out of the synovium and retinaculum at a distance away from the entry point. Again, this can be done with a metallic hook or a cautery. A holmium laser has also been used for this procedure. With a wave length of 2.1 microns, it readily goes through the soft tissues about the knee. It has the ability to cauterize small vessels and, on some occasions, can cauterize the superior geniculate vessels. In my experience, it does not do so on an absolutely consistent basis. Advances in the delivery of laser energy may change this.

Regardless of the technique used, it is important to cut the retinaculum with as few cuts as possible. One fell swoop with a Mayo-type scissors is probably best. Multiple small cuts with a small instrument may be more traumatic and may increase the risk of RSD (an unproved supposition on my part).

The arthroscopic approach has the advantage of minimizing scars—an obvious cosmetic benefit that has to be weighed against the factors listed above. As an aside, the patient who is overly concerned about a knee scar may not have enough disability to warrant surgery. What constitutes appropriate concern as opposed to excessive concern is a matter for the orthopaedic team to determine.

Complications

In addition to a hemarthrosis, other complications can occur. Excessive release—especially proximally into the vastus lateralis itself—can lead to medial subluxation of the patella.[15,16] An intraoperative test has been described by Cartier (personal communication), whereby with the knee in extension a medially directed force is applied to the patella. This effectively pushes the patella medially out of the trochlea onto the medial femoral condyle. The knee is then gently flexed. The patella should gradually glide back into the trochlea. If it suddenly snaps back into the trochlea, this suggests that the lateral release has been excessive. Should this be the case, the upper portion of the retinaculum should be reapproximated with sutures. This is easier to do when the procedure has been carried out in an open fashion rather than arthroscopically.

When carrying out the proximal part of the release, it is possible to drift toward the midline and section part of the quadriceps tendon. This is clearly not desirable, especially if the medial retinaculum release is divided as the initial part of a proximal realignment. The quadriceps tendon is placed at risk for rupture.

RSD is a risk associated with any surgical procedure and is described in Chapter 15.

Results

In the literature pertaining to the lateral release, all of the various techniques described above fall under the lateral release category; one often has to read the fine print to see exactly what technique was used. Needless to say, lumping the various techniques together and reviewing their success or failure as a whole may not be completely valid. The difference in results reported may be related to slight variations in technique. As of this writing, there are articles supporting the use of the isolated lateral release; articles suggesting that it does not work; articles suggesting that, even if it does work initially, results deteriorate with time; and an article (as noted above) suggesting that the procedure is indicated for patients with tilt alone (no clinical or radiological subluxation).

With a lateral retinacular release, more than with any other procedure, there is the question of whether one sees the glass as half empty or half full. Compared to other procedures such as hip and knee replacements, the results are unequivocally poor. But the lateral retinacular release is such an easy procedure.

Specifically, investigators have reported the following results:

- Aglietti et al[17] reported 60% good-to-excellent results (4-year average follow-up) in 20 knees with patellar pain and in 70% of 19 knees with instability. They went 4 cm proximal to the patella into the vastus lateralis muscle and included patients with patellofemoral arthritis.
- Dandy and Griffiths[18] performed the operation on 41 patients with patellar dislocation. The release went to the tibial plateau. Of the patients, 44% felt stable postoperatively;

32% dislocated at least once postoperatively, but 10 out of 13 "became stable and achieved a good result." The authors noted poor results when the patella subluxates in extension (*J* sign).

- Henry et al[11] evaluated 100 knees on which an open release had been performed for subluxation. In all cases, the patella could be medially tilted (medial side elevated) 90 degrees (turn-up sign). Follow-up averaged 3 years. Good results were reported in 90% of cases.
- In 1991, Jackson et al[19] reviewed 39 releases performed on patients over 30 years of age who were followed an average of 6 years and noted 56% good-to-excellent results.
- Fulkerson and colleagues have reported on a number of occasions that the best results are obtained in patients who have tilt alone with no other complicating factors such as an increased quadriceps (Q) angle or lateral displacement,[9,20,21] and they recommended adding other procedures to patients with any form of lateral displacement.[9,21] Fulkerson and Shea[9] found that at an average 40-month follow-up, 14 of 22 patients had a good or excellent result. Of note, 5 patients had a poor result. The technique used in these patients was an open procedure extending from "the fatty plane between the vastus lateralis and the more oblique fibers of the vastus lateralis obliquus" down to the tibial tuberosity. At the end of the procedure, the patella could be everted 90 degrees.
- Kolowich et al[22] reviewed 49 patients who were satisfied by their lateral retinacular release and 29 patients who required further surgery. They found the passive patellar tilt test (see Chapter 4) to be a good predictor of success.

Rehabilitation

Following lateral retinacular release, there is nothing to heal other than allowing the tissues to recover from the surgical procedure. As such, a physical therapy program can be instituted shortly after surgery without any limitation. This is particularly appealing to all concerned. Some patients recover quickly and uneventfully; however, enough patients require a few months of physical therapy and home exercise to warrant informing patients preoperatively that, although the operation is simple, it is not a quick fix.

Proximal Realignment

Overview

The medial retinaculum and medial patellofemoral ligament provide a passive medial restraint to lateral displacement of the patella, and the VMO is the major dynamic stabilizer of the patella (see Chapter 2). The presence of a Q angle imposes an automatic lateral vector to the patella when the quadriceps contracts. Opposing this tendency of the patella to track laterally is the VMO. Patients with tilt and/or subluxation often have a dysplastic VMO: instead of inserting one third to one half the way down the patella, it inserts near the proximal pole. Sometimes it does not even reach the proximal pole. Moreover, whereas the normal VMO forms an angle of approximately 50 degrees with the vertical, the dysplastic VMO can be much more vertical. The combination of these geometric factors significantly decreases the effectiveness of the VMO as a dynamic medial restraint. Considering the above factors, it is not surprising that a number of procedures have been developed to passively cinch down the medial side or increase the effectiveness of the VMO.

A common question is "If you pull the patella medially, are you not increasing the Q angle?" Because the answer is yes, the natural follow-up question is "Why would you perform any procedure that increases the Q angle because an increased Q angle can be part of the problem to begin with?" The solution to this paradox is simple: pulling the patella medially into the trochlea does not create an increased Q angle, it unmasks an increased Q angle. As noted in Chapter 3, the physiological Q angle has to be determined with the patella centered in the trochlea.

The simplest procedure in this category is the medial plication, as popularized in the United States by Hughston et al.[23] The medial retinaculum is divided as it inserts into the patella. It is then reattached more medially onto the patella itself in a "pants-over-vest" fashion. Hughston et al described pulling the superior part of the retinaculum (the "tendon of the VMO") in the direction of the VMO fibers (distomedially). Alternatively, the leading edge of the retinaculum can be excised and the remaining retinaculum reattached to the medial border of the patella. The net result is that the patella is passively pulled medially. Insall et al[24] described a "tube" realignment. Following the lateral retinacular release and the medial arthrotomy, the lateral border of the quadriceps tendon in continuity with a flap of lateral retinaculum is folded over medially to the midline and sutured to the medial border of the quadriceps tendon, which has been folded over laterally to the midline. The quadriceps tendon now has the appearance of a tube that envelops most of the patella. Insall and colleagues believed that this could medialize the pull of the quadriceps and, in effect, decrease the effective Q angle.

In addition to plicating the medial retinaculum, the VMO can be dissected free by dissecting along its insertion and then dissecting along its inferior border (Figure 14–1). The muscle can then be pulled in the direction of its fibers as far as one wishes onto the superomedial portion of the patella.[25,26] The inferior fibers can also be sutured more distally to "horizontalize" the VMO. The major limiting factor to this procedure is knee flexion; as the above maneuvers are carried out, it can become more difficult to flex the knee. For this reason, after the first few stitches are placed the knee should be flexed past 90 degrees. If the stitches pull out or break, the VMO has to be released back a bit. The procedure is repeated until the knee can be flexed without the stitches failing. Clearly, there sometimes has to be a compromise between optimal positioning of the patella and limitation of knee flexion.

Dissection of the VMO changes the rehabilitation considerably, since vigorous contraction of the muscle could conceivably pull the VMO out of its new position. (*Note*: A lateral release is carried out in conjunction with either of the above medial procedures.)

Indications

Indications for proximal realignment include moderate or severe patellar tilt, lateral translation of the patella (see Chapter 3), and subluxation (sensation of giving way).

Contraindications

This procedure is contraindicated by the presence of a grade IV chondral lesion on the medial half of the patella. Such a lesion might become more painful if subjected to increased forces, as might be expected to happen when the patella is "untilted" and medialized. A grade I or II lesion is a different matter. If those lesions are due to chronic hypopressure, restoring normal pressure may be harmless and perhaps even helpful. On the other hand, any kind of chondral abnormality may be a relative contraindication. This issue has not yet been resolved.

Surgical Approach

No compromise should be made with respect to surgical exposure. No patient will accept post facto a suboptimal result on the basis of the surgeon's unwillingness to make a bigger incision. However, surgery of the patella is often carried out in young patients, and it is reasonable to seek the most cosmetic incision. A midline incision gives easy access to both sides of the patella and does not compromise any future surgery. However, the incision may spread and remain quite visible. A subcuticular closure ("plastic surgery") can avoid the railroad track appearance, but it still spreads. A *medial parapatellar incision* approximately the length of the patella allows easy reconstruction of the medial side and, with some retraction of the patella medially, allows equally easy division of the lateral retinaculum. As one goes more medially with the incision, one increases the risk of injuring one of the branches of the saphenous nerve. This, in turn, can lead to a painful neuroma sometimes

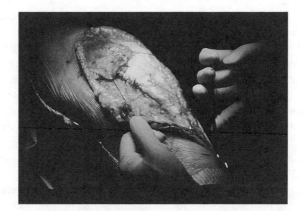

Figure 14–1 VMO Advancement. The advancement of the VMO is illustrated here in its most complete form. It is dissected free and advanced onto the patella. The knee is flexed 90 degrees to ensure that the sutures will not pull out. If they do, the surgeon must back off on the advancement. If they do not, the knee can be safely ranged in the immediate postoperative period.

misinterpreted postoperatively as patellar pain (see Chapter 8). A *lateral parapatellar incision* avoids this problem, but the incision needs to be longer than the others in order to gain adequate access to the medial side (the medial retinaculum requires greater exposure than the lateral retinaculum because of the stitching required on the medial side). *Arthroscopic medial plications* have been described. In this procedure, each stitch placement requires considerable time when compared to the open technique. Because stitches frequently have to be repositioned, this can be quite an onerous technique. I suspect that, as with the arthroscopic lateral release, arthroscopic medial plication is carried out with relatively little fine-tuning.

Complications

Because the origin of the VMO is posterior to the plane of the patella, concerns have been voiced with respect to creating a posterior vector on the patella. Will pulling or pushing the medial portion of the patella posteriorly increase pressure on the patella and increase pain? The answer to this question is unknown. In defense of the procedure, the patella is "pulled down" only as much as is needed to bring it back to a normal position.

Numbness can be a complication. Sensation about the knee comes to a large extent from branches of the saphenous nerve. This nerve sweeps around the medial aspect of the knee and fans around anteriorly. The skin incision interrupts some of these branches, and numbness lateral to the incision ensues. This numbness can resolve in time and usually does not interfere with everyday function. Patients undergoing patellar realignment should be willing to trade some pain for an element of numbness, which is not to say that the surgeon shouldn't try to minimize numbness. In my experience, patellar patients rate pain relief and cosmesis above sensation.

Rehabilitation

Following a simple medial plication, a standard patella rehabilitation program can be instituted as soon as the perioperative pain has subsided. The medial retinacular reconstruction is not put at risk with active range of motion exercises. Following dissection and advancement of the VMO, there has to be sufficient healing of the VMO to its new position before vigorous contractions of the VMO are allowed. To my knowledge, there has been no study to determine when such healing takes place, but I suspect that

6 weeks is a reasonable time limit. During that 6-week period, passive range of motion can and should be instituted and light quadriceps setting exercises are allowed. When the patient is coming off a bed, the patient should hook the good leg underneath the operated one and use active motion of the good leg to lift the operated one.

Casting is not used, but a knee immobilizer is used until the patient can easily perform a straight leg raise, holding the foot off the examining table for 10 seconds. If the patient has had a VMO advancement, this test is not usually performed until approximately 8 weeks postoperatively. Once the immobilizer is removed, the patient can be placed in a patella brace.

Literature Review

A number of investigators have looked at patients with patellar pain versus patients with instability and pain. Abraham et al[27] noted that they only had 55% good or excellent results at 5 to 11 years in patients without subluxation or dislocation. Cerullo et al[28] also noted inferior results in patients with stable (definition not given) patellae. Scuderi et al[29] did not find a correlation between results and the degree of chondral damage. Even patients with some erosion to bone obtained good results. Men did better than women, and patients did best when they were less than 20 years old.[29]

Distal Realignment Procedures

Elmslie-Trillat (Medial Displacement) Osteotomy of the Tibial Tuberosity

Overview. The concept of displacing the tibial tuberosity to affect patellar tracking goes back to the nineteenth century. Roux, from Switzerland, described in 1888 displacing the patellar tendon. He was also one of the first to write that patellar dislocation is a problem that occurs near extension (slight flexion).[30] People do not dislocate their patella going up and down stairs, but they readily dislocate with social dancing.

Elmslie popularized the procedure in Great Britain, and it was further popularized in the Western world by Albert Trillat from Lyon, France.[31] By transferring the tibial tuberosity medially, one decreases the Q angle. Accordingly, one decreases the bowstring effect of the quadriceps mechanism and, most significantly, the tendency of the patella to move laterally when the quadriceps contracts. Specifically, the tibial tuberosity is not transferred posteriorly (Figure 14–2). In this regard, the Elmslie-Trillat procedure is different from the Hauser procedure (Figure 14–3).

Indications. The presence of an increased Q angle is the prime indication for the Elmslie-Trillat procedure since the main effect of the operation is to decrease the Q angle. Some surgeons routinely perform this procedure, regardless of the Q angle. In such a situation, the Q angle is decreased to less than normal. How abnormally low the Q angle can be before it becomes a clinical problem is unknown (and, as with everything else, may vary from patient to patient). Conversely, because arthritis has been found in some patients who have undergone a tibial tuberosity transfer, some surgeons recommend avoiding the operation altogether.[32]

Contraindications. This procedure is contraindicated by an open apophysis at the tibial tuberosity. Premature closure of this apophysis can ensue with a resultant recurvatum deformity. A second contraindication is ligamentous laxity in combination with an out-toeing gait. As noted by Hughston and others, medial transfer of the tibial tuberosity decreases the internal rotation moment about the knee. As a result, the tibia is even more free to rotate externally than before, and the patient can end up with a Charlie Chaplin gait (not a crowd pleaser).[23,33]

Surgical Technique. A cut across the tibial tuberosity is made in the frontal plane. The distal portion of the tuberosity remains in the same location while the proximal portion is swung medially. The tuberosity is then affixed to the tibia. Variations include the following:

1. *The osteotomy.* The distal portion of the cut tuberosity can be cracked, in which case the tuberosity becomes a free frag-

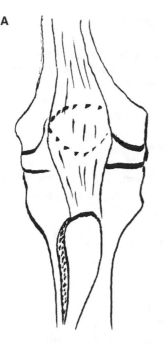
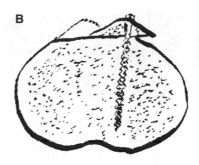

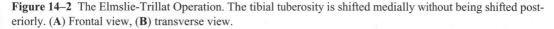

Figure 14–2 The Elmslie-Trillat Operation. The tibial tuberosity is shifted medially without being shifted posteriorly. (**A**) Frontal view, (**B**) transverse view.

ment completely detached from the tibia. It can also be left intact, in which case the tuberosity has to be bent ("greensticked") to get the proximal portion over medially. The former osteotomy is quicker but, because the tuberosity is a free fragment, greater attention must be paid to fixation. The latter osteotomy is more time consuming. Cortical bone does not readily bend. The base of the osteotomy must be nibbled with a small cervical rongeur until it is just thin enough to bend without breaking.

2. *The fixation.* Hughston originally described the use of the four-pronged Stone staple.[23] It does not provide compression across the osteotomy, and Hughston described putting patients in a cylinder cast postoperatively. Today, most surgeons use screws. Here again there are variations: one can use one or two screws, the screws can be cortical or cancellous, they can go through or just to the posterior cortex, and they can be aimed perpendicular to the tibial shaft or somewhat cephalad. If the distal cortex of the tuberosity remains intact, one screw probably suffices; it need not go through the posterior cortex, and I would favor a cancellous screw (countersunk). If the distal cortex is cracked and one is dealing with a free-floating fragment, I feel more secure with two screws (Shelbourne has reported using just one 4.0 cancellous screw aimed cephalad, even though the distal cortex of the shingle is cracked). If one of the screws goes through the posterior cortex, this provides optimal fixation; however, one has to keep in mind the presence of the femoral vessels even if the knee is flexed. Angling the screw somewhat medially can provide a measure of security in that respect. If the tuberosity fragment were to displace, it would do so in a ceph-

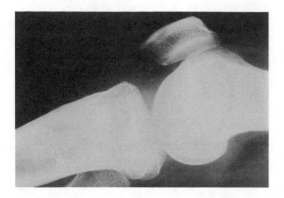

Figure 14–3 The Hauser Procedure. The tibial tuberosity is shifted medially, posteriorly, and distally. The Hauser procedure is associated with late arthritis and is no longer recommended.

alad direction. It is therefore recommended that the screw be angled slightly cephalad. Of course, the plateau has a posterior slope to it and, in angling the screw cephalad, one has to be careful not to violate the articular surface of the tibia.

3. *"Lock and key" osteotomy.* Instead of osteotomizing a shingle of bone, which includes the tibial tuberosity and tibial crest as described above, a trapezoidal piece of tuberosity can be freed up and slid along medially in a bony trough. This obviates the need for a screw. There is little room for error with this procedure; if the fixation is suboptimal the surgeon is left with only a small piece of bone to work with.

Complications. Loss of fixation is the most obvious complication but not the most serious. Excessive medialization can also be a problem. Some surgeons medialize the tibial tuberosity even in the presence of a normal Q angle, which leads to an abnormally low Q angle. Some investigators have disapproved of this practice. For example, Insall has stated that the quadriceps line of pull "should never be angled even minimally to the medial side."[34(p1)] Conceptually, I believe that this is correct because the main goal of surgery is to restore normal anatomy and function. But in some patients, medialization of the line of pull may be the best way to unload painful lateral lesions.

Vascular compromise from a screw or drill bit is possible when a screw is directed directly posteriorly through the posterior cortex. Surgery about the tibial tuberosity can lead to intra-compartmental pressure rises in the lower leg.[35] In more severe cases, full-blown compartment syndromes have been reported. Milder cases can manifest as a peroneal nerve palsy, subtle enough to present as no more than weakness of the extensor hallucis longus. I routinely perform a fasciotomy of the anterior compartment and have not had any palsies since doing so. Only the terminal branches of the peroneal nerve are located in this compartment, but decompression of this compartment alone appears sufficient in this particular setting.

Rehabilitation. The speed at which a full rehabilitation program can be instituted depends entirely on the perceived security of the fixation. When fixation is believed to be secure, active range-of-motion exercises and strengthening activities can be instituted as soon as they are tolerated by the patient. If the fixation is less than optimal, the surgeon must adjust the regimen accordingly. Partial weight bearing for 6 weeks is probably beneficial to minimize the risk of a tibial fracture.

Results. Cox reported 88% good or excellent results for "subluxation" in 1976.[36] In 1982, he reported 66% good or excellent results with a 7% incidence of return of this subluxation.[37] Fielding et al noted 73% good or excellent results in studies with an average follow-up of 3.5 years.[38,39] Riegler reported on 42 patients on whom he performed a tibial tuberosity transfer along with a lateral release and an occasional VMO advancement (not specifically described). He used a lateral parapatellar incision; transferred the tuberosity 8 to 15 mm; used cancellous screws (but not through the posterior cortex); and reported 6 excellent, 28 good, and 8 fair or poor results.[40]

Maquet Procedure

Overview. Anterior elevation of the tibial tuberosity (the site of the patellar tendon insertion) is referred to as the Maquet procedure. This is not a true realignment procedure, as it corrects neither the medial-lateral position nor the tilt of the patella. In 1963, Paul Maquet from Liège, Belgium, was one of the first to describe the procedure.[41,42] It is based on the concept that articular pressure (and therefore pain) can be diminished if the patella is elevated off the trochlea. Much has been published on the subject as a result of many in vitro and some in vivo studies. However, there is no agreement on the theoretical foundations, the exact surgical technique, or the clinical results of the procedure. The procedure differs conceptually from the operations described above to the extent that it makes no effort to create normal mechanics. In fact, it specifically changes the mechanics to diminish pain during activities of daily living. Few surgeons would suggest to a patient that they return to competitive athletics following a Maquet procedure.

Biomechanical (Mathematical and In Vitro) Studies. The numerous studies can be divided into those that support and those that refute the theoretical basis of the Maquet procedure. Pan et al[43] found a decrease in pressure, especially when a long (20 cm) tibial shingle was used. They only tested knee specimens at 15 and 30 degrees of flexion. Retaillaud et al[44] noted a significant decrease in pressure with just 1.25 cm of elevation. Nakamura et al[45] noted a considerable proximal shift in the contact areas of the patella and calculated that a 1-cm elevation is optimal. Using computer modeling, Cheng et al[46] did not find significant decreases in pressure. Ferrandez et al[47] have pointed out that pressure changes are not uniform throughout the patella. A decrease in pressure distally can be associated with an increase in pressure proximally, and Ferrandez and colleagues found this to be particularly true at higher elevations. Lewallen et al[48] found the procedure to be unpredictable. Singerman et al[49] investigated in vitro forces. They noted decreasing forces with increasing tibial tuberosity elevations. However, because changes in contact area were not factored into their study, no conclusion can be drawn with respect to changes in cartilage stresses (this again points to the impor-

tance of differentiating force from stress in evaluating biomechanical studies). Koshino[50] calculated that most patients with successful Maquet procedures had increased patellofemoral compressive forces (again, contact areas were not factored in).

The Maquet procedure is usually combined with a lateral release. Sorting out the benefits of the lateral release from those of the tuberosity elevation is therefore difficult.

Indications. The number of uses for this procedure appears to be decreasing. The most controversial use of this procedure is for "patellar pain" without arthritis. Proponents suggest that the mere change of stress distribution is beneficial, regardless of what that new distribution is. Detractors say that this shoot-from-the-hip approach is theoretically unsound and leads to a rather radical procedure just to a achieve a random alteration of mechanics. Less controversial is the use of this procedure for patellofemoral arthritis. However, not the entire articular surface of the patella is unweighed, only the distal portion. With elevations on the order of 2.5 cm (recommended by Maquet), one group of investigators has even suggested that the superior portion of the patella sees increased pressure.[47] If this theory is correct, patients with lesions in the proximal portion of the patella are not good candidates for the Maquet procedure. The least controversial use of the Maquet procedure is in arthritis involving only the distal portion of the patella. "Least" is used in a relative sense, because the procedure remains controversial even in this setting.

Contraindications. Raising the tibial tuberosity places some increased tension on the overlying skin. Unhealthy skin of any kind is therefore a relative contraindication for this type of operation. Because the tuberosity is raised and becomes more prominent, kneeling can remain painful after surgery. Patients whose jobs or hobbies involve much kneeling are at particular risk for this. Global patellofemoral arthritis, as noted above, is probably a contraindication for the procedure. Some believe that the desire for a good cosmetic result is a contraindication for the Maquet procedure, but I disagree. Although it is normal for a patient to be concerned about the appearance of the leg, the surgeon should beware of exaggerated concern about appearance. By the time a patient is considered for a salvage procedure, he or she should be mostly focused on pain relief. More significantly, vertical incisions over the tuberosity and tibial crest usually heal with a fine scar, whereas incisions directly over the patella tend to widen with time.

The elevation can create a very visible bump at the front of the knee, but certain technical modifications can minimize this (see discussion of surgical technique below). Adding a Maquet procedure to any kind of proximal realignment need not significantly worsen the cosmetic results.

Surgical Technique. The original technique calls for a tuberosity elevation of 2.5 cm. Since the publication of Ferguson's in vitro work in 1979,[51] some surgeons[52] prefer to raise the tuberosity no more than 1.5 cm and others find more consistent results with the full elevation[53-56] (Figure 14–4). Schepsis et al[57] recommended an elevation of 1.6 to 1.8 mm, with the expectation that there will be 2 to 3 mm of settling. Heatley et al[58] elevated the tibial tuberosity by 1.5 cm to 2 cm. The original impetus for a smaller elevation related to attempts at decreasing wound healing problems.

With the patient supine on the operating table and the leg held in neutral rotation, a horizontal cut is made through the tibial tuberosity and proximal tibial crest. A narrow osteotome is then slipped between the tuberosity and the underlying bony bed. As the osteotome is rotated, the tuberosity is elevated. The longer the bony shingle, the greater the tuberosity elevation one obtains for a given degree of angular elevation. Similarly, the longer the shingle, the more gradual the elevation becomes and the less visible and palpable the bump becomes. The longer the shingle, the smaller the angle created between the patellar tendon and the tuberosity. This may decrease the odds of the patient developing tendinitis (unproved hypothesis). A 9-cm shingle is usually a good length in a patient of average size. Longer shingles (12 to 15 cm) do have biomechanical support.[43]

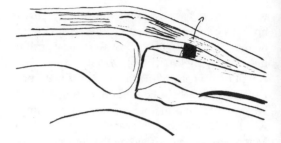

Figure 14–4 The Maquet Operation. This procedure elevates the tibial tuberosity anywhere from 1.5 to 2.5 cm. The graft can be obtained from a number of sources including the upper tibia. It may increase pressures in the proximal patella and is relatively contraindicated when chondral lesions are present proximally.

Once the tuberosity is elevated, it must be maintained in its elevated position. The original technique called for an iliac crest bone graft to be wedged under the tuberosity. Iliac bone is strong and plentiful. However, because this requires another surgical incision and this second wound can be more painful than the operated knee itself, surgeons have looked for other substances to wedge under the tuberosity. These have included bone from the upper tibia and allograft (cadaveric) bone. Unlike allograft, bone from the upper tibia does not represent a foreign body, but the quantity that can be harvested is limited.

Ideally, the base of tuberosity/tibial crest shingle is thinned out just enough to allow the tuberosity to be elevated but not enough to crack the base upon elevation of the tuberosity. If this condition is realized, the elastic properties of bone tend to make the tuberosity regain its original position, thus compressing the graft and keeping it in its place. This is a stable construct and no added fixation is required. When the base is cracked, fixation is required. If the surgeon chooses screw fixation, he or she then has the choice of one or two cortical or cancellous screws. Cortical screw fixation through the posterior cortex offers probably the strongest fixation; however, even with the knee flexed, the surgeon must be mindful of the popliteal vessels directly behind the tibia. If a cancellous screw is used, it is a good idea to try to countersink it and to use a washer. One group has strongly denounced the use of any screw, preferring K-wires instead.[58]

Postoperatively, the patient is placed in either a cast or a knee immobilizer.

Complications. Wound healing is the complication traditionally associated with the Maquet operation. Maquet himself recognized this problem in his original works.[41,42] Healing problems can be minimized by using a lesser elevation or by using a long shingle.[59] Early range of motion is probably not a good idea either. With the patient in a cast or immobilizer this is usually not an issue.

Subsidence of the graft with loss of the tuberosity elevation is a complication particular to this procedure. The graft has to be sufficiently strong to avoid being crushed. Pressure on the graft has to be great enough to keep the graft in place, but not so strong as to crush the graft or cause it to subside into the underlying cancellous bed. Goutallier has successfully used a block of polymethylmethacrylate in opening wedge osteotomies of the tibia, and consideration could be given to using such a material instead of a bone graft.

Tendinitis (pain at the patellar tendon insertion) has been reported following the Maquet procedure. It may be due to altered mechanics, an altered angle between the tendon and the tuberosity, or both.

Rehabilitation. This is one of the few knee procedures that requires some form of postoperative immobilization. Such immobilization is required to protect both the graft and the skin. Quadriceps setting can be instituted shortly after surgery. The start of active and passive range-of-motion exercises has to be individualized to each patient based on the progress of graft and skin healing. Ferguson noted that return to full function averaged 6 months.[60]

Results. Heatley et al[58] noted that after 6 years, patients with severe arthritis did worst, whereas patients with minimal degenerative changes did best. Conversely, Jenny et al[61] found that patients with grade 4 changes (Outerbridge) did best. Most patients reported good pain relief, although only slightly more than half resumed nearly normal athletic activity. Schmid[56] followed 35 arthritic knees an average of 16 years and noted poor results only in patients whose tibial tuberosity was elevated less than 1.5 cm. Osteoporosis was noted in the operated patellae. Schepsis et al followed 97 knees a mean of 7 years and obtained approximately 70% good-to-excellent results.[57]

Anteromedialization Osteotomy

Overview. The Elmslie-Trillat osteotomy and the Maquet osteotomy represent simple, one-plane mobilizations of the patellar tendon insertion (tibial tuberosity); the former medializes and the latter elevates ("anteriorizes" or "ventralizes"). The tibial tuberosity can also be osteotomized in such a way as to provide a measure of both medialization and elevation. For example, a *V*-shaped cut can be made in the tuberosity. By modifying the two limbs of the *V*, the tuberosity can be preferentially displaced in one direction or the other. The simplest way of combining elevation with medialization is to angle one straight cut. The cut is the same as for an Elmslie-Trillat, except that it is angled in an anteromedial to posterolateral direction. Thus, when the tuberosity is displaced medially, it is also displaced anteriorly.[62] The amount of medialization is equal to the displacement times the cosine of the angle, and the amount of elevation is equal to the displacement times the sine of the same angle. When the cut is angled 45 degrees, the medial and vertical displacements are the same (one half the absolute displacement). In the United States, this procedure has been popularized by Fulkerson and called the anteromedialization (AMZ) osteotomy[63] (Figure 14–5).

The advantage of the AMZ osteotomy is that with one cut, both medialization and elevation can be obtained. No bone graft is needed (although it can be added for increased elevation). The disadvantage is that one loses correction

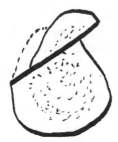

Figure 14–5 The Anteromedialization (AMZ) Operation. This procedure, popularized by Fulkerson,[63] is a combination of the Elmslie-Trillat and the Maquet procedures. The slope of the cut determines the proportion of medial versus anterior displacement.

relative to one-plane osteotomies. For example, a 1-cm displacement along a cut angled 45 degrees leads to ½ cm of medialization and ½ cm of vertical displacement. A fortuitous byproduct of this osteotomy is that screws placed perpendicular to the osteotomy are aimed away from the popliteal vessels. This osteotomy most likely unloads the distolateral aspect of the patella and loads its superomedial aspect.

Indications. Broadly speaking, the AMZ osteotomy is indicated whenever both elevation and medialization are desired. For example, a patient with a high Q angle and a distolateral lesion might benefit from such a displacement. Broader indications (as advocated by Fulkerson) would be patellar subluxation or dislocation. I have been concerned about medializing a tuberosity in the face of a normal Q angle or elevating out of the trochlea a patella that is already unstable. But judging by Fulkerson's results, these concerns may be unfounded.

Contraindications. Poor skin anteriorly is a relative contraindication. Elevations obtained with the AMZ procedure tend not to be as high as with the pure (2.5 cm) Maquet elevation, and as such may be safer in this setting. Superomedial articular cartilage lesions contraindicate the AMZ osteotomy because the procedure places increased loads on this portion of the patella (Fulkerson has noted less satisfactory results in this situation[63]).

Surgical technique. The technique for the AMZ osteotomy is similar to the Elmslie-Trillat procedure. Starting on the medial side of the tuberosity, the cut is directed posteriorly. The greater the angle (ie, the steeper the cut) the greater the relative elevation and the smaller the relative medialization. As described in the Maquet procedure, a longer shingle has advantages over a shorter shingle with respect to cosmesis and with respect to the new angle formed between the patellar tendon and the tuberosity. At the proximal portion of the tuberosity, the obliqueness of the cut leads the blade of the saw or osteotome into the upper tibia proper. Therefore, a cut must be made on the medial aspect of the tuberosity (about 45 degrees from the vertical) to "intercept" the osteotomy and prevent propagation of the cut into the upper tibia.

Complications. The complications associated with the AMZ osteotomy are similar to those listed for the Elmslie-Trillat and the Maquet procedures. Wound healing is somewhat less of a problem than with the standard Maquet because elevations are smaller. Loss of fixation has been known to occur, and Fulkerson has recently recommended partial weight bearing until healing has occurred.

Distal Transfer of the Tibial Tuberosity

In situations where the patella is riding high (patella alta), consideration can be given to lowering it. This can be done by osteotomizing the tibial tuberosity, freeing it up on three sides (medial, lateral, and distal), removing a portion of the tuberosity at its lower end, and transferring the remainder of the tuberosity distally into the underlying bony bed. The patella ought to be brought distally enough to allow engagement of the articular surface into the trochlea upon early knee flexion. Caton et al[64] have reported on a series of 61 patients with patella alta, 8 of whom initially had surgery that did not involve lowering of the patella. These 8 patients only got better after a second operation in which the patella was lowered. Simmons and Cameron[65] also reported on patients with patella alta whose symptoms resolved after lowering of the patella.

Unfortunately, this procedure is often confused with the Hauser operation, developed in the 1930s by Emil Hauser from Chicago to address patellar dislocation.[66] The Hauser operation transferred the patella distally, medially, and—by virtue of the triangular shape of the tibia—posteriorly. The purpose of the operation was to cinch down an extensor mechanism viewed as being too lax and too lateralized. The operation was a success with respect to correction of dislocation but a failure with respect to long-term function. In the long run, the tightened extensor mechanism led to patellofemoral arthritis.[67] Surgeons should seriously consider transferring back the tibial tuberosity of patients with a Hauser procedure if the patients demonstrate patellar symptoms.[68]

Naturally, one can voice a similar concern with any lowering of the tuberosity. Will the lowering not tighten the extensor mechanism, increase articular pressures, and lead to arthritis? Straightforward, single-plane lowering of the tuberosity differs in two ways from the Hauser operation. (1) The tuberosity is not brought posteriorly. Thus no reverse Maquet effect is created. (2) The indication for the procedure is patellar instability with severe patella alta, not simple instability. The patient selected for tibial tuberosity lowering is already very disabled from patella alta. At least one study has reported that the patient's symptoms will not improve until the tuberosity is brought closer to its normal position.[64] None of this ensures that the patient will stay arthritis free, but the surgeon has little choice. It is better to risk arthritis in the future than to guarantee disability in the present.

Miscellaneous Soft Tissue Transfers

Overview

Just about any medial soft tissue structure can (and has) been used to pull the patella medially. In addition to the VMO (see discussion of proximal realignment above), the pes tendons (semitendinosus and gracilis) have been released proximally, woven through a patellar tunnel, and reattached at the level of their insertion on the upper medial tibia. For example, the semitendinosus can be woven about the patella as a static medializing force in a procedure attributed to Galeazzi in 1921.[13] This can be of use in the pediatric population where one is reluctant to work on the tibial tuberosity for fear of causing premature closure of the apophysis (with resultant recurvatum deformity).

A portion of the patellar tendon can be used to stabilize the patella. The medial third of the tendon can be detached with a wafer of bone and transferred medially (Figure 14–6). This has been reported to be successful in at least one review of a pediatric cohort.[69]

The lateral third of the tendon can be detached and reattached medially. When it is passed under the remaining portion of the tendon, the procedure is referred to in the United States as the *Roux-Goldthwait operation*. In other locales it is simply called the *Goldthwait procedure*. The procedure, described by Joel Goldthwait in 1904, was developed to address dislocation and what we would today call an increased Q angle.[70] In 1904 the concept of patellar tilt had not yet been introduced, and the possible effects on patellar tilt were therefore not a concern.

The procedure is effective in medializing the resultant forces on the patella, but it increases patellar tilt. You can see this for yourself by looking at the back of your hand, then pulling your little finger to your thumb. This brings the ulnar side of your hand down and the radial side up. Likewise, the Goldthwait procedure pulls down the lateral border of the patella, thus increasing tilt. Although some surgeons continue to advocate its use,[12,71] I believe that the Goldthwait operation joins the Hauser operation as one of the few procedures that should no longer have a place in the surgeon's armamentarium. As noted above, the medial portion of the patellar tendon can be transposed with essentially the same stabilizing effect.

Complications

Flandry and Hughston[14] have noted that the detached portion of tendon must be very pre-

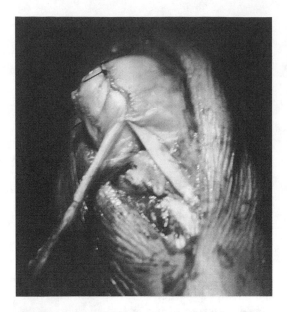

Figure 14–6 Medial Transposition of the Medial Third of the Patellar Tendon. This is a reasonable alternative to the Roux-Goldthwait procedure, which transposes the lateral third and increases the tilt of the patella.

cisely tensioned. In revisions of failed Goldthwait procedures, they have noted that the split portion of the tendon is severely compromised (detached, ruptured, or even autolyzed). Templeman and McBeath[72] noted that in one of their two Roux-Goldthwait revisions, the transferred portion of the ligament was scarred in with the main body of the tendon requiring transfer of the entire tendon insertion.

Other Information from the Literature

Roux's name is often used in different contexts. As is common in the field of patellofemoral disorders, the same term or eponym has different meanings in different parts of the world. Thus, it is instructive to review exactly what Roux wrote.[30] He described the use of an osteotome to peel the patellar tendon off the tibial tuberosity. The tendon was then trans-

ferred to a preroughened portion of upper medial tibia and fixed with two smooth nails placed through the skin. (This article is truly a classic—often quoted but rarely read.)

Brief[73] has described a procedure for patients who exhibit a combination of instability and hypermobility, whereby the patellar tendon is sutured to the capsule and to the tibial periosteum.

Miscellaneous Bony (Patellar) Procedures

Patellar thinning operations have been described, whereby the subchondral bone is removed along with the remaining articular cartilage.[74,75] The term *spongialization* has been used by some to describe this removal of all subchondral bone down to cancellous ("spongy") bone. When the cartilage is viable, a layer of bone can be removed from the center of the patella much like removing the ham from a sandwich. The goal is to decrease the stress on the patella when the knee is flexed. Both the removal of the layer and the reattachment of the two remaining portions may be technically difficult, especially because care has to be taken not to injure the articular surface. Nerubay et al[76] performed the procedure in Israel on 15 patients with malalignment; the patients were followed an average of 3 years, with 12 obtaining good to excellent results. Vaquero[77] described the use of a double saw to remove 7 mm of bone from the center of the patella, using Fuji film to validate this approach. With this procedure, there may not be much bony bed left for a prosthetic replacement if needed at a later time.

Triangular wedges of bone (based dorsally) have been taken out in order to decrease venous pressure. Macnicol[78] has described performing this procedure without regard to chondral lesions or malalignment, and has described the "unstable temperament" of the patella.

Complete excision of the diseased medial portion of the patella (a form of partial patellectomy) was described by Sachs,[79] but Weaver et al[80] obtained 0 good results in 12 knees.

Operations on the Trochlea

On occasion, the surgeon may believe that the trochlea itself is the problem. This is the case when the trochlea is dysplastic (ie, relatively flat). This dysplasia is quite variable. In extreme cases, the trochlea can even present an area of convexity giving the trochlea a "fried egg" profile. These are among the most difficult cases to address surgically. Trochleoplasties have been attempted, in which a wedge of bone is placed within one or both condyles in an attempt to crank up the condyle(s) and provide a deeper trochlear groove. This is actually one of the oldest patellofemoral procedures, going back to Albee's 1915 report.[81] Unfortunately, the articular cartilage of the patella then no longer matches that of the trochlea, and early arthritis has been reported with this approach. Masse's trochleoplasty,[82] which involved scooping out bone from under the cartilage, also led to poor results—perhaps due to the direct blows applied to the cartilage in an attempt to keep it affixed to its new subchondral bed. Kobayashi made use of both patellar and trochlear wedges. Most recently, Dejour and his team have used Masse's trochleoplasty with a more gentle approach to cartilage fixation.

Patellofemoral Replacement

Overview

When a joint is severely worn out and severely painful, it is reasonable in this day and age to seek to "replace" it (ie, resurface it with prosthetic components). This has been done with the patellofemoral joint—a procedure that is even more controversial than the ones listed above.

Indication

The indication for patellofemoral replacement is isolated patellofemoral *osteo*arthritis, which includes arthritis secondary to malalignment or trauma. Inflammatory arthritis can initially affect just the patellofemoral joint, and a basic rheumatological workup is indicated for most patellofemoral replacement candidates. Because the patella articulates with the femoral condyles, a worn out patella can damage these condyles. Thus, in time, patellofemoral arthritis can lead to femorotibial arthritis. On the other hand, prior to the onset of severe patellofemoral arthritis, surgeons are reluctant to perform an arthroplasty. Therefore, there is a small window of opportunity to perform this procedure; the patellofemoral arthritis should be severe, but the femorotibial compartments should be spared.

History

All knee arthroplasties began with the concept that the worn out compartment(s) should be resurfaced while leaving uninvolved compartments and both cruciates intact. While a femorotibial replacement was being developed in the 1950s, a patellar replacement was also being developed.[83] The first replacement, which was metallic, was reported on in 1955 by Duncan and McKeever.[83] There was no femoral (trochlear) component, and the implant was fastened to the patella via a transverse medial-lateral screw. In 1973, Vermeulen et al[84] reported on 10 cases, 9 of which had 8- to 10-year follow-up. All patients were women, and their average age was 61 years. No knee had required re-operation, and it appeared that the trochlear cartilage tolerated the metal well. Pickett and Stoll[85] reported on 46 knees with such a prosthesis that were followed 1 to 22 years (average not stated). Some of these procedures were combined with a femorotibial resurfacing. Of the cases, 39 were found to be "satisfactory" to both patient and surgeon. This implant was last discussed in the English language by Harrington[86] in 1992; he reported acceptable results in patients with degeneration limited to the patella. Specifically, he reported on 24 young patients (average age 36 years), 24 of whom were followed a mean of 5 years and 16 of whom were followed a mean of 8 years. At 5 years, 17 of the 24 results were good to excellent. The poor results tended to be in older patients who had signs of osteoarthritis in the other compartments. Aglietti et al[87] reported on a poly-ethylene patellar component in 1975, and Worrell[88] reported on a cobalt-chrome patellar prosthesis with very short-term follow-up in 1979.

Lubinus[89] and Blazina et al[90] also reported in 1979 on true patellofemoral replacements. In the latter study, the patients were young (average age 39) and the follow-up short (average less than 2 years). Both studies featured a polyethyl-ene patellar button and a metallic trochlear im-plant. In 1988, Tisserand and Aubaniac[91] re-ported good results in 63 patients who were followed 1 to 4 years. In 1990, Cartier et al[92] re-ported on 72 replacements that were followed 2 to 12 years (average 4 years); by arthroplasty standards, these patients were doing well at this short- to medium-term follow-up. As of this writing, Cartier still considers this the most reli-able procedure for severe patellofemoral arthri-tis (Figure 14–7).

Surgical Technique

The patellar button is placed as would be the button of a total knee replacement. If there is a proximal to distal ridge on the button, care must be taken to align this ridge with the trochlea (when the patella is everted, its longitudinal axis can be rotated—making this part of the proce-dure less easy than one would expect). The me-tallic trochlea is placed along the condyles, which may have to be chiseled to deepen a dys-plastic trochlea. It is also important to remove the osteophytes from the distal trochlea to avoid impingement of the tibial spines and to avoid placing the trochlear component too low (dis-tally).

Cartilage Grafting

A biological approach to the worn-out articu-lar cartilage is to transplant a source of cells that can develop into cartilage. This represents the holy grail of arthritis surgery and has been tried a number of ways.[93] Cartilage can be harvested from the patient, cultured in vitro, and reim-planted (currently, this exciting but expensive approach is receiving the greatest publicity). Other approaches involve harvesting periosteum from the tibia, iliac crest, or ribs and placing this periosteum into the cartilage defect. In 1990, Hoikka et al[94] reported on the 8-month to 9-year (3.8-year average) follow-up of 13 patients who had a periosteal graft harvested from the anterior tibia and sutured to the patellar defect (cambium layer against subchondral bone). These investi-gators found that all but one patient had satisfac-tory pain relief.

To date, the long-term follow-ups have been nonexistent or the results have been disappoint-ing. Even though the cartilage that is formed can appear normal to visual inspection, it is still not clear that it is normal. Biomechanical testing has not been performed on these regenerated carti-lage matrices. Clearly, it is reasonable to pursue these exciting approaches, but when the cost is high it is unreasonable to promote them until long-term results are available.

Patellectomy

Overview

Removal of the patella is tantamount to a re-section arthroplasty of the patellofemoral joint. Its appeal lies in its perceived relative simplicity compared to other procedures. Moreover, by simply removing the patellar half of the painful patellofemoral joint, it can be reasoned that the pain will disappear. On the down side, there is always the concern that the patient will develop thigh weakness or an extensor lag due to the loss of the patella's lever function. By increasing the force of the quadriceps contractions (to offset this lack of a lever), the forces across the femo-rotibial are increased—possibly leading to femorotibial arthritis. Denham and Bishop[95] found a 14% increase in compressive forces across the femorotibial joint and a 250% in-crease in "tangential" forces. Patellar pain is a complex issue and, interestingly enough, re-moval of the patella does not automatically eliminate the pain. If the patient has had pain from instability, removal of the patella does not

A

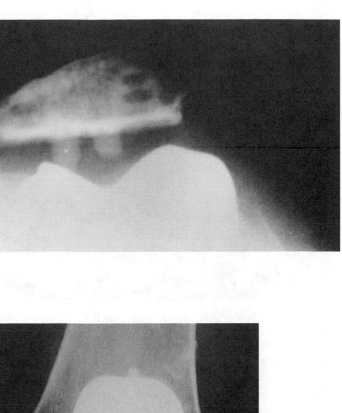

B

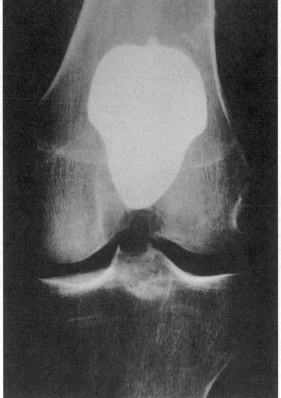

Figure 14–7 Patellofemoral Replacement. (**A**) Axial view, (**B**) frontal view.

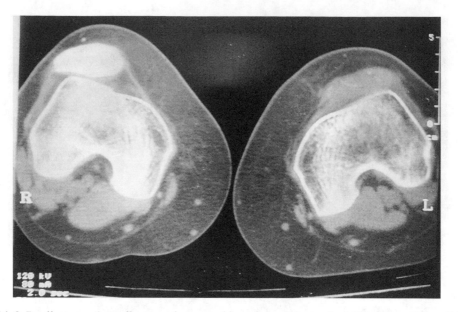

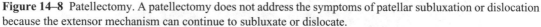

Figure 14–8 Patellectomy. A patellectomy does not address the symptoms of patellar subluxation or dislocation because the extensor mechanism can continue to subluxate or dislocate.

correct this problem. The quadriceps tendon may continue to subluxate or dislocate (Figure 14–8). Finally, a patient requiring total knee arthroplasty is at some disadvantage if he or she has had a patellectomy.

History and Results

Putz is reported to have performed a patellectomy in 1860.[96,97] Since then, the popularity of the procedure has gone through cycles. Heineck[98] in 1909 condemned it. Brooke[99] in 1937 reported on good results in 30 cases, and Hey-Groves[100] supported him. In 1948, McFarland[101] went so far as to recommend the procedure for simple, recurrent patellar dislocation. But in 1949, Scott[102] reviewed 101 patella fractures treated with patellectomy and reported that 60% of patients reported giving way and 90% of patients still had pain. Since then, there have been both favorable and unfavorable reports. Haggart,[103] Haliburton,[104] Geckeler,[105] Boucher,[106] Stougard,[107] Burton,[108] and Kelly[109] have reported good success rates for the arthritic patellofemoral joint.[96]

In 1969, Castaing et al[110] reported 62% good to very good results in 61 patients followed an average of 5 years. Overall, residual pain, quadriceps strength, active range of motion, and knee stability were acceptable. Stair descent tended to be a source of problems. Reossification ("patellar regeneration") about the patellectomy site was noted twice with no correlation with results. Recovery tended to be long, and a number of patients continued to note improvement over time.

On the other hand, Ackroyd[111] noted in 1978 a good result in only about half his cohort of 87 knees followed an average of 6½ years (including a subgroup of 40 knees followed an average of 10½ years). A variety of surgical techniques had been used. The results were probably skewed by patients with femorotibial arthritis who predictably did not have as good results (the article does not state how many such patients were present).

Compere et al[112] reported on 29 knees followed an average of approximately 7 years. This was a young group of patients (average age 43.5 years). Of the knees, 90% were rated good to excellent. One patient developed "symptomatic calcification in the patellar tendon," which was surgically removed and had an excellent eventual result.

De la Cafiniere[113] in 1985 noted good results in young patients (30 to 60 years of age) and also noted that final quadriceps strength could not be assessed before 2 years.

In 1988, Baker et al[114] noted satisfaction after an average of 14 years with 19 of 20 knees operated on with a Miyakawa technique.

Lennox et al[115] found that a patellectomy worked best in patients with pain without arthritis (75% reported good results, 10% of patients were worse than they were preoperatively). When the procedure was done for arthritis, 54% of patients reported good results and 27% felt worse than they felt preoperatively. Not only can there be a correlation between technique and results, there can be a correlation between underlying etiology and results. Not all investigators have the same mix of patients. For example, De la Cafiniere's cohort consisted of patients with severe (pathological) chondromalacia,[113] Castaing's patients had mostly fractures,[110] and West's patients were dislocators.[116] Baker et al[114] note some of the late complications including persistent malalignment of the extensor mechanism.

It appears that a patellectomy can work well in certain patients but not predictably so. The last word on the best technique and specific indications has not been written.

Surgical Technique

A number of techniques have been described for patellectomy. At least two problems need to be addressed:

1. By removing the patella, there is a functional lengthening of the extensor mechanism, which is therefore rendered more lax. This can lead to extensor weakness and an extensor lag (inability to actively straighten the knee). Therefore, the extensor mechanism needs to be tightened somehow to compensate for this.

2. If there was an element of malalignment to begin with, it needs to be addressed at the time of the patellectomy. If not, the malalignment will persist and the patient may have pain despite the patellectomy.

West[116] made a relatively transverse, *C*-shaped skin incision and cut the quadriceps expansion over the lower third of the patella, again in a transverse manner. Following removal of the patella, the proximal portion of the quadriceps expansion is pulled distally over the distal portion to restore tension to the extensor mechanism. The VMO is detached and advanced laterally as needed.

Steurer et al[117] and Ziran et al[118] have described enucleation of the patella followed by a cruciform repair where the VMO is advanced after all other limbs of the repair have been sutured.[116–119] The cruciform repair gives some bulk to the area where the patella used to be (thus tightening the extensor mechanism some) and suturing the VMO last allows fine-tuning of the quadriceps' direction of pull.

The Miyakawa and related techniques[13,110] address the lengthening of the extensor mechanism by folding a tongue of quadriceps tendon distally onto the area where the patella used to be. They do not address malalignment of the extensor mechanism.

The Compere technique[112] involves a medial and lateral arthrotomy and a suturing together of the newly created medial and lateral borders of the extensor mechanism. The extensor mechanism takes on the appearance of a tube. Any remnant of the patella is incorporated into the tube. The VMO is detached and advanced as needed, and an excessive Q angle is addressed distally.

ANESTHESIA

Because the surgeon is attempting to correct a dynamic situation, it is tempting to perform the realignment operation in such a way as to allow the patient to contract the quadriceps muscles during the actual procedure. The use of local anesthesia has been reported in soft tissue procedures about the knee.[72] Another option is a selective epidural. The patient is given just enough anesthetic to eliminate pain but not enough to block motor control. In my experience, this is easier said than done, but in select cases it may be a goal worth shooting for.

AUTHOR'S OPINION

As stated at the beginning of the chapter, the surgeon's goal is to

* Correct position/tracking, with respect to 6 degrees of freedom (3 in translation, 3 in rotation, eg, tilt and height).
* Address dysplasias.
* Unload/resurface chondral lesions.

Achieving these goals requires an appreciation of the tilt, retinacular tightness, medial-lateral position, and height of the patella, as well as recognition of the nature and location of chondral lesions. Although this can sometimes be determined through the physical and radiographic examination, there are times when only the arthroscopic examination can provide some of this critical information (especially pertaining to chondral lesions).

As a rule, I am less sanguine about the lateral retinacular release than most surgeons. The patients that I consider good candidates for the procedure usually recover with the nonoperative modalities described in the prior chapters. If a patient has failed a good nonoperative regimen

and I do not think that the pain is mostly biological or psychogenic, my indications for the lateral retinacular release include patients with mild to moderate tilt, no apparent lateral displacement, a normal Q angle, and no open lesions about the medial aspect of the patella.

If these conditions are not met, I add a proximal-medial soft tissue procedure and/or a displacement of the tibial tuberosity. If the Q angle is normal and there are no significant chondral lesions, I plicate the medial retinaculum or advance the VMO. If the Q angle is increased, I add an Elmslie-Trillat procedure. If there are medial lesions, I am more inclined to eliminate the VMO advancement and perform an anteromedialization of the tibial tuberosity.

If the patella is well aligned but painful because of distal lesions on the patella, a Maquet is a reasonable salvage (limited goals) procedure. Proximal lesions on the patella or trochlear lesions are relative contraindications for a Maquet procedure.

If lesions are extensive, I prefer a patellofemoral replacement over a patellectomy.

If the patella is high, it is brought distally (but not posteriorly).

If the trochlea presents a convex area, this is a most troublesome scenario. Current techniques of trochleoplasty do not work, but this remains a fertile area for investigation.

For patients who present with pain following any kind of patellar surgery, I follow the principles listed in Chapter 15.

REFERENCES

1. Cotta H. Zur therapie der habituellen patellarluxation. *Arch Orthop Unfall Chir*. 1959;51:265.

2. Carson WG Jr, James SL, Larson RL, et al. Patellofemoral disorders: physical and radiographic evaluation, I: physical examination. *Clin Orthop*. 1984; 185:165–177.

3. Merchant AC, Mercer, RL. Lateral release of the patella. *Clin Orthop*. 1974.103:40–45.

4. Ficat P, Ficat C, Bailleux A. Syndrome d'hyperpression externe de la rotule. *Rev Chir Orthop*. 1975;61:39–59.

5. Fulkerson JP, Grossling HR. Anatomy of the knee joint lateral retinaculum. *Clin Orthop*. 1980;153:183.

6. Horner G, Dellon L. Innervation of the human knee joint and implications for surgery. *Clin Orthop*. 1994; 301:221–226.

7. Dellon AL, Mont MA, Mullick T, Hungerford DS. Partial denervation for persistent neuroma pain around the knee. *Clin Orthop*. 1996;329:216–222.

8. Nove-Josserand L, Dejour D. Dysplasie du quadriceps et bascule rotulienne dans l'instabilité rotulienne objective. *Rev Chir Orthop*. 1995;81:497–504.

9. Shea KP, Fulkerson JP. Preoperative computed tomography scanning and arthroscopy in predicting outcome after lateral retinacular release. Arthroscopy. 1992; 8:327–334.

10. Marumoto JM, Jordan C, Akins R. A biomechanical comparison of lateral retinacular releases. *Am J Sports Med.* 1995;23:151–155.

11. Henry JH, Goletz TH, Williamson B. Lateral retinacular release in patellofemoral subluxation. *Am J Sports Med.* 1986;14:121–129.

12. Fondren FB, Goldner JL, Bassett FH. Recurrent dislocation of the patella treated by the modified Roux-Goldthwait procedure. *J Bone Joint Surg.* 1985; 67A:993–1005.

13. Baker RH, Carroll N, Dewar FP, et al. The semitendinosus tenodesis for recurrent dislocation of the patella. *J Bone Joint Surg.* 1972;54B:103–109.

14. Flandry F, Hughston JC. Complications of extensor mechanism surgery for patellar malalignment. *Am J Orthop.* 1995;24:534–543.

15. Hughston JC, DeLee M. Medial subluxation of the patella as a complication of lateral release. *Am J Sports Med.* 1988;16:383–388.

16. Shellock FG, Mink JH, Deutsch A, et al. Evaluation of patients with persistent symptoms after lateral retinacular release by kinematic magnetic resonance imaging of the patellofemoral joint. *Arthroscopy.* 1990; 6:226–234.

17. Aglietti P, Pisaneschi A, Buzzi R, et al. Arthroscopic lateral release for patellar pain or instability. *Arthroscopy.* 1989;5:176–183.

18. Dandy DJ, Griffiths D. Lateral release for recurrent dislocation of the patella. *J Bone Joint Surg.* 1989; 71B:121.

19. Jackson RW, Kunkel SS, Taylor GJ. Lateral retinacular release for patellofemoral pain in the older patient. *Arthroscopy.* 1991;7:283–286.

20. Krompinger WJ, Fulkerson JP. Lateral retinacular release for intractable lateral retinacular pain. *Clin Orthop.* 1983;177:176.

21. Fulkerson JP, Schutzer SF, Ramsby GR, Bernstein RA. Computerized tomography of the patellofemoral joint before and after lateral release or realignment. *Arthroscopy.* 1987;3:19.

22. Kolowich PA, Paulos LE, Rosenberg TD, Farnsworth S. Lateral release of the patella: indications and contraindications. *Am J Sports Med.* 1990;18:359.

23. Hughston J, Walsh WM, Puddu G. *Patellar Subluxation and Dislocation.* Philadelphia: WB Saunders; 1984. Saunders Monographs in Clinical Orthopaedics, no. 5.

24. Insall JN, Bullough PG, Burstein AH. Proximal "tube" realignment of the patella for chondromalacia patellae. *Clin Orthop.* 1979;144:63–69.

25. Madigan, R, Wissinger HA, Donaldson WF. Preliminary experience with a method of quadricepsplasty in recurrent subluxation of the patella. *J Bone Joint Surg.* 1975;57A:600–607.

26. Mansat CH, Bonnel F, Jaeger JH. *L'Appareil Extenseur du Genou.* Paris: Masson; 1985.

27. Abraham E, Washington E, Huang TL. Insall proximal realignment for disorders of the patella. *Clin. Orthop.* 1989;248:61.

28. Cerullo G, Puddu G, Conteduca F, et al. Evaluation of the results of extensor mechanism reconstruction. *Am J Sports Med.* 1988;16:93.

29. Scuderi G, Cuomo F, Scott WN. Lateral release and proximal realignment for patellar subluxation and dislocation. *J Bone Joint Surg.* 1988;70A:856.

30. Roux C. Luxation habituelle de la rotule: traitement operatoire. *Rev Chir.* 1888;8:682–689.

31. Trillat A, Dejour H, Couette A. Diagnostic et traitement des subluxations récidivantes de la rotule. *Rev Chir Orthop.* 1964;50:813–824.

32. Grana WA, Krieghauser LA. Scientific basis of extensor mechanism disorders. *Clin Sports Med.* 1985;4:247–256.

33. Andrews JR, Thornberry R. The role of open surgery for patellofemoral joint malalignment. *Orthop Rev.* 1986; 15:72.

34. Insall JN, Falvo KA, Wise DW. Chondromalacia patellae—a prospective study. *J Bone Joint Surg.* 1976; 58A:1

35. Wall JJ. Compartment syndrome as a complication of the Hauser procedure. *J Bone Joint Surg.* 1979; 61A:185–191.

36. Cox JS. An evaluation of the Elmslie-Trillat procedure for management of patellar dislocations and subluxations: a preliminary report. *Am J Sports Med.* 1976;4:72.

37. Cox JS. Evaluation of the Roux-Elmslie-Trillat procedure for knee extensor realignment. *Am J Sports Med.* 1982;10:303–310.

38. Fielding JW, Liebler WA, Urs D, et al. Tibial tubercle transfer. *J Bone Joint Surg.* 1974;56A:1315–1316.

39. Fielding JW, Liebler WA, Urs D, et al. Tibial tubercle transfer: a long-range follow-up study. *Clin Orthop.* 1979;144:43–44.

40. Riegler HF. Recurrent dislocations and subluxations of the patella. *Clin Orthop.* 1988;227:201.

41. Maquet P. Considérations biomécaniques sur l'arthrose du genou. Un traitement biomécanique de l'arthrose femoropatellaire: l'avancemenent du tendon rotulien. *Rev Rheum.* 1963;30:779–783.

42. Maquet P. Advancement of the tibial tuberosity. *Clin Orthop.* 1976;115:225–230.

43. Pan HQ, Kish V, Boyd RD, et al. The Maquet procedure: effect of tibial shingle length on patellofemoral pressures. *J Orthop Res.* 1993;11:199–204.

44. Retaillaud JL, Darmana R, Devallet P, et al. Etude biomécanique expérimentale de l'avancement de la tubérosité tibiale. *Rev Chir Orthop*. 1989;75:513–523.

45. Nakamura N, Ellis M, Seedhom BB. Advancement of the tibial tuberosity: a biomechanical study. *J Bone Joint Surg*. 1985;67B:255–260.

46. Cheng CK, Yao NK, Liu HC. Computer surgery simulation and its biomechanical evaluation of the anterior displacement of the tibial tubercle. *Trans Orthop Res Soc*. 1992:476.

47. Ferrandez L, Usabiaga J, Yubero J, et al. An experimental study of the redistribution of patellofemoral pressures by the anterior displacement of the anterior tuberosity of the tibia. *Clin Orthop*. 1989;238:183–190.

48. Lewallen DG, Riegger CL, Myers ER, Hayes WC. Effects of retinacular release and tibial tubercle elevation in patellofemoral degenerative joint disease. *J Orthop Res*. 1990;8:856.

49. Singerman R, White C, Davy DT. Reduction of patellofemoral contact forces following anterior displacement of the tibial tubercle. *J Orthop Res*. 1995;13:279–285.

50. Koshino T. Changes in patellofemoral compressive force after anterior or anteromedial displacement of tibial tuberosity for chondromalacia patellae. *Clin Orthop*. 1991;266:133–138.

51. Ferguson AB Jr., Brown TD, Fu FH, et al. Relief of patellofemoral contract stress by anterior displacement of the tibial tubercle. *J Bone Joint Surg*. 1979;61A:159–166.

52. Leach RE, Paul GR, Yablon IG, et al. Anterior displacement of the tibial tubercle: the Maquet procedure. *Contemp Orthop*. 1981;3:119–123.

53. Hirsch DM, Reddy DK. Experience with Maquet anterior tibial tubercle advancement for patellofemoral arthralgia. *Clin Orthop*. 1980;148:136–139.

54. Mendes DG, Soudry M, Iusim M. Clinical assessment of Maquet tibial tuberosity advancement. *Clin Orthop*. 1987;222:228–238.

55. Radin EL. The Maquet procedure—anterior displacement of the tibial tubercle: indications, contraindications and precautions. *Clin Orthop*. 1986;213:241–248.

56. Schmid F. The Maquet procedure in the treatment of patellofemoral osteoarthrosis: long-term results. *Clin Orthop*. 1993;294:254–258.

57. Schepsis AA, DeSimone AA, Leach RE. Anterior tibial tubercle transposition for patellofemoral arthrosis. *Am J Knee Surg*. 1994;7:1320.

58. Heatley FW, Allen PR, Patrick JH. Tibial tubercle advancement for anterior knee pain: a temporary or permanent solution. *Clin Orthop*. 1986;208:215–224.

59. Radin EL, Labosky DA. Avoiding complications associated with the Maquet procedure. *Complications in Orthop*. March-April 1989;48–57.

60. Ferguson AB Jr. Elevation of the insertion of the patellar ligament for patellofemoral pain. *J Bone Joint Surg*. 1982;64A:766–771.

61. Jenny JY, Sader Z, Henry A, et al. Elevation of the tibial tubercle for patellofemoral pain syndrome. *Knee Surg Sports Traumatol Arthrosc*. 1996;4:92–96.

62. Lord G, Samuel P, Gory M. L'ostéotomie tibiale en "crosse de hockey": traitement des chondromalacies ouvertes et des arthroses fémoro-patellaires avec désaxation de l'appareil extenseur. *Rev Chir Orthop*. 1977;63:397–401.

63. Fulkerson JP. Anteromedialization of the tibial tuberosity for patellofemoral malalignment. *Clin Orthop*. 1983;177:176.

64. Caton J, Mironneau A, Walch G, et al. La rotule haute idiopathique chez l'adolescent: a propos de 61 cas opérés. *Rev Chir Orthop*. 1990;76:253.

65. Simmons E Jr, Cameron JC. Patella alta and recurrent dislocation of the patella. *Clin Orthop*. 1992;274:265.

66. Hauser EDW. Total tendon transplant for slipping patella. *Surg Gynecol Obstet*. 1938;66:199.

67. Hampson WGJ, Hill P. Late results of transfer of the tibial tubercle for recurrent dislocation of the patella. *J Bone Joint Surg*. 1975;57B:209.

68. Nogalski MP, Bach BR. Treatment of failed Hauser procedures via modified Maquet procedure. *Am J Knee Surg*. 1995;8:71–76.

69. Bonnard C, Nocquet P, Sollogoub I, et al. Instabilité rotulienne chez l'enfant. *Rev Chir Orthop*. 1990;76:473–479.

70. Goldthwait JE. Slipping or recurrent dislocation of the patella: with the report of eleven cases. *Boston Med Surg J*. 1904;150:169–174.

71. Bentley G, Dowd G. Current concepts of etiology and treatment of chondromalacia patella. *Clin Orthop*. 1984;189:209.

72. Templeman D, McBeath A. Iatrogenic patella malalignment following the Roux-Goldthwait procedure, corrected by dynamic intraoperative realignment. *J Bone Joint Surg*. 1986;68A:1096–1098.

73. Brief P. Lateral patellar instability: treatment with a combined open-arthroscopic approach. *Arthroscopy*. 1993;9:617–623.

74. Beltran JE. Resection arthroplasty of the patella. *J Bone Joint Surg*. 1987;69B:604–607.

75. Ficat P, Gédéon P, Léger M, Bausssaton M. Résultats des arthrolyses externes et des spongialisations. *Rev Chir Orthop*. 1980; 66:268–272.

76. Nerubay J, Katnelson A. Osteotomy of the patella. *Clin Orthop*. 1986;207:103–107.

77. Vaquero J, Arriaza R. The patella thinning osteotomy. *Int Orthop.* 1992;16:372–376.

78. Macnicol, MF. Patellar osteotomy for intractable patellar pain. *Knee.* 1994;1:41–45.

79. Sachs J. Semipatellectomy, an operation for chondromalacia of the knee joint. *South African Med.* 1962; 36:518.

80. Weaver JK, Wieder D, Derkash RS. Patellofemoral arthritis resulting from malalignment. *Orthop Rev.* 1991;20:1075.

81. Albee FH. The bone graft wedge in the treatment of habitual dislocation of the patella. *Med Rec.* 1915; 88:257–258.

82. Masse Y. La trochléoplastie: restauration de la gouttière trochléene dans les subluxations et luxations de la rotule. *Rev Chir Orthop.* 1978;64:3–17.

83. Duncan C, McKeever DC. Patellar prosthesis. *J Bone Joint Surg.* 1955;37A:1074–1084.

84. Vermeulen H, De Doncker E, Watillon M. Les protheses rotuliennes de MacKeever [sic] dans l'arthrose femoropatellaire. *Acta Orthop Belg.* 1973;39:79–90.

85. Pickett JC, Stoll DA. Patellaplasty or patellectomy. *Clin Orthop.* 1979;144:103–106.

86. Harrington KD. Long-term results for the McKeever patellar resurfacing prosthesis used as a salvage procedure for severe chondromalacia patellae. *Clin Orthop.* 1992;279:201–213.

87. Aglietti P, Insall JN, Walker PS, Trent P. A new patella prosthesis. *Clin Orthop.* 1975;107:175.

88. Worrell RV. Prosthetic resurfacing of the patella. *Clin Orthop.* 1979;144:91–97.

89. Lubinus HH. Patella glide bearing total replacement. *Orthopedics.* 1979;2:119.

90. Blazina ME, Fox JM, Del Pizzo W, et al. Patellofemoral replacement. *Clin Orthop.* 1979;144:98–107.

91. Tisserand PT, Aubaniac JM. Notre experience de la prothèse trochleo-rotulienne: a propos de 106 cas. *Rev Chir Orthop.* 1988;74(suppl. 2):186. Abstract.

92. Cartier P, Sanouiller JL, Grelsamer RP. Patellofemoral arthroplasty: 2–12 year follow-up study. *J Arthroplasty.* 1990;5:49.

93. Mow VC, Newton PM, Grelsamer RP. Biomechanics of articular cartilage and meniscus. In: Fu FH, Harner CD, Vince KG, eds. *Knee Surgery.* Baltimore: Williams & Wilkins; 1994.

94. Hoikka VEJ, Jaroma HJ, Ritsila. Reconstruction of the patellar articulation with periosteal grafts. *Acta Orthop Scand.* 1990;61:36.

95. Denham RA, Bishop RE. Mechanics of the knee and problems in reconstructive surgery. *J Bone Joint Surg.* 1978;60B:345.

96. De Maio M, Drez DJ Jr. Patellectomy. In: Fox JM, Del Pizzo W, eds. *The Patellofemoral Joint.* New York: McGraw-Hill; 1993:259–272.

97. Cohn BNE. Total and partial patellectomy: an experimental study. *Surg Gynecol Obstet.* 1944;79:526.

98. Heineck AP. The modern operative treatment of fractures of the patella. *Surg Gynecol Obstet.* 1909;9:177.

99. Brooke, R. The treatment of fractured patella by excision: a study of morphology and function. *Br J Surg.* 1937;24:733.

100. Hey-Groves EW. A note on the extension apparatus of the knee joint. *Br J Surg.* 1937;24:747.

101. McFarland B. Excision of patella for recurrent dislocation. *J Bone Joint Surg.* 1948;30B:158.

102. Scott JC. Fractures of the patella. *J Bone Joint Surg.* 1949;31B:76.

103. Haggart GE. Surgical treatment of degenerative arthritis of the knee joint. *N Engl J Med.* 1947;236–971.

104. Haliburton RA, Sullivan CR. The patella in degenerative joint diseases: a clinicopathologic study. *Arch Surg.* 1958;77:677.

105. Geckeler EO, Querenta AV. Patellectomy for degenerative arthritis of the knee—late results. *J Bone Joint Surg.* 1962;44A:1109.

106. Boucher HH. Patellectomy in the geriatric patient. *Clin Orthop.* 1958;11:33.

107. Stougard J. Patellectomy. *Acta Orthop Scand.* 1970; 41:110.

108. Burton VM, Thomas HM. Results of excision of the patella. *Surg Gynecol Obstet.* 1972;135:753.

109. Kelly MA, Insall JN. Patellectomy. *Orthop Clin North Am.* 1986;17:289.

110. Castaing J, Castellani C, Plisson JC, et al. La patellectomie totale: technique et resultats. *Rev Chir Orthop.* 1969;55:259–278.

111. Ackroyd CE, Polyzoides AJ. Patellectomy for osteoarthritis: a study of 18 patients followed from two to 22 years. *J Bone Joint Surg.* 1978;60B:353.

112. Compere CL, Hill JA, Lewinnek, GE. A new method of patellectomy for patellofemoral arthritis. *J Bone Joint Surg.* 1979;61A:714–719.

113. De la Cafiniere JY. In: Mansat C, Bonnel F, Jaeger JH, eds. *L'Appareil Extenseur du Genou.* Paris: Masson; 1985:232–236.

114. Baker CL, Hughston JC. Miyakawa patellectomy. *J Bone Joint Surg.* 1988;70A:1489–1494.

115. Lennox IAC, Cobb AG, Knowles J, Bentley G. Knee function after patellectomy—a 12 to 48 year follow-up. *J Bone Joint Surg.* 1994;76B:485.

116. West FE. End result of patellectomy. *J Bone Joint Surg.* 1962;44A:1089–1108.

117. Steurer PA Jr, Gradisar IA Jr, Hoyt WA Jr, et al. Patellectomy: a clinical study and biomechanical evaluation. *Clin Orthop.* 1979;144:84-90.
118. Ziran BH, Goodfellow DB, Deluca LS, Heiple KG. Knee function after patellectomy and cruciform repair of the extensor mechanism. *Clin Orthop.* 1994; 302:138–163.
119. Soto-Hall R. Traumatic degeneration of the articular cartilage of the patella. *J Bone Joint Surg.* 1945; 27:426.

ADDITIONAL READINGS

Chaimsky G, Milgrom C. Modification of the Maquet barrel-vault osteotomy. *Orthop Rev.* 1987;16:113–116.

Galeazzi R. Nuove applicazioni del trapianto muscolare e tendineo. *Archivio di Ortopedia.* 1921;38.

Grelsamer RP. Patellofemoral arthroplasty. *Techniques in Orthopaedics.* 1997;12:200–204.

Lund F, Nilsson BE. Anterior displacement of the tibial tuberosity in chondromalacia patellae. *Acta Orthop Scand.* 1980;51:679–688.

Meister K, James SL. Proximal tibial derotation osteotomy for anterior knee pain in the miserably malaligned extremity. *Am J Orthop.* 1995;24:149–155.

O'Neill DB. Open lateral retinacular lengthening compared with arthroscopic release: a prospective randomized outcome study. *J Bone Joint Surg.* 1997;79A:1759–1769.

Pidoriano AJ, Weinstein RN, Buuck DA, Fulkerson JP. Correlation of patellar articular lesions with results from anteromedial tibial tubercle transfer. *Am J Sports Med.* 1997;25:533–537.

Stetson WB, Friedman MJ, Fulkerson JP, et al. Fracture of the proximal tibia with immediate weight-bearing after a Fulkerson osteotomy. *Am J Sports Med.* 1997;25:570–574.

Vaille R, Beddouk A, Cronier P, Fournier D. Prevention des complications hemorragiques de la section du retinaculum patellaire lateral. *Rev Chir Orthop.* 1997;83:665–669.

CHAPTER 15

The Failed Patella

OVERVIEW

The discouraging term *failed patella* is borrowed from the world of spine surgery, where the term *failed back* has been used to designate the wide range of conditions that can lead to persistent pain after back surgery. The patient who still has pain following patellar surgery presents one of the greatest diagnostic dilemmas in orthopaedics.

The orthopaedist's first task lies in determining whether the patient's pain is mechanical, biological, or emotional. Because these three categories of pain can coexist, sorting the relative contributions of each is a formidable, time-consuming endeavor.

MECHANICAL PAIN

Mechanical pain can fall into three categories:

1. pain not related to patella malalignment
2. pain resulting from persistent patella malalignment
3. pain from chondral lesions

Pain Not Related to Patella Malalignment

Pain not related to patella malalignment can be from any of the conditions listed in Chapter 8. The orthopaedist must look at the patient with a fresh perspective, keeping in mind the possibility that the patient's symptoms are coming from another part of the knee. If the patient is com-

plaining mostly of instability, the orthopaedist must consider the possibility of an anterior cruciate ligament tear, quadriceps atrophy (unrelated to any patellar pathology), or a loose body. The quadriceps atrophy is particularly difficult to factor into the equation because it can be either the cause or the result of the patient's problem. If the complaint is pain, all the conditions listed in Chapter 8 (ie, neuroma, anterior cruciate ligament tear, plica syndrome, meniscal tear, osteochondritis dissecans, tumor infection, iliotibial band tendinitis, referred pain, rheumatological conditions) are possible suspects until proven otherwise.

Pain from Persistent Patella Malalignment

Pain from persistent patella malalignment falls into two categories:

1. pain from insufficient correction of the original pathology
2. pain from overcorrection of the initial malalignment (It is possible for a patella to translate medially in excessive fashion and/or be subject to excessive medial pressure. This can happen if the lateral retinacular release is too extensive,[1,2] the tibial tuberosity transfer is too large, and/ or the medial plication/advancement is too significant. Overcorrection can easily happen because the titration of patellar alignment can be quite difficult.)

Pain from Chondral Lesions

A well-aligned patella can be painful if there are significant chondral lesions. "Significant" varies from patient to patient, and it is not always clear preoperatively whether realignment of a malaligned patella will alleviate all symptoms. Fibrillation and small, focal lesions do not cause significant pain in most patients with well-aligned patellae. If patients with such lesions are experiencing severe pain, the practitioner should consider the biological causes of knee pain. For obvious reasons, it is critical to differentiate between pain from chondral lesions and pain from biological causes. Too many patients are told that if the lateral release did not work they probably need a transfer of the tibial tuberosity. Although this is occasionally true, it is not automatically so.

Case Histories

Case 1

BF is a 27-year-old woman who has right knee pain 18 months following a lateral retinacular release carried out for persistent anterior knee pain. She does not recall feeling better at any time after surgery. The knee also tends to give out on occasion. Examination of the right knee reveals a well-healed, nontender scar. Pushing the patella medially is very uncomfortable. The patient exhibits 2 cm of atrophy 10 cm above the superior pole of the patella. Examination of the other knee reveals a normal extensor mechanism. She is not flatfooted or loose-jointed. Plain radiographs are unremarkable.

Assessment. The patient probably did not have patella malalignment to begin with because (1) patella malalignment is usually bilateral (even if only one side is symptomatic), (2) the patient has abnormal medial play, and (3) she now feels unstable. Although the instability could be secondary to the atrophy, in this case it is probably the other way around. One has to consider the other possible causes of anterior knee pain and consider reapproximating the lateral retinaculum. Discussions with the patient should remain tactful.

Case 2

AM, a 21-year-old aspiring model, has persistent anterior knee pain following a car accident, an arthroscopic debridement of her patella, and a plica resection. Repeat magnetic resonance imaging and technetium bone scan are unremarkable. On examination, she has exquisite tenderness at the anteromedial joint line away from the arthroscopy portal. Mere pinching of the skin causes pain. Her symptoms resolve with a subcutaneous injection of lidocaine.

Assessment. The patient probably has a saphenous neuroma. (It is questionable whether the surgery and imaging workup were necessary.)

Case 3

JR, a 28-year-old man, notes pain and giving way that persist even after a lateral retinacular release. He undergoes a tibial tuberosity transfer. The symptoms of giving way lessen but are still present. Examination reveals a dysplastic vastus medialis obliquus (VMO), considerable lateral tilt, and a lower than average quadriceps (Q) angle. The Q angle on the opposite side is within normal limits. He has had an appropriate course of nonoperative management.

Assessment. Assuming the presence of normal articular cartilage on the medial aspect of the patella, the patient may need plication or advancement of the superomedial structures in addition to a second release of the retinaculum that has surely reformed. The tibial tuberosity can probably be left in its place, although the surgeon can consider putting it back in its native (normal) position.

BIOLOGICAL PAIN—REFLEX SYMPATHETIC DYSTROPHY AND RSD-LIKE CONDITIONS

Biological pain is pain that is due solely to inflammation and/or irritation of one or more soft tissues about the knee—without a mechanical component. This includes the inflammatory arthritides, sympathetically maintained pain, Lyme disease, and infection. Referred pain might also be included in this category.

RSD—Definition and Pathophysiology

Reflex sympathetic dystrophy (RSD) is a condition that causes severe pain far out of proportion to the underlying mechanical condition. There are often associated vasomotor, thermoregulatory, and/or neurotrophic changes.

RSD and related conditions fall into the category of "nerve pain," although no specific nerve around the knee need be injured for the conditions to be present. RSD has gone by many names since it was coined *causalgia* by Mitchell[3] in 1872 (Exhibit 15–1). *Reflex* reflects the thinking that the condition is an involuntary neurological response to a stimulus. *Sympathetic* refers to the autonomic nerves most implicated, and *dystrophy* is what can eventually happen to the involved joint or limb.

Unlike pregnancy, RSD is not an "either you have it or you don't" situation. It is rather like a flu virus, the symptoms of which can vary significantly from case to case. The symptoms can be very mild to the point of being missed altogether or, at the other extreme, can be very disabling. Because of this variability, it is difficult to say just what the prevalence of RSD is among patients with knee pain.

The nerves involved are the "sympathetic" nerves, which are part of the autonomic nerve system. Along with the parasympathetic nerves, they control involuntary body functions such as heart rate, intestinal mobility, blood vessel constriction, and dilation (ie, skin color and temperature)—to name but a few. They respond to pain, and it has been suggested that the sympathetic fibers can themselves carry pain impulses via afferent fibers in the sympathetic chain.[9] The autonomic system consists of a central and a peripheral component. The central component consists of the hypothalamus. The peripheral component consists mainly of afferent sensory fibers and efferent motor fibers to all tissues except skeletal muscle. They synapse in ganglia on either side of the spinal cord. Of particular pertinence to the patella and lower extremity, the lumbar sympathetic chain is "formed by the anterior (ventral) divisions of the first, second, third and fourth lumbar nerves, with a branch

Exhibit 15–1 Partial List of Names for Reflex Sympathetic Dystrophy

- causalgia
- shoulder hand syndrome
- acute atrophy of bone[4]
- Sudeck's atrophy
- osteodystrophy
- reflex dystrophy of the extremities[5]
- algodystrophy
- reflex sympathetic dystrophy[6]
- sympathetically maintained pain[7,8]

from the twelfth thoracic nerve and the fifth lumbar nerve. It is located anterior to the transverse processes of the respective lumbar vertebrae."[9]

In RSD, the nerves are not doing anything abnormal. Normally, pain is transmitted via A delta and the smaller C fibers, which enter the spinal cord through the dorsal roots (as noted above, afferent sympathetic fibers may also transmit pain). The pain impulses are then transmitted (1) cephalad to the somatosensory cortex where pain is "felt," (2) to the anterior horn where a motor reflex may be initiated (eg, removing a hand from a hot stove), and (3) to the sympathetic chain. Nerves leaving the sympathetic chain then produce vasoconstriction followed by vasodilation. Again, it must be emphasized that this is normal. What is abnormal is for the vasoconstriction to persist. This condition can lead to ischemia, which leads to even more pain, more sympathetic stimulation, and so on. The dysfunction therefore consists of a sustained and exaggerated variation on normal physiology—the nervous system's equivalent of violent, repeated sneezes. The sensitivity of nociceptors is enhanced by the ischemia itself; changes in vascular permeability; smooth muscle contraction about the nociceptors; and local release of norepinephrine, substance P, prostaglandins, and bradykinin.[9]

The specific cause of the persistent sympathetic irritation and exaggerated response is unknown. Melzack and Wall[10] have proposed the "gate control theory": the "gate" that modulates the inhibition and facilitation of pain impulses is dysfunctional in the sense that the pain impulses are not shut out after a normal period of time. This results in a persistent painful stimulus and a reverberating cycle of pain and sympathetic response. Spontaneous depolarization at the exposed, regenerating surfaces of injured nerves[11] has been proposed (when there has been nerve injury) as has a receptive field expansion of the pain-contributing neurons in the dorsal horns of the spinal cord.[8,12] It remains common teaching that there is an emotional predisposition to RSD. Anxious, depressed, laconic, flat-affect women are at particular risk, according to this theory. There is no proof of this theory, and chronic pain makes almost anyone anxious and depressed. Most series do report a preponderance of women in their cohorts. Various pain pathways can even exist in a given patient, which would explain why symptoms can recur even after complete surgical sympathectomy.[8,13] In any case, the condition eventually affects the bone (osteoporosis), vasculature (vasodilation and constriction), and all soft tissues in the affected area.

Signs and Symptoms

In classic RSD, the patient early on feels a constant, burning pain, the affected joint is stiff, and the skin is warm (decreased sympathetic activity) and mottled. Light touch is extremely painful (allodynia). In later stages, the skin is cool and shiny. Eventually the joint develops contractures and becomes atrophic. However, not all of these signs and symptoms are present in all cases, and the symptoms vary over time.

The stiffness that occurs is also seen in arthrofibrosis, a condition in which for no apparent reason the joint is unable either to fully extend, to fully flex, or both. Arthrofibrosis is very poorly understood. It is possible that RSD and arthrofibrosis are related, although arthrofibrosis has a greater component of fibroblast stimulation.[14]

RSD can occur almost anywhere in the body, and it has even been reported in the back following spine surgery. It can exist in children.[15]

Etiology

RSD requires an inciting agent; this agent is usually, but not necessarily, trauma. The trauma need not be severe and, in fact, is usually relatively mild.[9,14,16–18] A simple wrist sprain, for example, can trigger RSD. Surgery is a form of trauma and, not surprisingly, a source of RSD. Although long, complex operations can cause RSD, short, outpatient procedures can also be the cause.[17] This is consistent with the concept that the inciting trauma is usually minimal. As noted, there need not be any trauma at all: a number of medical conditions have been documented to cause RSD, most notably myocardial infarction but also pneumonitis, carcinoma, embolism, infectious diseases, and thrombophlebitis.[9]

At this point, it appears that patient predisposition is the major factor with respect to the development of RSD.

Testing

There is no easy, risk-free, accurate test. X-rays classically show a patchy osteoporosis, but pain and disuse following surgery can also produce this picture. A sympathetic block comes closest to being the definitive test for the condition: anesthetizing the lumbar sympathetic chain provides significant pain relief for the duration of the block—but only in patients with RSD. Failure to obtain pain relief with such a block suggests that the patient does not have RSD.[19] However, because some sympathetic fibers can bypass the sympathetic chain, failure of a block still does not automatically rule out RSD. Sympathetic blocks have their downsides. They are costly and invasive; and, for the test to be meaningful, care must be taken not to inadvertently anesthetize the somatic nerves. Therefore, the decision about whether to perform a block can be difficult when the patient does not have all the classic RSD symptoms. Consultation with an anesthesiologist from a pain service can be useful.

Prior to the advent of sympathetic blocks, technetium bone scanning was favored. This involves the injection of the radioactive material technetium into an arm vein. The technetium is picked up by bone everywhere in the body. An area of increased bone activity is read as "hot" on the scan that is carried out a few hours after the injection. A scan is often "hot" in patients with RSD. Unfortunately, technetium bone scans are neither sensitive nor specific enough to provide a definitive diagnosis.[8,14] A hot scan need not be present for the patient to have RSD. Indeed, patients with RSD go from a hyperemic stage to a stage of decreased flow. Thus, at some point in the transition the blood flow must be normal. Scanning in this period yields a normal exam. Conversely, a hot scan does not automatically imply that the patient has RSD, as a number of conditions can cause hyperemia.

Because a hot scan leads the doctor to order a sympathetic block, and a cold scan in a patient suspected of having RSD also leads the doctor to order a sympathetic block (see above), scanning is in my opinion rarely warranted.

It is not uncommon for anesthesiologists from pain services to turn patients down for sympathetic blocks on the grounds that the patients have insufficient findings of RSD to warrant the risks and expense of such testing. In such situations, I may institute some other aspects of the RSD treatment.

Treatment

If the patient is found to have RSD, a multidisciplinary team is often assembled, including an orthopaedist, an anesthesiologist, a physical therapist, and sometimes a psychiatrist to address the depression that can be associated with the condition. Treatment consists of chemically blocking the sympathetic nerves. This is done via injections in the sympathetic chain just lateral to the spine or, on occasion, via oral medication. Many injections can be required.[14,17] Alternatives include peripheral intravenous injections (Bier blocks) of guanethedine, reserpine, or bretylium. An oral, nonsteroidal anti-inflammatory medication can be added, as can a tricyclic antidepressant such as amitriptyline[8] and/or a fentanyl patch. More recently, the use of an indwelling epidural blockade has been suggested.[20] This provides around-the-clock protection to the knee. It may be more effective than repeated injections, especially when no single treatment is long-lasting enough to "hold" the patient until the next injection.

Recovery can take months or years, especially if the condition is severe and the diagnosis is made long after the onset of the condition. Because RSD can be very subtle in its presentation and there is no simple, risk-free, reliable test, it is not uncommon to detect RSD after it is in its chronic stage.

There is a fine line between too much and just enough physical therapy. The joint must be mobilized—but not too aggressively. Cold in the early phase can be soothing, but extreme cold may be harmful. Gentle massage can be pleasant, but deep-friction massage may lead to histamine release from mast cells and stimulation of inhibitory fibers.[17]

In a chicken-and-egg situation, a mechanical problem can contribute to a continuation of RSD. It may then be necessary to perform surgery in the presence of known RSD. This would seem to be contraindicated, because surgery (as well as any trauma) can exacerbate RSD. Fortunately, if the patient is known to have RSD, epidural medications administered during a surgical procedure can successfully address the problem.[14]

RSD-Like Conditions

To make life even more difficult, there are, I believe, pain conditions that are not RSD. They do not necessarily involve the sympathetic nerves and they do not respond to a sympathetic block. Nevertheless, the patient feels a constant pain not related to a mechanical problem and not caused by localized inflammation of a single nerve as one might see with a neuroma.

EMOTIONAL PAIN

There are patients whose pain is psychogenic. It is beyond the scope of this book to discuss the differential diagnosis of psychogenic pain, but it is important for the treating doctor to recognize it. This is easier said than done. The long list of possible diagnoses discussed in this book must be ruled out before a patient can be said to have "emotional" problems or to be malingering. Making the diagnosis particularly difficult is the fact that the patient with psychogenic pain may well have a mechanical or biological cause for his or her pain. The pain is then greatly exaggerated by the psychological component or the thought of emotional or financial secondary gain. The mere suggestion that the pain could be psychogenic is often enough to send the patient scurrying elsewhere. The doctor must therefore summon up all of his or her interpersonal skills to suggest psychological problems in an effective manner.

One way to determine the presence of emotional pain or RSD is to perform a differential sympathetic block.[9,18] The block has three components: (1) the injection of saline, (2) the injection of just enough anesthetic to block the sympathetic nerves (10 cc of 0.25% procaine), (3) the injection of added anesthetic to block the sensory and motor nerves. Patients responding to the second injection have RSD. Patients responding only to the third injection usually have nonneurogenic pain (eg, arthritic pain or pain from patella malalignment). Patients who claim to have sustained pain relief from the saline injection and patients who say that they still have pain after their entire leg has been anesthetized have bought themselves a one-way ticket out of the orthopaedist's office. (The operative word here is *sustained*. Due to the placebo effect, up to one third of patients may report transient improvement[18] for 10 to 30 minutes.)

REFERENCES

1. Hughston JC, DeLee M. Medial subluxation of the patella as a complication of lateral release. *Am J Sports Med*. 1988;16:383–388.
2. Shellock FG, Mink JH, Deutsch A, et al. Evaluation of patients with persistent symptoms after lateral retinacular release by kinematic magnetic resonance imaging of the patellofemoral joint. *Arthroscopy*. 1990;6:226–234.
3. Mitchell SW. *Injuries of Nerves and Their Consequences*. Philadelphia: JB Lippincott; 1872.
4. Sudeck P. Über die acute entzundliche Knochenatrophie. *Arch Klin Chir*. 1900;62:147.
5. De Takats G, Miller BS. Post traumatic dystrophy of the extremities: a chronic vasodilator mechanism. *Arch Surg*. 1943;46:469.
6. Evans JA. Reflex sympathetic dystrophy: a report on 57 cases. *Ann Intern Med*. 1947:26;417.
7. Roberts W. A hypothesis on the physiological basis for causalgia and related pains. *Pain*. 1986;24:297–311.
8. Ngeow, JY. Reflex sympathetic dystrophy of the knee. In: Scuderi GR, ed. *The Patella*. New York: Springer-Verlag; 1995:333–339.
9. Raj P, Calodney A, Janisse T, et al. Reflex sympathetic dystrophy. In: Browner BD, Jupiter JB, Levine AM, Trafton PG, eds. *Skeletal Trauma*. Philadelphia: WB Saunders Co; 1992:471–499.
10. Melzack R, Wall PD. Pain mechanisms: a new theory. *Science*. 1965;150:971.
11. Devor M. Nerve pathophysiology and mechanisms of pain. *J Auton Nerv Syst*. 1983;7:371.
12. Woolf C, King A. Dynamic alterations in the cutaneous mechanoreceptive fields of dorsal horn neurons in the rat spinal cord. *J Neurosci*. 1990;10:2717–2726.
13. Price D, Bennett G, Raffii A. Psychophysical observations on patients with neuropathic pain relieved by a sympathetic block. *Pain*. 1989;36:273–288.
14. Cooper DE, DeLee JC. Reflex sympathetic dystrophy of the knee. In: Fu FH, Harner CD, Vince KG, eds. *Knee Surgery*. Baltimore: Williams & Wilkins; 1994:429–442.
15. Wilder R, Berde C, Wolohan M, et al. Reflex sympathetic dystrophy in children. *J Bone Joint Surg*. 1992;74A:910–919.
16. Bryan AS, Klenerman L, Bowsher D. The diagnosis of reflex sympathetic dystrophy using an algometer. *J Bone Joint Surg*. 1991;73B:644–646.
17. Vince KG, Eissmann E. Stiff total knee arthroplasty. In: Fu FH, Harner CD, Vince KG, eds. *Knee Surgery*. Baltimore: Williams & Wilkins; 1994:1529–1538.
18. Neuschwander D, Drez D, Heck S. Pain dysfunction syndrome of the knee. *Orthopedics*. 1995;19:27–32.
19. Schutzer SF, Gossling HR. The treatment of reflex sympathetic dystrophy: current concepts review. *J Bone Joint Surg*. 1984;4:625.
20. Cooper D, DeLee J, Ramamurthy S. Reflex sympathetic dystrophy of the knee: treatment using continuous epidural anesthesia. *J Bone Joint Surg*. 1989;71A:365–369.

ADDITIONAL READINGS

Ficat C, Nedjar C, Sarre J, Villa PL. [Treatment of reflex algodystrophy by intravenous reserpine block.] *Rev Chir Orthop Reparatrice Appar Mot.* 1983;69(suppl 2):83–88.

Lindenfeld TN, Bach BR, Wojtys EM. Reflex sympathetic dystrophy and pain dysfunction in the lower extremity. *J Bone Joint Surg.* 1996;78A:1936–1944.

Nedjar C, Ficat C. [Importance of intravenous reserpine in the treatment of reflex sympathetic dystrophy.] *Aggressologie.* 1982;23:317–320.

Index

EWU LIBRARIES
CHENEY, WASHINGTON 99004

This material is due on the last d'